Functional Visual Behavior

A Therapist's Guide to Evaluation and Treatment Options

Michele Gentile, MA, OTR/L
Editor

D1605226

The American Occupational Therapy Association, Inc.

The American Occupational Therapy Association, Inc., Mission Statement

The mission of the American Occupational Therapy Association is to support a professional community for members, and to develop and preserve the viability and relevance of the profession. The organization serves the interest of its members, represents the profession to the public, and promotes access to occupational therapy services.

Disclaimers

"This publication is designed to provide accurate and authoritative information in regard to the subject matter covered. It is sold or distributed with the understanding that the publisher is not engaged in rendering legal, accounting, or other professional services. If legal advice or other expert assistance is required, the services of a competent professional person should be sought."

　　—*From the Declaration of Principles jointly adopted by the American Bar Association and a Committee of Publishers and Associations*

It is the objective of the American Occupational Therapy Association to be a forum for free expression and interchange of ideas. The opinions expressed by the contributors to this work are their own and not necessarily those of either the editors or the American Occupational Therapy Association.

AOTA Director of Nonperiodical Publications: Frances E. McCarrey
AOTA Managing Editor of Nonperiodical Publications: Mary C. Fisk
Designed by WorldComp, Inc.

ISBN 1-56900-071-9

Printed in the United States of America

Table of Contents

Foreword

In the pages that follow, an impressive array of clinical talent has been assembled for the purpose of bringing together diverse and considerable skills and experience in working with individuals who have deficient and/ or dysfunctional visual information processing abilities. You, the reader, will be treated to explorations of a widely diverse range of treatment options, all the way from the application of optical correction devices to training of orientation-mobility type compensatory skills to functional neurorehabilitation restoration of visual function. This collection of treatment options, written by clinicians from numerous disciplinary backgrounds, will give you an extensive menu of possibilities from which to choose in your own clinical setting.

Burpee opens a window on the sensory integration approach to visual function/dysfunction, while Chaikin and Downing-Baum explore an optometric functional vision approach to a broad range of "common" visual problems (such as general binocular dysfunction, strabismus, and amblyopia). Erhardt and Duckman take a combined optometric-occupational therapy look at issues of visual-perceptual-motor dysfunction, while Loikith examines a more psychological, cognitive view of visual-perceptual function/dysfunction. Frymann injects a genuine breath of fresh air into the offerings with an introduction to the cranial-sacral rhythm and an osteopathic approach to treatment of compromised visual capacity. Gianutsos and Padula and Connor provide two different looks at the value of the optometric-occupational therapy alliance in neuro-rehabilitation treatment of individuals with neurological impairment, while Gianutsos examines the relationship between visual information processing and cognitive impairment. The final section of six chapters takes a varied and in-depth look at the many ways of approaching the treatment of individuals with low vision dysfunction.

The richness and enormous clinical value of this sort of a widely ranging approach is that you will be exposed to a wide array of valuable, clinically tested treatment options. However, this widely ranging approach also brings with it some inherent caveats for the reader. Because of the wide diversity of views, philosophies, and approaches represented here, you also will find a wide range of what might be called "levels of discourse." Some of the chapters are written with a very strong bias toward the "scientific data-point" approach to conveying information, with a great deal of emphasis on tracts and pathways and on neurological centers and networks believed to be responsible for vision. In other chapters, the writing is very much from a "clinical language" approach, with the emphasis on clinical actions and efficacy in the treatment of visual dysfunction. In still other chapters, there is a mingling of both of these levels of discourse. Both levels are, of course, valuable parts of the discussion. However, too often, especially in the latter half of the 20th century, we are prone to favor anything couched in "scientific" terminology over those things communicated in "clinical" terminology, or vice versa. In the former case, it's often a case of the "demand" for scientific credibility and validation, while in the latter case it's often a case of believing that the "ivory tower scientific types" really do not have a good grasp of the clinical realities of life.

To put this into a slightly different frame of reference, I would like to borrow from Joseph Campbell (1988, 1989). Campbell's professional life centered on the study of mythology and the examination of the common body of truth found in the mythologies of varied times and cultures. He effectively redefined "myth," not as fiction, fantasy, or made-up story, but as truth told in the language of metaphor when no "scientific data-point" language was available. Often, he said, people would approach him and challenge this assertion, on the basis that "metaphor" was just another way of saying that something "is a lie." In one of his last recorded interviews, when confronted with this same challenge, Campbell put it in very concrete terms, Suppose, he suggested, that you know someone named John, who is a fleet and agile runner of the high hurdles. You could probably do a good job, Campbell said, of giving a "scientific data-point" explanation of John's running and jumping abilities (e.g., you could talk of skeletal mechanics, muscle-skeletal biomechanics, neuro-muscular physiology, respiratory physiology and biochemistry, cardio-vascular physiology and biochemistry). However, asked Campbell, suppose that you live in a time and/or place when/where you do not have access to that scientific data-point language, could you simply say, "John is a deer?" Wouldn't you communicate a great deal about John's running and jumping abilities with that statement? Yet, if you demand that the metaphoric statement be interpreted at the level of the scientific data-point language, then it does become a lie. John is verifiably not a deer. He has 46 chromosomes and all of the other characteristics that make him a human being, not a deer. However, Campbell extols us, if you allow yourself the freedom to communicate at both the metaphoric level of discourse and the scientific data-point level of discourse, then your understanding will be further enriched and expanded beyond what would be communicated by either level of discourse alone.

It is my belief that most of the important discoveries about human biology are made by clinicians in their day-to-day interaction with that human biology. However, in most instances, there is little or no scientific data-point language available to the clinician to be able to describe and explain his or her discoveries to others. Therefore, the clinician resorts to using what, by analogy, I would call the language of "clinical metaphor." Too often, however, in the last half of this century, that sort of explanation has been challenged as "a lie," with such statements as, "Where's the scientific proof?" or "There's no scientific evidence to support that." If we can accept Campbell's challenge of allowing ourselves the freedom to shift between levels of discourse, we then gain a much fuller, broader understanding of the "truths" under discussion. I want to urge you, then, to read the chapters that follow with your best "clinical metaphor" and your best "scientific data-points" hats on. Allow yourselves the freedom to see "truth" in both levels of discourse, and you will, I believe, be much richer for your efforts.

Finally, there is one other issue for the reader of this book that I would like to call to your attention. There are nearly as many definitions (both implicit and explicit) of "vision" in this books as there are authors. Each chapter is written from a different understanding of what vision is. Some consider vision to be what takes place in the tracts and pathways of the neuroanatomy of the visual system. Other emphasize vision as what takes place in the brainstem/mid-brain centers. Still others are certain that vision is what takes place in the cortical centers of the brain. Some treat vision as cognitive information processing. Others treat visions as a reflexive, automatic response to light stimulation. Some view vision as the registration of light stimulation in the visual pathways. Others view it as the extraction of information from the light-induced stimulation of the pathways.

Thus, you must be wary as you read this book, lest you think that every time the terms "vision" or "visual perception" or "visual information processing" or other apparent "synonyms" are used that the writers are meaning the same thing. You must take care with each chapter to ferret out (either from explicit statement or from implicit context) what each author means when he or she says "vision." If you can continually be aware of that caveat as you read this set of 16 essays, you will become aware of the rich variety of ideas that people have about what vision really is and you will be clinically enriched. You also will be clinically enriched with respect to a wide array of potential assessment and intervention strategies. In the end, you should have an expanded awareness of the many potential professional alliances and partnerships there are for you.

In spite of the lack of language and definitional consistency and integration from one essay to another, you nonetheless will be treated to a broad smorgasbord of clinical assessment and intervention strategies and philosophies. When you have finished with this reading, I would like to challenge you to write yourself a short essay entitled "Vision is. . . ." What you believe vision to be will definitely determine how you practice and how you will apply the techniques, procedures, and approaches presented in these essays. You owe it to yourself and to your clinical clientele to make that "vision is. . ." definition explicit to yourself and to your practice.

Happy reading!
Steven J. Cool, PhD, FAAO

Reference
Campbell, J., & Moyers, B. (1988). *The power of myth*. New York: Doubleday.

Preface

With the creation of this insightful multidisciplinary text, devoted to the dynamics of the process of vision, including both functional and dysfunctional outcomes, Michele Gentile takes the reader on a tour de force of the visual system, mapping out its integral relationship with man's "Total Action System."

This work literally breathes life into the integrative processes of vision and sensorimotor input from the perspective of occupational therapists, physical therapists, optometrists, and other individuals involved in visual function, while at the same time acknowledging the nature of our present understanding of the emergent visual system. It is my expectation that the reader will gain an expanded view of what vision is and does, and how visual dysfunction can be treated in a multimodel and collaborative fashion.

The editor of this significant collaboration is to be congratulated for illuminating the complex while setting this stage for productive communication, particularly between the professions of occupational therapy and behavioral optometry. Here indeed are the words that provide a vital communication bridge between these dynamic professions.

I highly recommend it for students and practitioners alike.

Robert E. Titcomb, OD
Behavioral Optometrist
Virginia Beach, Virginia

Acknowledgments

This book is the result of a tremendous amount of time, effort, and care provided by many people. I would like to thank everyone involved for help in bringing this book to completion. I thank Dr. Steven Schiff, who spent countless hours introducing me to developmental optometry and who co-created the original idea for this book. I thank Renee Okoye and Dr. Rosamund Gianutsos for nurturing and broadening the original concept and for giving me sufficient encouragement and support to pursue my goal. Thanks to Frances McCarrey, for without her problem-solving skills this book would not have come to be. Thanks to Jennifer Cusumano for developmental writing, for lending her organizational skills, and for supporting the creative effort involved. A special thanks to Joanne and Charlie Davolio, who provided technical assistance at a moment's notice. Thanks to all of the authors who contributed to this text and who are listed on the authors' page. Thanks to those individuals whose names do not appear on the authors' page but who shared their expertise and information along the way. Among them are Nancy Alwais, Carla Brown, Patti Collins, Bonnie Hanschu, Cindy MacMurdo, Dr. Neil Rubin, Dr. Israel Greenwald, Dr. John Streff, Dr. Irving Peiser, and D. Zinsida Pekley. A heartfelt thanks to David and Joshua Gentile for their patience with the process of creating a book, and to the rest of my family members for their support and encouragement. Finally, a very special thanks to Dr. Robert Titcomb, who assisted in all of the above as well as in picking up the ball and carrying it across the finish line.

Authors

Shannon Downing-Baum, MS, OTR/L
Private Occupational Therapy Practice, Phoenix, AZ
Vision Therapist (COVTT), 1994
National Conference Presenter and Author: *Vision Rehabilitation in Occupational Therapy*

Jeannetta D. Burpee, MEd, OTR/L
Director
Jeannetta D. Burpee Institute, Blue Bell, PA
Conference Presenter: *Sensory Integration*
Professor Emeritus, Sensory Integration International
SIPT Certified

Laurie Efferson Chaikin, OD, MS, OTR
Developmental Optometrist, Clinical Associate
Primary Eyecare Optometrics, San Lorenzo, CA
Conference Presenter: *Vision Screening, OT and OD, Visual Dysfunction and Head Injury*
Chapter Author: Disorders of Vision and Visual Perceptual Function

Maureen Connor, OTR/L
Director, Outpatient Services
Central Jersey Rehabilitation Services, Inc., Toms River, NJ
Conference Presenter

Robert H. Duckman, OD, FAAO
Professor, College of Optometry
Chief, Childrens Special Needs Services
State University of New York, New York, NY

Rhoda P. Erhardt, MS, OTR, FAOTA
Consultant in Pediatric Occupational Therapy
Maplewood, MN
NDT Trained
National Conference Presenter and Author: *Prehension, Vision, Eye-Hand Coordination, Feeding Problems, Perceptual Problems*

Eleanor E. Faye, MD, FACS
Ophthalmological Consultant
The Lighthouse Center for Education, New York, NY

Michael Fischer, OD, FAAO
Director of Low Vision Services
The Manhattan and Queens Lighthouse, New York, NY
Author: *Low Vision*

Viola M. Frymann, DO, FAAO, MB, BS, M.F. Hom. (England)
Osteopathic Center For Children
College of Osteopathic Medicine of the Pacific, La Jolla, CA

Tricia Geniale, Grad. Dip., OT, NDT
New South Wales Department of Community Services
Ryde Community Services Centre, Epping, Australia
Author: *Low Vision and Child With Cerebral Palsy*

Rosamond Gianutsos, PhD
Neuropsychologist
Director, Cognitive Rehabilitation Services, Sunnyside, NY
Adjunct Associate Professor, College of Optometry
State University of New York, New York, NY
Research Associate Professor, Psychiatry
New York University Medical Center, New York, NY
Adjunct Professor, Occupational Therapy
Touro College, Dix Hills, NY

Beverly P. Horowitz, DSW, OTR/L
Associate Professor, Department of Occupational Therapy
Touro College, Dix Hills, NY
Private Practice Specializing in Gerontic Occupational Therapy,
 Huntington, NY
Author: *Gerontic OT Practice*

Carol Coté Loikith, MA, OTR
President
OT Ideas, Inc., Randolph, NJ

Tressa Kern, MS, OTR/L
Director of Occupational Therapy, Medical Coordinator
Visions Services for the Blind and Visually Impaired, New York, NY
Conference Presenter and Author: *Low Vision*

Nancy D. Weber Miller, MSW
Executive Director
Visions Services for the Blind and Visually Impaired, New York, NY
Adjunct Faculty, Post Masters Certificate in Gerontology Program
Hunter College, New York, NY

Linda Baker-Nobles, MS, OTR
Assistant Professor of Occupational Therapy
Rockhurst College, Kansas City, MO
Conference Presenter and Author: *Pediatric Low Vision*

Renee Okoye, MS, OTR, BCPOT
Board Certified Pediatric Occupational Therapist
Certified in Sensory Integration
Director
Dove Rehabilitation Services, Wantagh, NY
Conference Presenter and Author: *Computer Applications, Sensory
 Integration*

Bruce Rosenthal, OD, FAAO
Chief of the Low Vision Programs
The Lighthouse, Inc., New York, NY
Adjunct Professor
Mt. Sinai Hospital, New York, NY
Adjunct Distinguished Professor, College of Optometry
State University of New York State, New York, NY

William V. Padula, OD, FAAO
President
Shoreline Vision Rehabilitation Associates, Guilford, CT
Past President, Ncuro-Optometric Rehabilitation Association
Author: *Neuro-Optometric Rehabilitation*

Steven Schiff, OD
Developmental Optometrist
Deer Park, NY
Conference Presenter: *Vision Screening, OT/OD Collaboration*

Robert E. Titcomb, OD
Developmental Optometrist
Haygood Medical Center, Virginia Beach, VA
Conference Presenter: *Receptive Integration Dysfunction*

Part I.   Developmental Aspects
of Vision

1 Introduction to the Dynamic Process of Vision

Robert E. Titcomb, OD, and Renee Okoye, MS, OTR, BCPOT, with Steven Schiff, OD

The visual system is a kind of meeting ground ... where the electrodynamic forces that culminate in adaptive behavior ... are organized.

Arnold Gesell
(Hoopes & Hoopes, 1979)

Why should a therapist concern himself or herself with learning more about the visual system? There are several reasons. The most important, perhaps, is that the human visual system serves as a dynamic synthesizer of the body's motor action systems. Dr. Josephine C. Moore captures the essence of this concept in "Vision: Our most important sense" (see Figure 1.1) and in so doing breathes life into Dr. Gesell's "meeting ground." A second reason is that the human visual system by its very nature and complexity often embodies many dysfunctional skills that severely affect its effectiveness and efficiency as a vehicle for information processing. Together with its potential for internal problems, the human visual system may be affected by the numerous

3

Of all of our receptors or senses vision is the only one that integrates, or enables us to make sense of, all of our other sensorimotor systems. Hence vision is *the unifying system that integrates all other systems* and enables us to learn about, interact with and survive[1] in our world.

To survive, *distant receptors* are vital. Only the visual and auditory systems endow us with these senses. Of the two, vision is far superior in alerting us to pleasure, danger, or that which attracts our attention.

Movement detection is also necessary for survival. The visual system has the fastest fibers, synapses, and circuits of all of our senses and gives us advanced warning of movement around us as well as informing our CNS about our own *spatiotemporal movements, posture and balance.*

Vision plays the most critical role in *attentive functions*, i.e. awake, alert, and attending to that which is most important for learning, communicating, interacting with, and adapting to our ever-changing environment.

Vision is the primary sense that we use for *understanding non-verbal communication.* (Gesture or non-verbal "language" comprises about 70% of all communication between individuals, while only 30% is actually verbal language).

Vision endows us with the unique ability to "pick up" *subliminal perceptions or clues* from our environment, all of which reinforce the anticipatory capabilities of our nervous systems and hence our survival and adaptive skills.

Last but not least, *visual-manual skills*, or eye–hand coordination, along with our amazing brains, have endowed us with the exceptional ability to continually create, invent, and discover new things. We have moved from being simple tool users with "primitive" language abilities to computer, fax, and satellite communicators, moving about in cars, planes, and "space ships." Yet, in spite of all of our advances in technology and science we still have to depend upon our basic visual-manual skills for learning about and using the "tools" that we create.

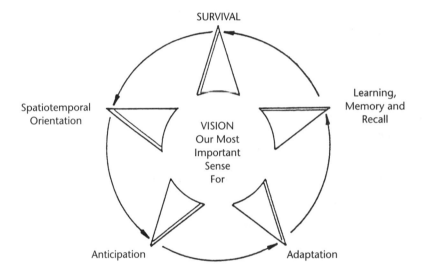

SURVIVAL:
Of our two distant receptors, vision is our primary early alerting system, especially for movement detection, with the auditory system second. All other receptors are contact receptors.

SPATIOTEMPORAL ORIENTATION:
Peripheral vision is critical for orientation and movement in space, together with the vestibular and proprioceptive systems of the neck and body. These senses enable us to maintain dynamic postures, balance, complex movement patterns, and move *freely* in the environment.

ANTICIPATION or the ANTICIPATORY NERVOUS SYSTEM:
Vision, being our most far-reaching sense, plays the major role in the anticipatory NS's planning and programming the complex postures and movements necessary for obtaining goals. Vision is the only sense capable of constantly updating the CNS about our ever-changing environment thus enabling the NS to respond appropriately to all ongoing changes.

ADAPTATION:
To cope with an ever-changing environment we must constantly adapt, and adapting depends upon planning ahead and being prepared. The visual system enables us to be constantly aware and updated about the context of the environment and leads other senses in telling the CNS how best to adapt to complete a task or survive.

LEARNING, MEMORY and RECALL:
Learning is contextual and most of our learning and memory is obtained through our visual system. Memories are best recalled when one is in the context or visual surroundings where the learning occurred. When out of context and trying to recall a memory (person, place, or thing) visual searching and "mind-pictures" usually precede recall.

[1]The term "survive" is used in its broadest sense and includes learning, playing, working, sleeping, interpersonal relations, and all activities of daily living.

Figure 1.1 Vision: Our most important sense, by Josephine C. Moore, PhD, OTR, DSc (Hon).

neurological conditions for which we are already treating our patients. This is covered in detail in several chapters in this book, particularly in part II. A third reason is that treatment of the visual system through the use of lenses, prisms, and other visual therapies alone or in conjunction with other sensorimotor treatment modalities can affect muscle tone, posture, movement, visual-motor, visual-spatial, visual-perceptual, and cognitive functioning. Visual therapies are prescribed and administered by an appropriate eye care professional—generally a behavioral or neuro-optometrist. A recent trend has been for these optometrists to work in collaboration with physical and occupational therapists with greater bene-fit to the patient as optimum visual input improves motor function and motor function enhances visual functioning. The foundation for understanding the neurological relationship of vision and motor abilities is addressed in this chapter and in more detail in chapter 9.

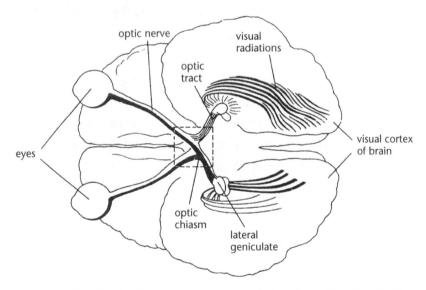

Figure 1.2 Brain with visual pathways shown from below. From *Your Eyes: An Owner's Manual* by J. F. Collins. Copyright by Prentice-Hall Publishers. Reprinted with permission.

Vision: Beyond 20/20 Sight

In this chapter, we will discuss how *vision* is more than 20/20 *sight*. We will explain the process by which we see and will describe the anatomical structures involved in vision. We will provide the neurological foundation for understanding how vision is integrated with other sensorimotor systems and how this integration results in adaptive visuomotor behaviors.

As you can see in Figure 1.2, the eyes are actually an extension of the brain with the retina composed of nervous system tissue. The significance of the "in-house" nature of the eye as an extension of the brain will become apparent as the leadership role of vision in man's "total action system" of visuomotor behaviors emerges. The term *total action system* refers to the blending of proprioceptive, vestibular, and visual processing into a dynamic system of data processing that summates new visual and motor input, compares it to previously stored data, then, in the twinkling of a millisecond, instructs one's body how to react appropriately, be it with hand, foot, leg, or total body. This is what is meant by *vision* being more than 20/20 *sight* and what Gesell referred to as "the meeting ground," where vision and motor become as one.

A holistic, functional view of the visual system goes far beyond optics and begins with an understanding that vision does not function in isolation; rather, it integrates with the rest of the nervous system for optimal visuomotor functioning. Indeed, to realize optimal visuomotor function, there must be a blending of adequate distance optics with visual and visual-sensorimotor integrative skills.

The Components of Vision

Optics (static in nature) (a) involves distance acuity and defines best static sight with refractive correction, (b) provides a stable foundation for the development of visual skills.

Visual Skills (dynamic in nature) involve the moving parts of the eye (the extraocular muscles and the lens), as well as knowledge from prior experience (e.g., understanding of depth perception and cognition). These skills are developmental in nature. The motor visual skills can also be affected by muscle tonus imbalances from central nervous system (CNS) disorders as well as being affected by fluctuations in homeostatic balance of the autonomic nervous system, particularly in young children. The visual skills are as follows:

Fixation. The coordinated aiming of the eyes while shifting rapidly from one object to another (e.g., shifting gaze from word to word or groups of words when reading a printed line). Cognitive decoding occurs during these rapid "pit stops."

Tracking/Pursuits. The description of the eye's ability to follow a target being moved in the cardinal positions (left to right, up and down, and the diagonals). The ability of the eye to follow a target in a circular path, typically at near point, is called *rotation*.

Note: In both rotation and tracking/pursuits, fixation should never be lost. However, it is not uncommon for the developmentally delayed or neuromotor challenged child to exhibit midline jump as well as regressions and loss of fixation when attempting to track.

Saccade. The ability of the eye to *change* fixation from point to point. These are the eye movements used during reading.

Accommodation. The neuromuscular act describing the innervation of the ciliary body within the eye that causes this intraocular muscle to alter the shape of the eye's crystalline lens. This act results in the altering of the eye's focal distance; e.g., shifting the gaze from chalkboard to book.

Particularly important is an individual's facility of focus that allows rapid shift from far to near as well as near to far.

Binocular Vision. The combining of information received through the visual pathway of each eye to make one single mental mind's eye picture. Using one eye while shutting off the other involuntarily is called *suppression*.

Convergence is the turning of the eyes inward as the object of regard moves toward the observer. This skill could involve changing convergence angle while tracking an incoming ball as well as sustaining a fixed angle of inward gaze as in the act of reading.

Coordination of Accommodation and Convergence is a neurological symbiosis between these two functions. For every unit of accommodation, a corresponding unit of convergence occurs. The ratio of these exact amounts is known as the Accommodating Convergence (ACA) ratio and differs from individual to individual. While it is often assumed that the child is properly coordinating the convergence and focusing of his or her eyes at a target in the appropriate manner, in reality, this coordination often does not occur. For instance, if the target is at 12 in., the eyes may indeed be converging at a distance inappropriate to the task such as at 8 in. or 14 in., resulting in a doubling or near-doubling of the target. This can cause visual-spatial confusion, headaches, as well as overall reduced visual efficiency affecting all the individual visual skills.

Stereopsis is monocular or binocular depth perception or an egocentric appraisal of the depth of an object within the totality of an individual's visual space. This skill originates from both an individual's sense of stored memory relating to object distance and separations as well as from the *active* input of *retinal disparity*, which is the visual system's egocentric device of judging retinal image separation relative to the fovea centralis. Monocular perception of depth is not a true indicator but rather an estimate made on the basis of previously stored information.

Form Perception is the recognition and organization of visual sensation produced by differing patterns of lines, shapes, and contours. Especially important in developing a sense of ordered arrangement (e.g., was and saw, 21 and 12, b and d), form perception depends on the eyes' ability to point or converge appropriately as well as the development of an individual's sense of laterality and directionality, which ensures consistency in replicating the appropriate left and right orientation of the shape in question.

Field of Vision is a measure of an individual's ability to detect light and movement in his or her superior, inferior, right, and left fields of vision as well as central field, while maintaining central fixation. This static measurement of visual function represents the sum total of the optic media, retina, optic nerve, visual pathway, and visual cortex.

In functional or behavioral terms the field of vision also includes the ability of the individual to *interact* with stimuli in the peripheral visual field while maintaining central fixation. A child who bumps into things may be having difficulty with this area of visual function. Such a child may be visually centered inward with the potential for ignorance of his or her peripheral environmental input. Visual treatment of this dysfunction might include use of yoked, base-down prisms to facilitate an awareness of peripheral space as well as it is related in office therapy.

Note: All of the above skills are considered reflective of the individual's adaptive development. However, through appropriate visual therapy, errant relationships and misbehaviors of the mechanisms of vision can be brought into balance by stimulating the individual's innate visual feedback mechanisms, which facilitates self-correction. In dealing with the mechanisms of changing present visual patterns, recall the "in-house" nature of the visual system and that it is part and parcel of the brain itself. All of the visual skills listed employ oculomotor feedback circuits that continually compare the brain's "view" of the input it is receiving to what previously has been stored. For example, when focusing at near, the brain expects clear, well-defined input, thus it regulates and re-regulates how much or how little focusing effort is required by the ciliary body producing focus. The same is true for convergence; the brain strives for a single, unified image by converging the two eyes appropriately. A simplified way of viewing this feedback process is to understand it as the brain's circuitry to effect a fine-tuning process. In approaching these problems in a child's early years, the plasticity of the developing nervous system allows for easier correction compared to attempting to stimulate correction of an embedded pattern.

Visual and Sensorimotor Integration involves the integration of visual skills with the body's other sensorimotor systems of proprioception; kinesthesia; tactile, auditory, and vestibular processing (as well as other information that is described later in this chapter) for the development of functional skills of orienting reactions; protective reactions; reflexive postural movements; spatiotemporal orientation; perceptual skills; academic functioning; and eye–hand, eye–foot, and eye–body coordination.

Just as the visual skills, as previously defined, provide the foundation for visual integrative function, the other sensorimotor skills can enhance the development of visual skills. Motor challenges (e.g., working on a walking rail or balance board) that are appropriate to the skill level of the individual can improve attending and can heighten an individual's innate feedback mechanisms that can, in turn, improve an individual's eye–hand–body functioning. In the absence of adequate results, however, a consultation with an eye care professional who specializes in functional vision (e.g., a developmental or behavioral optometrist) is recommended to obtain an assessment of the individual's functional and dysfunctional areas. Possible reasons for integrative difficulties could stem from excessive refractive error, a pronounced difference of refractive error between the two eyes, excessive under- or over-convergence as well as a host of other problems addressed under visual skills.

The Process of Vision

Sight begins when light rays are reflected into our eyes from a surface that is illuminated in some manner (see Figure 1.3). These incoming rays enter the eye through the cornea, where they are refracted or bent; they then pass through the aqueous humor to the crystalline lens, where they are further refracted or bent, passing through the vitreous humor to focus on the retina. This portion of sight, focused in the area of the retina identified as macula and para-macula, is known as *central* or *focal* with its locus being in the functional center of the retina known as the fovea. The image thus found on the retina at the fovea is optically inverted; fortunately, this detail is handled quite nicely by the brain's capacity for conditioned learning. Through this, we human organisms learn that by cortically reinverting the image, we are able to function appropriately. Sight formed from the area of the retina peripheral to the macula and para-central area is known as *peripheral* or *ambient*.

Neural Processing of Vision

Reception

The newly formed electrical signals representing our retinal image are projected through at least three major neural pathways. One large pathway

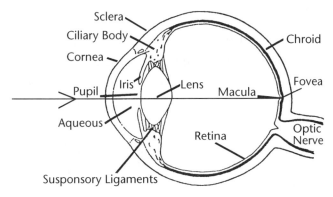

Figure 1.3 Light rays entering the eye begin the process of sight.

provides for reception of the retinal image in the primary visual cortex where neurons respond only to visual stimuli. A second group of tiny but mighty pathways provides for integration of the retinal image with postural mechanisms and orientating reactions. A third pathway of parallel-distributed processing fibers provides for perception of the retinal image by ascribing meaning to it. Functional vision is dependent on the dynamic interaction of these three major systems of interrelated pathways.

Once an image reaches the retina, the eyes shift from their optical mode to one of neurological transmission by synaptically transferring the light image into chemical energy. Both the rods and the cones in the retina contain chemicals that decompose on exposure to light and, in the process, excite the nerve fibers leading from the eye. The pathway of fibers that provide for reception of visual stimuli in the primary visual cortex diverge in partial decussation at the optic chiasm, which is located at the base of the brain (below and slightly in front of the hypothalamus, on about the same level as the rostral pons). Fibers arising from the nasal halves of each retina cross to the opposite side, while fibers arising from the temporal halves of each retina remain uncrossed. This means that half of the visual information conveyed in the optic tracts projects to cortical regions that are contralateral to the field from which the stimulus arose. Visual information received from the right nasal visual field is projected to the left visual cortex before it is distributed, and information received from the left nasal visual field is projected to the right visual cortex before it is distributed. Sometimes a clinical manifestation of this may be observed with patients who have unilateral visual field deficits, or visual neglect following a cerebral vascular accident (CVA) where often their field of visual neglect is contralateral to the involved side. When this finding is not seen, it generally is a diagnostic sign that the CVA occurred at a level above the optic chiasm. After the fibers from this pathway pass through the optic chiasm, they continue to the lateral geniculate body that is a principal relay nucleus for the pathway concerned with the reception of primary vision. The fibers for this pathway terminate in a point-to-point projection upon layers of the lateral geniculate body of the thalamus. The efferent fibers from the lateral geniculate body form a wide, flat band termed the optic radiations. Fibers from this wide band terminate in the primary visual region, the calcarine sulcus, of the cerebral cortex. The precise name for these fibers, the *geniculocalcarine tract*, indicates that they arise in the geniculate body and terminate in the calcarine sulcus. A precise point-to-point projection from the retina to the lateral geniculate body is found, and from the latter to the various aspects of the calcarine sulcus. As the retinal image is received in the visual cortex along these pathways, the neural signals are rapidly projected along parallel-distributed fibers (see Figure 1.4) to visual association, somatosensory, auditory, motor, and frontal regions of the cortex, where the impulses are compared with previous sensory memories in order for the eyes to garner meaning from their sense of sight.

Integration

There is a tiny but powerful group of pathways that provides for integration of the retinal image with postural mechanisms, as well as functioning to integrate incoming visual stimuli with the other sensorimotor systems. These pathways that receive their input from visual fibers arising from the lateral geniculate body serve to integrate the signals sent from the rods and cones with the brain's dynamic movement-oriented components. Hence, the importance of the term *functional vision*, which is reflective of the brain's ability to synthesize sight with movement. The end product thus innervated then forms the basis for a person's total action system.

The principal relay structure responsible for integrating vision with other sensorimotor systems is the superior colliculus, which is the tectum or the roof of the midbrain. This major integrative center is concerned with relaying information between incoming visual stimuli with ongoing

PARALLEL-DISTRIBUTED PROCESSING of the VISUAL SYSTEM

Sequence of synaptic and axonal flow in the cerebral cortex: input into 1° and 2° visual cortex, then via several parallel-distributed pathways and circuits:

1. Superior circuit ➡ superior parietal lobe and prefrontal lobe + FEF[1].
2. Inferior circuit ➡ post. temporal lobe and prefrontal lobe + FEF[1].
3. To limbic cortex especially temporal lobe components[2] and cingulate gyrus.
4. To the kinetic system to obtain a visual-manual and/or visual-motor program.
5. To the synergic system to obtain coordinated-sequencial programs for desired (goal oriented) movements involved in activities including visual movements.

[1]Prefrontal lobes: anticipatory executive, including judgement, of the CNS including frontal eye fields for controlling visual movements in all skilled activities.

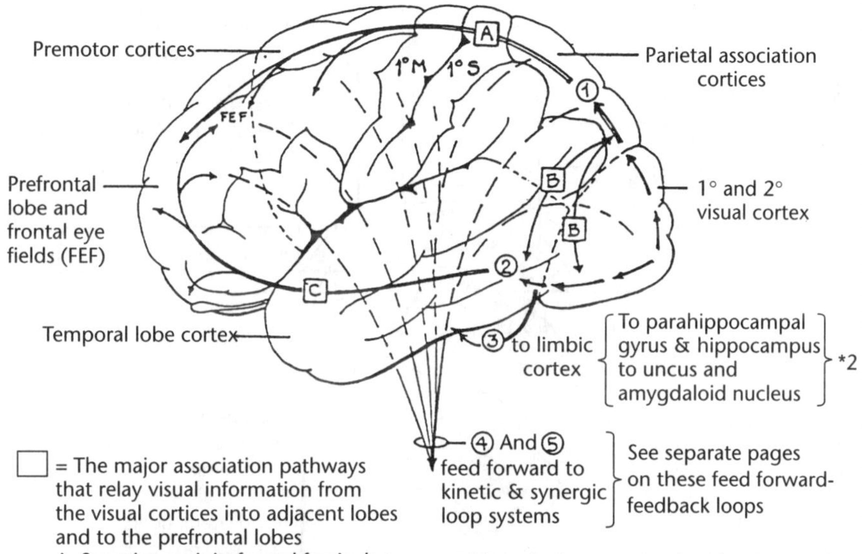

Premotor cortices

Parietal association cortices

Prefrontal lobe and frontal eye fields (FEF)

1° and 2° visual cortex

Temporal lobe cortex

③ to limbic cortex

To parahippocampal gyrus & hippocampus to uncus and amygdaloid nucleus] *2

☐ = The major association pathways that relay visual information from the visual cortices into adjacent lobes and to the prefrontal lobes
   A. Superior occipitofrontal fasciculus.
   B. Parietotemporal & parieto-occip. fascic.
   C. Inferior occipitofrontal fasciculus.

④ And ⑤ feed forward to kinetic & synergic loop systems

See separate pages on these feed forward-feedback loops

Note: Brain stem circuitry that is critical for normal vision is not illustrated.

Area ① noted above is in the post. part of the superior parietal lobule: *major functions* include visuospatial orientation, sensory appreciation of the external environment including an internal memory map of the environment and body-image map plus movement detection. Area ② noted above is in the posterior temporal lobe: *major functions* include visuo-object and color recognition, orientation of objects and detailed serial processing of environment stimuli.

Figure 1.4 Parallel-distributed processing and the visual system. Copyright Josephine C. Moore. Reprinted with permission.

background neural activity occurring in the cortical systems; visual, auditory, and vestibular systems; reticular system; kinetic (basal ganglion), synergic (cerebellum), and somatosensory (spinotectal and trigeminotectal) systems that provide input to the brainstem. Figure 1.5 illustrates these systems of integrative relay that pass between the paired superior colliculi and the functional systems they interact with. All this occurs prior to the incoming visual information reaching the visual cortex.

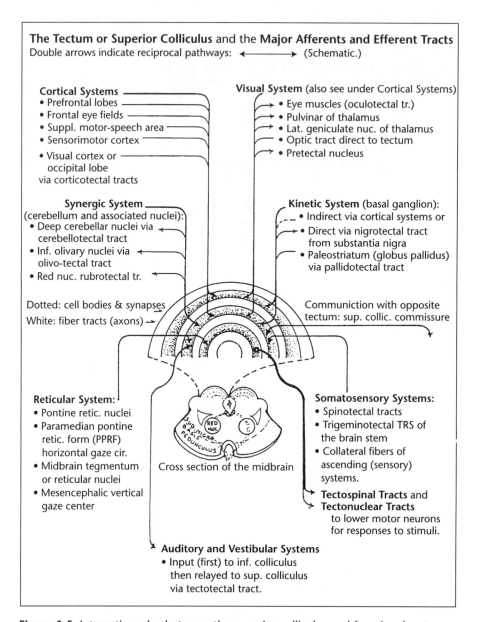

The Tectum or Superior Colliculus and the **Major Afferents and Efferent Tracts**
Double arrows indicate reciprocal pathways: ←———→ (Schematic.)

Cortical Systems ————
• Prefrontal lobes ————
• Frontal eye fields ————
• Suppl. motor-speech area ——
• Sensorimotor cortex ——
• Visual cortex or
  occipital lobe
via corticotectal tracts

Visual System (also see under Cortical Systems)
• Eye muscles (oculotectal tr.)
• Pulvinar of thalamus
• Lat. geniculate nuc. of thalamus
• Optic tract direct to tectum
• Pretectal nucleus

Synergic System ——
(cerebellum and associated nuclei):
• Deep cerebellar nuclei via
  cerebellotectal tract
• Inf. olivary nuclei via
  olivo-tectal tract
• Red nuc. rubrotectal tr.

Kinetic System (basal ganglion):
• Indirect via cortical systems or
• Direct via nigrotectal tract
  from substantia nigra
• Paleostriatum (globus pallidus)
  via pallidotectal tract

Dotted: cell bodies & synapses
White: fiber tracts (axons) →

Communiction with opposite
tectum: sup. collic. commissure

Reticular System:
• Pontine retic. nuclei
• Paramedian pontine
  retic. form (PPRF)
  horizontal gaze cir.
• Midbrain tegmentum
  or reticular nuclei
• Mesencephalic vertical
  gaze center

Cross section of the midbrain

Somatosensory Systems:
• Spinotectal tracts
• Trigeminotectal TRS of
  the brain stem
• Collateral fibers of
  ascending (sensory)
  systems.

Tectospinal Tracts and
Tectonuclear Tracts
to lower motor neurons
for responses to stimuli.

Auditory and Vestibular Systems
• Input (first) to inf. colliculus
  then relayed to sup. colliculus
  via tectotectal tract.

Figure 1.5 Integrative relay between the superior colliculus and functional systems.
Copyright Josephine C. Moore. Reprinted with permission.

Cortical systems linked with the superior colliculi serve to integrate vision with cognitive processes via corticotectal fibers. Cortical processes involved with directing eye gaze and providing visual vigilance needed for daily living activities, such as reading, shaving, applying make-up, and so forth, are carried out through these corticotectal pathways. Cortical processes involved with thinking about or visualizing the mental manipulation of concepts and objects also stimulate eye movements through corticotectal pathways that arise from respective functional areas of the cortex and project to the superior colliculi. For example, when thinking through the correct spelling of a word containing the "ie" combination, one-to-one correspondence of the letters in proper sequential order is generally needed. This process of visualization involves eye movements even though the image is not actually seen, but rather "visualized." These eye movements would generally be paired with relays from the auditory, visual, and motor speech regions of the cortex. Another example would be the eye movements that accompany the task of mentally rearranging the furniture in a room.

The synergic system with its cerebellar relays and pathways to associated nuclear centers in the brainstem is linked with the superior colliculi and serves to integrate eye movements with other synergistic movements of the body (e.g., coordinating inversion and adduction of the eyes with flexor synergies of the trunk and extremities). For example, neural pathways that project from the medullary, pontine, and midbrain portions of the reticular system to the superior colliculi serve primitive protective functions by bringing about sudden turning of the eyes to the side when a flash of light or some other sudden visual stimulus occurs on that side. These pathways involving the synergic system are also responsible for fixing the eyes on important highlights in the visual field. This action can be seen as protective as well.

Input to the superior colliculi from the auditory and vestibular systems is indirectly handled by pathways that first project to the inferior colliculi before being relayed to the superior colliculi via the tectotectal tract. These relays originate from the inferior colliculi and terminate in the superior colliculi. They provide ongoing information about the external environment and integrate these data with input from the visual system. One functional example of the result of such integration is the clinical behavior we term "orienting reactions"—those rapid, combined movements that provide for eye gaze and head turning toward the source of external stimuli. One of the principal functions of the superior colliculi is to participate in the control of orienting reactions. These orienting reactions are affected in part through the tectotectal relays through the collicular levels of the tectum.

The visual system constitutes the most substantial and highly organized projections from the cortex to the superior colliculi. These projections originate from the visual cortex and pass to the superior colliculi via the brachium. The superior colliculi receive additional input from the visual system from the pulvinar and lateral geniculate body of the thalamus, the oculomotor nuclei, along with fibers from the optic tract and the pretectal nucleus. These latter projections serve to integrate field and movement specificity. They are involved in coding the location of an object in the visual field relative to the fovea and in eliciting saccadic eye movements that produce foveal acquistion of the object (Carpenter, 1991). The projections from the pulvinar and lateral geniculate body of the thalamus serve to integrate images from the *quadrants* and *hemifields* of vision. They also provide relays to the visual association areas of the cortex (areas 18 and 19) where the data are compared with previously acquired sensory memories.

The kinetic system, which includes the basal ganglion and related nuclei, is linked with the superior colliculi via tracts that project from these nuclei to the tectum. Relays from the substantial nigra and the globulus pallidus provide the visual integrative center of the brainstem an efference copy of the "movement to come," thereby appraising the visual system of gross stereotypical movement patterns that are imminent and those that are underway. This early warning of movement to come is timed in advance of the "smoothing" available from the synergic and cortical systems. The visual system and other cortical systems can then initiate any last-minute corrections necessary to guide the body parts so that the final motor pattern can be fluidly executed.

Afferent fibers of the somatosensory system involved with neural communication at the level of the superior colliculi serve to mediate reflexive postural movments in response to visual and auditory stimuli. These include spinotectal and trigeminotectal tracts that convey general sensory components to the superior colliculi. Tectospinal and tectonuclear tracts project motor impulses from the deep zones of the superior colliculi to the upper levels of the cervical cord. These tracts convey small amounts of potential and do not terminate directly upon alpha motor neurons. Instead, they help to provide for the background postural adjustments necessary to praxis, by stimulating interneurons in laminae VII and VIII of cervical cord segments in response to incoming auditory, visual, and vestibular stimuli.

One primary integrative performance component of functional vision behavior is the provision of spatiotemporal orientation. The ability to orient oneself in space and time is foundational to many facets of human behavior. Social functions, such as being able to make an appointment to meet someone in a specific place at a specific time, being able to dance with a partner, and even such elementary behaviors as learning to share and take turns, require the ability to function within a spatiotemporal orientation. Vocational functions, such as not losing one's orientation when moving through the community; operating a motor vehicle; using revolving doors, escalators, or elevators; or using a map for public transportation, require the ability to function within a spatiotemporal orientation. This ability touches on academic performance in skills, such as spelling (i.e., serial ordering of letters and sounds), history (i.e., ordering of events and people in time and place), scientific inquiry (i.e., ordering elements of chemical equations in spatial orientation), and geometric equations and calculations (i.e., ordering spatial relationships of figures within a sequence of operations). These abilities all depend heavily on fairly sophisticated spatiotemporal orientation. Emotional well-being suffers when we cannot explore and learn about our environment because of deficits in spatiotemporal orientation.

Components of functional vision that allow for emergence of the sophisticated adaptive behavior we term spatiotemporal orientation are closely intermingled in terms of their neural pathways. Spatiotemporal orientation requires the ability to interdigitate three key factors: (a) the ability to maintain foveated gaze, (b) the ability to compare incoming visual data with speed and direction of head movement, and (c) the ability to compare movement of the body with incoming visual data. Integration of these three key components is referred to as the vestibulo-oculo-cervical triad by Moore (personal communication, August, 1996) (see Figures 1.6 and 1.7).

A functional skill of daily living that illustrates the work of this triad in a dynamic way is the ability to walk off an escalator that is moving down. (Note that walking onto an escalator that is moving up is not

NOTES CONCERNING SPATIOTEMPORAL ORIENTATION

- Orientation in space and time is the foundation of all human behavior. Without orientation we cannot become bipedal, move, explore and learn about our environment. In reality, we cannot survive unless cared for.

- Abnormal function in any one component of the vestibulo-oculo-cervical triad interferes with normal function in the other components, resulting in insecurities, postural and balance impairments and changes in muscle tone, thus compromising ones' ability to explore, manipulate and learn from interacting with the environment.

- Of the three components of the vestib-oculo-cervical triad which one is most important? They are all of equal importance as no one component can function normally without the other. For example:

  - The vestibulocerebellum (aka archicerebellum) is vitally necessary for keeping the eyes foveated on a target during all head and body movements. This system is also responsible for gravity detection, balance or posture and muscle tone during all activities of daily living.

  - The visual component (ocular system) especially peripheral or ambient vision is vital for orientation in space, movement detection and a global awareness of space and time. The foveal (macular) vision is essential for learning details (reading, driving, writing, etc.) as well as saccadic and smooth pursuit movements used in all learning and activities of daily living.

  - The rostral neck (cervical) receptors orient the head in space along with all special senses including the ocular and vestibular systems. The rostral cervical levels of the neck prove to be the vital link between the rest of the body and the head enabling the entire body/head to function together as an integrated whole.

and the
VESTIBULO-OCULO-CERVICAL TRIAD

- VOR = Maintains a foveated gaze on a target during all head movements, especially during fast, brief head movements. This is a compensatory mechanism (reflex) which moves the eyes equal and opposite to the head movements thus keeping the eyes foveated (focused) on a target.

- OVR = Feedback circuit of VOR (or eyes to vestib. nucleus). Relays data informing vestib. nuc. if eyes are on target (a match) or off-target (mis-match) and needs correcting.

- COR = A back-up system for VOR (may account for 25% of VOR function), especially utilized for slow, sustained movements of the neck/head. Same functions as VOR, plus links head and body together as a unified whole.

- OCR = Voluntary or involuntary (reflexive) eye movements as in supra- or infraversion or levo- or dextroversion. Increases muscle tone in muscles "looked at" which in turn extends, flexes, or rotates the neck in the gaze direction, and reciprocally reduces tone in the opposite group of muscles, thus reinforcing movement in direction of gaze.

- VCR = Functions with above reflexes for equilibrium, antigravity muscle tone and informing the rostral cervical area about the moment to moment (milliseconds) state of the vestibulocerebellum and ocular system.

- CVR = Feedback to vestibulocerebellum for correcting or reinforcing neck movements in relation to head and body balance/posture, gravity, muscle tone of all movements.

- VSR = Functions with all above for body parts in relation to balance, gravity, movement and orientation of body in space. Involved in tonic and dynamic responses, especially of limbs.

- SVR = Feedback to vestibulocerebellum to correct or enhance body posture and movements, especially with the limbs.

Figure 1.6 Notes on spatiotemporal orientation and the vestibulo-oculo-cervical triad.

Copyright Josephine C. Moore. Reprinted with permission.

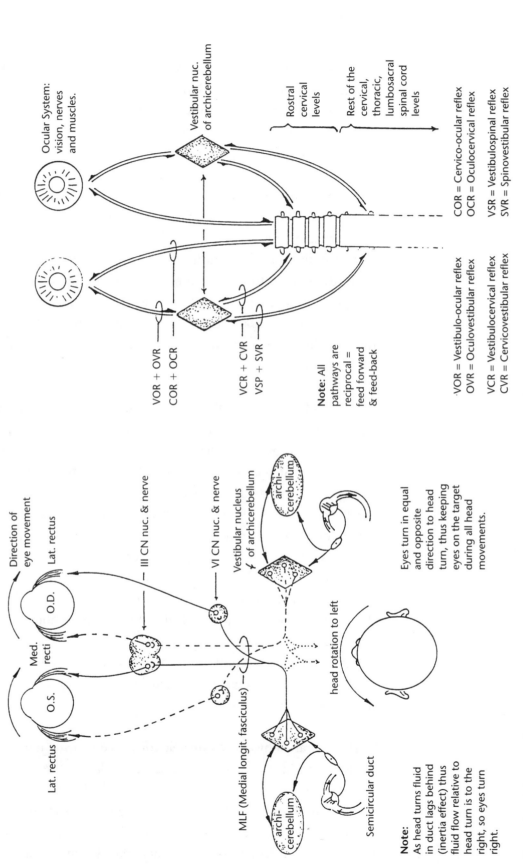

Figure 1.7 Schematic diagram of spatiotemporal orientation, vestibulo-ocular-reflex, and the vestibulo-oculo-cervical triad. Copyright Josephine C. Moore. Reprinted with permission.

19

nearly so tricky as walking off a downward moving stairway for most people.) Consider (a) the need to maintain foveated gaze on the upcoming floor and the gap between moving and nonmoving supporting surfaces that become the visual target. Now consider (b) the ability to compare the efference copy of movement of the visual field arising from the foveated gaze with the efference copy of speed and direction of movement of the head in space arising from incoming vestibular data. Next, hold that thought while (c) the visual and vestibular efference copies of movement are compared with incoming kinetic data arising from the proprioceptors in the neck that apprise the individual that the body is involved in steady-state postural adjustments and is working on "standing still." Temporospatial orientation provides for resolution of movement equations in time and space, among other things, and enables a person to time the integration of body movement with the location of sensory events in the environment.

The vestibular ocular reflex (VOR) is the neural mechanism responsible for (a) the ability to maintain foveated gaze. Relays between the vestibular nuclei and the nuclei of the extraocular muscles project through and around the medial longitudinal fasciculus (MLF) to produce compensatory eye movements in response to head movements. These eye movements help to stabilize the visual image on the retina. Feedback from the oculomotor nuclear complex is accomplished via reciprocal interneural pathways. These pathways link the functions of the vestibular and oculomotor complexes and complete the loop by keeping the vestibular nuclei apprised of the movement occurring in the eye muscles. The portion of the loop that provides feedback directly to the vestibular nuclei from the oculomotor complex is termed the oculovestibular reflex (OVR). Integration of data from both of these circuits serves to accomplish (b) the ability to compare incoming visual data with speed and direction of head movement.

The neural pathways responsible for (c) comparing movement of the body with incoming visual data, consist of relays between the interstitial nucleus of Cajal, the oculomotor nuclear complex, and the spinal cord. These circuits provide both feed-forward and feedback mechanisms and are termed the oculocervical reflex (OCR) and the cervico-ocular reflex (COR). Efferent fibers from this functional system of relays descend to the spinal cord as the interstiospinal component of the MLF and provide synergistic changes in muscle tone to complement movement in the direction of eye gaze.

Reflexive pathways linking the superior colliculus and the spinal cord via the interstiospinal component of the MLF, reticulospinal, vestibulospinal, tectospinal, and fastigiocerebellar relays constitute the vestibulocervical reflex (VCR) and vestibulospinal reflex (VSR). The VCR and VSR serve as the final link in the vestibulo-oculo-cervical triad by interfacing postural support mechanisms with visual and vestibular efferences. Their interaction complements the work of the COR and OCR by adjusting postural tone to support the "movement to come." The action of the VCR and VSR is modified by their feedback loops that arise from upper cervical segments of the spinal cord and project to the superior colliculus, cerebellum, and vestibular nuclear center via spinotectal, spinocerebellar, spinovestibular, and spinorecticular fibers.

This roundabout network of integrated reflexes and interneural relays represents a total action system that provides postural support for praxis, eye–hand teaming, and spatiotemporal orientation, all of which are significant components of functional vision. Functional vision thus defines the ultimate marriage of vision and movement, encompassing a vast network of related pathways whose influence extends throughout the neuraxis. Correspondingly, disruption along any of these pathways brings with it the very real potential of disrupting some aspect of functional visual behavior.

Perception

Neurological support mechanisms for cognitive visual perception begin as the retinal image is received in the visual cortex. The neural signals are then rapidly projected along parallel-distributed fibers that often are referred to as *association connections* to visual association, somatosensory, motor and premotor cortices, auditory, and frontal regions of the cortex where the impulses are compared with previous memories.

Neurons in the primary visual cortex (area 17) respond to visual stimuli. However, neurons located in the secondary and tertiary zones of the occipital lobe (areas 18 and 19) are more multimodal in nature. This means that they respond to more than one mode of sensory stimulation and can be excited by signals arising from visual, auditory, or somatosensory neurons and especially tactile information. Two short association pathways project from the visual cortex to nearby cortical fields. The pathway projecting from the inferior or ventral primary visual cortex to areas 18 and 19 and the inferior temporal cortex are mainly concerned with the analysis of form and color and are crucial for recognition of objects. When this pathway is interrupted, an object agnosia results and the patient is not able to recognize objects when presented visually. When such patients are subsequently allowed to handle the objects, they are able to recognize and demonstrate appropriate use of the objects they were unable to recognize visually.

The second short pathway of visual association fibers projects from the superior or dorsal areas 18 and 19 to somatosensory regions in the parietal cortices and is involved with visuomotor performance, spatial recognition, and the analysis of visual motion. When this pathway is interrupted, a visuodyspraxia (also termed constructional apraxia) results and the patient is not able to recognize how objects and movements are related in space. For example, the patient may be unable to recognize how holes in the shirt or pants are related to the spatial orientation of the body parts so that the head is now thrust into the armhole of the shirt when the patient is dressing; the patient who was a proficient homemaker before CVA may now be unable to assemble the inner parts of a drip coffeemaker.

Association fibers of intermediate length project from the visual cortices to the frontal and temporal lobes. The fibers that project from the visual cortices to the motor and premotor regions are mainly concerned with integrating the cortical recognition aspects of incoming visual stimuli with the kinetic system. When this pathway is interrupted, an apraxia (sometimes termed an *ideamotor apraxia*) results, and although the ideatory phase of movement remains intact, the patient is unable to visually monitor motor output, and performance is clumsy, inefficient, and marked with errors in visually mediated sequencing of coordinated movements. For example, when dressing, the patient may expend a great deal of energy turning the body and clothing about but grasp and hand-turning components will be inefficient. When asked to change position, the patient will be unable simply to shift spatial orientation. The patient will have to get up and move his or her entire body around.

Other pathways of intermediate length that project from the visual cortices to temporal areas are concerned with linking incoming visual data with language functions. When these pathways are interrupted, visually mediated forms of aphasia, dysgraphia, and dyslexia result. For example, the patient may be unable to recognize or interpret the meaning of symbols, facial expressions, written language, and so forth.

Visual guidance of motor activities provides the final link in the reverberating neural circuits that constitute functional vision. Visual guidance allows us to respond to our perceptions of the retinal image (see Figure 1.8). Cortical control of eye movements is accomplished through reciprocal pathways among three cortical centers: (a) the frontal eye fields (area 8), responsible for cortical control of eye gaze; (b) the supplemental eye fields (area 6, medially located), responsible for purposeful, anticipatory, saccadic eye movements to targets of behavioral importance, and (c) the posterior eye fields (area 39), responsible for smoothing out eye movements. Disturbance of these pathways is implicated in ideational apraxia while disturbances of motor planning results when circuits linking visual, premotor, and motor speech areas are interrupted (see Figure 1.9).

Functional vision is, therefore, dependent on neural interaction of circuits that allow for reception of retinal image, integration of that image with subcortical mechanisms of postural control, balance and anticipatory sensorimotor relays, perception of the retinal image through parallel-distributed processing at the various cortical levels or centers, and finally, the ability to use cortically controlled direction of eye gaze to plan a response to the retinal image or vice versa (i.e., the eyes can move first to find a specific retinal image).

Functional vision thus encompasses a vast network of related pathways whose influence extends throughout the neuraxis. Disruption due to trauma, developmental delay, or congenital abnormalities along any of these pathways brings with it the potential to disrupt some aspect of

HOW VISUAL CLUES DIRECT MOTOR MOVEMENTS

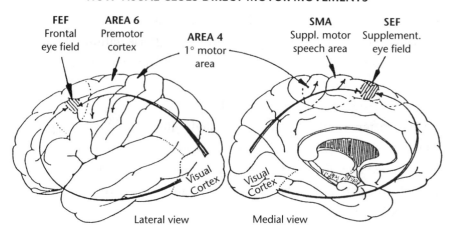

1. Direct pathways from visual cortices to areas noted above.

2. Concurrently (via dentatothalammocortical circuits) input from the neocerebellum reaches areas **6** and **4** for coordinating all synergic movements = direction, extent, force, timing and (muscle) tone of intended movements.

3. **FEF** and **SEF** send fibers directly and indirectly to saccadic generator centers of brain stem, hence to CN. Nuc. of III, IV and VI to move eyes to guide movements.

4. Final commands for movements from areas **6** and **4** descend via corticospinal and corticonuclear TRS. to LMNs involved in performing skilled sequential movements.

MOVEMENT PROGRAM GENERATOR CENTERS ENGAGED IN MENTAL PLANNING OF A MOVEMENT SEQUENCE

SEF (Supplementary eye field) is believed to be the *program generator center* for *saccadic eye movements* accompanying all preplanned or anticipatory eye movements. This center is active prior to any actual movements of the eyes. **SEF** has reciprocal connections and functions with the **FEF**, **PEF** (posterior eye field in rostral area 39 of the angular gyrus and intraparietal sulcus) and the **DLFPC** (dorsolateral prefrontal cortex), all centers involved in cortical control of saccadic eye movements, etc. Hence, **SEF** is active even during mental imagery and mental planning of a movement sequence prior to the actual movement taking place.

SMA (Supplementary motor-speech area) is believed to be the *program generator center for anticipatory or preplanned* (i.e. mentally thinking through a movement sequence) *"motor"* behaviors.

Area **4** (1° motor) and area **6** (premotor cortex) are active during the actual performance, having been signaled to act by the program generator centers **SEF** and **SMA**.

Persons with bradykinesia, hypokinesia or akinesia as seen in Parkinson's disease and Parkinsonism, demonstrate the phenomenon of "can't get started" syndrome due to loss of dopaminergic input to **SMA** and other cortical/subcortical areas. However a patient can use vision as a "starter" if a definite area (hallway, room, walk) is clearly marked off with high contrast guidance lines on the floor.

Figure 1.8 How visual clues direct motor movements. Copyright Josephine C. Moore. Reprinted with permission.

CIRCUITRY INVOLVED IN MENTAL PLANNING OF AN ACTIVITY

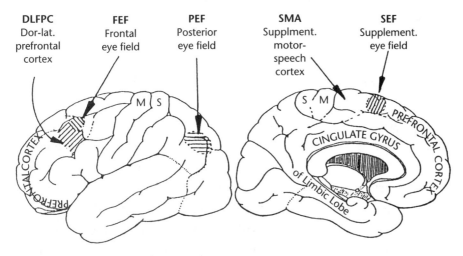

DLFPC	FEF	PEF	SMA	SEF
Dor-lat. prefrontal cortex	Frontal eye field	Posterior eye field	Supplment. motor-speech cortex	Supplement. eye field

1. From all neocortical areas and limbic cortex & especially FEF, DLFPC, PEF, and *SEF* (program generator center for saccadic eye movements) and *SMA* (program generator center for face/body movements).

2. Via corticostriatal TRS to caudate nuc., putamen and ventral striatum and substantia nigra. (all are nuclei of basal ganglia.)

3. Nigrostriatal feedback pathway (dopaminergic system).

4. From basal ganglia nuc. (see #2) via thalamus to cortical areas SMA, and concurrently via thalamic nuclei (centromedian, vent. lat. and vent. post. nuc.) to sensorimotor cortices, the prefrontal cortex and the cingulate gyrus of the limbic lobe via sub. nigra, dor-med. and ventral medial thalamic nuclei.

5. Above represents circuitry involved in "setting up" a preplanned or anticipated sequence of skilled activities.

CIRCUITRY INVOLVED IN VOLUNTARY CONTROL OF GAZE AND INITIATION OF EYE MOVEMENTS

1. From all cortical areas and especially SEF, FEF, DLPFC and PEF. (See illustration this page.)
2. Via corticostriatal tracts to caudate nucleus, putamen, ventral striatum and relay to paleostriatum.
3. To substantia nigra (of midbrain) with parallel distribution to striatum (feedback), to sup. collic. (tectum) of midbrain and to saccadic generator CTRs.
4. Parallel distribution from tectum (sup. collic) to:
   - Cranial nerve nuc. of III, IV and VI.
   - PPRF (paramedian pontine reticular formation) for horizontal gaze and saccadic movements.
   - RIMLF (rostral interstitual nuc. of medial longitudinal fasciculus) for vertical gaze and saccadic movements.
   - Hence to cranial n. nuclei III, IV and VI and to their respective eye muscles controlling horizontal and vertical eye movements.
   - Tectoreticular input to reticular formation of the medulla. Hence reticulospinal tracts to LMNs of the body.
   - Tectonuclear and tectospinal TRS to LMNs of face/body for coordinating eye movements with facial (head) and body movements.

Note: The circuits of the synergic system (cerebellum, et al.) are not included but are engaged in all facial/body actions including mental planning, etc.

Figure 1.9 Circuitry involved in mental planning of an activity. Copyright Josephine C. Moore. Reprinted with permission.

functional vision behavior, with its resulting impact on the body's total action system.

Development of Visual Integrative Abilities

Clearly one does not spring forth with a fully developed, homeostatically balanced visual system. Rather, one must move slowly and sometimes laboriously through both the development and integrative processes of the feedback mechanisms of *vision, proprioception, balance, touch,* and *audition.* Pause for a moment to reflect on the systems and development involved for a major league baseball player to make a seemingly impossible acrobatic catch. Now think back to the first attempt of the preschooler to catch a ball gently tossed. How did each get from A to Z? Remember also the confusion of the 6-year-old ballerina as she struggled to keep from being lost in space. Contrast this individual with the extraordinary grace shown by the same person just a few years later. Vision and integration of motor skills are indeed *emergent.*

In defining the process, Arnold Gesell stated, "For the child, the space world is not a fixed and static absolute. It is a plastic domain, which he manipulates in terms of his nascent powers. He was born with a pair of eyes, but not with a visual world. He must build that world himself through a series of positive acts" (Gesell, Ilg, & Ames, 1946).

Thus, the function of a child's developmental vision years is to establish the foundation of sensory information and experience needed to direct movement (e.g., the "positive acts" referred to by Gesell). Each time the young child makes a foray into space, the visual system is directing the exploration. The proprioceptive, kinesthetic, tactual, vestibular, olfactory, auditory, gustatory, and visual sensory experiences thus garnered through the movement itself and through interaction with objects in the environment are returned to the visual system where they are integrated and stored. The action years between 1 and 6 are particularly responsible for the developmental integration of these systems. During this time, the organism is driven to explore and experiment with its motor systems, resulting in the formation of the ability to interact with stimuli within arm's length, as well as garnering an understanding of how to project and localize objects outside arm's length. Therein lies the definition of the term *visual space world*.

Dr. John Streff (1971) explained the creation of this space world as follows:

> Every time the visual system receives a stimulus it analyzes and matches it against the memory banks of cumulative experience of the whole body/mind system. Accordingly, the way it integrates ("sees") that stimulus or image is conditioned by the previous experience of the whole organism. At the same time the new stimulus is added to and synthesized with the old experience, becoming a part of the analyzing, matching mechanism that is applied to the next stimulus.

Visual skills (as described above) as well as visual integrative abilities are inherent to the system of the developing child. The newborn open their eyes, and the process of visual ability development begins. However, even though the intact child comes with muscles, neural connections, and integrative pathways the degree to which these structures are *efficient* and *integrated* with each other as well as their integration with the other sensory systems becomes a developmental question. Some children develop normally and enjoy well-coordinated eye–hand–body skills; some become good athletes; while other individuals, either on their own or through various therapy modalities, develop and integrate their skills to an even higher level with the ability to perform extraordinary feats, such as the type of skills and abilities demonstrated by a Top Gun pilot.

Some children, though, will have difficulty developing their visual skills and integrative abilities in an efficient manner. This is especially true of children with developmental delays and nervous system disorders restricting their development of orderly movement patterns. As a consequence of their compromised or delayed nervous systems as explained in the section on neural processing of vision, they may have a reduced opportunity for accurate feedback opportunities on which to build a foundation for optimal functional sensorimotor integration. These delayed and compromised children are also at great risk for dysfunction within their visual systems.

While, in one sense, the visual system could exist isolated from the potential of the other sensorimotor systems, the individual's visual abilities would develop without the benefit of the input of the other sensorimotor systems. Potentially, the individual's visual abilities then would not develop as efficiently or completely as would occur in a normally functioning system. Conversely, in an individual with a normally functioning sensorimotor system, any visually directed act carried out in the presence of bodily movement or involving eye–hand–body response to expected or unexpected external stimuli would then be representative of the integration occurring in the total action system.

Although this chapter does not specifically address treatment, it is important that remediation of the sensorimotor system be conducted in concert with an individual's visual skills so that optimal integration can be achieved. Specifically, the visual skills of tracking, saccades, pursuits, convergence, divergence, and accommodative flexibility are notably enhanced when the variables of proprioception and vestibular input (e.g., walking rail, balance board) are added to the equation.

Conversely, the introduction of *visual variables* when working on a child's sensorimotor integrative abilities opens up multiple new ways for the child to experience eye, hand, and body activities. The visual variables in any particular equation are produced by the use of lenses and prisms that do not clear or blur sight but more importantly the individual's perception of stimuli location. Yoked-prism glasses (glasses made with the base of the prism in the same location on both eyes—both have base down or base up) are especially useful for this purpose.

This information is only the tip of the iceberg of potential dynamic interaction among the professions of occupational therapy, physical therapy, and behavioral optometry. It suggests the enormous benefits to each that result from sharing their respective expertise.

In defining the above visual abilities, we have only obliquely touched on the relevance to learning. However, the degree of an individual's clear, stable, efficient, comfortable vision impacts directly on his or her attention span and should be explored when evaluating the child with learning dysfunction.

Visual Dysfunctions

Now that we have an insight into the many components that determine the process of vision, we can begin a discussion of what can go wrong with the visual system. This section is intended as an overview or framework for understanding the nature of various visual dysfunctions. Dysfunctions will be categorized as pathological, refractive, and physiological.

Pathological Dysfunction

This category refers to ocular disease or problems with ocular health. A description of the ocular structures and associated pathologies are included in Appendixes A and B, respectively.

Refractive Dysfunction

This category refers to problems with visual acuity, or optical errors. A description of optics follows.

Light rays enter the eye and pass through several transparent ocular structures and undergo a process of bending known as *refraction*. Refraction makes it possible for light from a large area to be focused on a very small area (the retina) where the photoreceptors (rods and cones) are found.

The cornea and crystalline lens are the primary ocular structures responsible for refraction. The cornea is very powerful, but because the corneal focus is fixed, the cornea cannot adjust to view objects at variable distances. The internal lens of the eye generally provides the fine tuning. The focusing power of the eye must be exactly matched to the length of the eye for clear vision to be present.

Refractive errors occur when a deviation occurs in the course of the light rays as they pass through the eye, thus preventing sharp focus on the retina. The three primary refractive errors are myopia, hyperopia, and astigmatism.

Myopia, or nearsightedness, is the condition characterized by an eye with too much focusing power, as a result of the cornea or crystalline lens having excessively curved or the globe itself being too long. As a result, light rays entering the eye are focused in front of the retina and the retinal image is blurred. Near objects, which require the most focusing power, can be seen clearly, but distant objects are blurred. This condition is remedied by interposing a concave lens in front of the eye. This type of lens, also known as a "minus lens," is thinnest in the center and has a divergent, or "spreading" effect on incoming light rays.

Hyperopia, or farsightedness, is a type of refractive error in which the eye, as a result of insufficient curvature of the cornea or crystalline lens, and/or because the eyeball itself is too short, possesses insufficient refracting power. The focal point in these cases (or the locus where incoming light rays come to focus) is behind the retina, because light rays cannot bend sharply enough to focus on the retina. The closer an object is placed to the eye, the greater the retinal blur becomes; thus, the farsighted individual sees more clearly at far distance than at near. It must be noted that a person with a significant degree of farsightedness (and insufficient focusing ability) may focus inadequately even for distant objects and would, therefore, have blurred vision at both distant and near viewing. This condition is remedied by convex lenses, which are also known as "plus" lenses. Convex lenses are thicker in the center than at the edges and cause a convergent effect on light rays.

Astigmatism can be described as a "warpage" of the eye's optics caused by the cornea being steeper in certain directions, or meridians as well as the lens and globe itself having the potential for asphericity, or lack of roundness. These irregular curvatures result in a distortion of the image, causing light rays to be spread out along a blurred line, rather than achieving a pinpoint focus. This condition is remedied by the use of a "toric" aspherical lens, which has varying amounts of power in different meridians. With astigmatism, objects both near and far may be blurred.

Presbyopia, while not a refractive error per se, is the decreased ability to change the focus of the crystalline lens because of a loss of elasticity. This "hardening" of the lens occurs gradually throughout life but becomes apparent at about age 40. Patients of this age and older generally require spectacles for reading to compensate for this condition.

Physiological Dysfunction

This category refers to the mechanics of the autonomic nervous system and its impact on visual skills. It may surprise the reader to learn that the visual system is influenced by the autonomic nervous system, which can impact heavily on the visual development of the school-age child, whose nervous system is still quite immature. Prior to the completion of the myelinization process of the CNS by approximately age 15, the child can experience inconsistencies in homeostatic CNS balance because of a lack of balanced control between the sympathetic and parasympathetic nervous systems. This imbalance can result in inconsistencies in visual function, especially with regard to focusing because the ciliary body that controls focusing is under both sympathetic and parasympathetic control.

To further explain, accommodation is "owned" and innervated by *two masters* within the autonomic nervous system. The parasympathetic nervous system commands "Focus" by causing the ciliary bodies to focus the lenses of the eyes and the sympathetic system commands "Do not focus" by causing the ciliary bodies to unfocus the lenses of the eyes. Hence the individual, especially in the age group between kindergarten and grade 3, may not automatically focus correctly or in a stable manner, resulting in intermittent blurring or poor resolution of detail that can cause the child to slow his or her reading rate in order to achieve optimum reception of the visual stimulus. Such children then perform as word readers rather than being able to group words together. They may lose their place when reading and have difficulty when shifting from one line of print to another. They often go up or down a line inappropriately. They may also have difficulties in spatial organization in pencil-and-paper tasks.

Note: Difficulties in adequate focusing with accompanying poor resolution of detail can also cause children to manifest ciliary body spasm as they attempt to self-correct. This in turn causes frontal headache or eye ache.

These deficiencies in accommodative innervation in the developing child can often be traced back to sympathetic override of the parasympathetic nervous system balance. The developing visual system is extremely dependent on the developing nervous system. In a sense, especially in the developmental years of 4 to 8, the dynamic skills of the visual system are hostage to the inconsistencies of an individual's developing nervous system. The term *sympathetic override* refers to the adrenalin-infused sympathetic side of the ANS striving for attention at the expense of the calming control of the parasympathetic system being denervated. Emotional stress also can create sympathetic override. Imagine the stress a child with learning disabilities experiences on a daily basis in school. Although a controversial idea, evidence suggests that sugar ingestion in children, particularly between the ages of 5 and 7 years, can create an adrenalin-induced response, resulting in sympathetic override. When under visual stress, the fallout is that visuospatial organization can suffer, color vision can suffer, and visual fields can constrict, all of which typically goes unreported and unnoticed (Streff, 1962).

Another visual deficit results from the neural control mechanisms that supply feedback to the visual skills of coordination of convergence and accommodation. It is very important that the relationship of these skills be precisely balanced to ensure comfortable, efficient vision. Consider, for example, the havoc that can result if the eyes converge at one distance while they are attempting to focus at another distance. Actually this is a very common problem that can result in an uncomfortable visual mismatch, a short attention span, and problems with reading and comprehension.

Consider that in reading, a data link between the book and the cognitive area of the brain is established. If the receptive nature of this data link is erratic because of problems associated with the visual skills of pointing, focusing, and tracking (saccades), then the data link becomes flawed. In the case of the child who is learning to read, this flawed data link has been shown to cause slow vision. For example, the child can call out single words when learning to read, but when tasked to group or combine words (essential for comprehension) he or she experiences problems because of the visual skills responsible for a larger *visual capture* not supporting the task. In other words, because of the flawed receptive quality of the incoming visual signal, the cognitive aspect can then remain limited or dysfunctional.

The importance of the individual's visual skills influencing his or her ability to maintain a stable data link without regressions or loss of fixation cannot be overstated. At the very least, it calls into question the reliability of reading testing in grades K-3 without proper visual skill assessment and remediation if warranted.

Fortunately, the profession of behavioral optometry has a body of knowledge regarding both the differential diagnosis and treatment of these above-mentioned visual misbehaviors. Specifically, lenses and prisms that alter an individual's vergence pattern (by producing either additional convergence or divergence) in spectacle-mounted form can be worn to reskew an individual's visual input into the proper balance and comfort zone. Likewise, lenses that balance an individual's focusing needs are also prescribed. Behavioral optometry in fact refers to remedial lenses or training lenses as those lenses (often spectacle mounted) whose purpose is to help the whole body and mind system work toward better balance, alignment, and coordination. Additionally in- or out-of-office therapy may be suggested to augment the skewing action of the lenses.

Assessment of Vision

To begin this complex process, the practitioner starts the examination of the optical functioning of the eye with a measurement of unaided visual acuity. This refers to the smallest line of letters that can be read on an eye chart with the naked eye. Almost everyone is familiar with the standard Snellen eye chart designations of 20/20, 20/30, 20/40 on up to 20/200. These measurements actually express the individual's ability to *resolve detail*, using letters, numbers, or figures of various sizes on an eye chart positioned at 20 feet. The 20/20 line has characters of a size that, when resolved to their correct detail, represents an optical system in good working order. In other words, an individual with no major refractive error or a corrected refractive error in place, no abnormalities of the optical media, and good retinal function accompanied by a healthy optic nerve would be expected to see the 20/20 line.

Having thus defined a measure of an individual's sight, which is called *acuity*, we can see little about the definition that is dynamic or involves function. Herein lies the root of the common misconception that 20/20 is perfect vision.

As an example, while 20/20 acuity is helpful for passing the Department of Motor Vehicles' acuity test, it does not provide a measure of an individual's visual abilities that allow him or her to dynamically act and interact with the environment—the real test of driving ability. Just as passing the Department of Motor Vehicles' acuity test does not assess the actions and reactions that define being a good driver, neither does the distance Snellen chart address the individual's *visual abilities* that allow him or her to dynamically interact with the environment.

A thorough, primary care vision examination would include at least a determination of acuities at both far and near, an assessment of ocular motility, cover test (for assessment of over- or under-convergence tonicity), pupillary responses, and assessment of refractive status, eye pressures, confrontational visual fields, as well as an assessment of internal and external eye health.

It should be noted that while the above primary care procedures satisfy the medical and legal requirements of an eye examination, they do not necessarily include the functional evaluation of an individual's dynamic visual abilities or skills, especially at near point. As you have seen, visual skills are extremely important and should be assessed. It should be further noted, however, that while the assessment of visual skills is extremely important to an understanding of visual function or dysfunction, this area is usually not probed in detail by eye care professionals other than behavioral optometrists.

Eye Care Specialists

Having outlined the various visual dysfunctions, we will describe the specialists involved in treating the various dysfunctions. Traditionally, a discussion of vision has invoked the image of the three "Os": ophthalmology, optometry, and opticianry. Previously, the definitions were clear-cut; however, because of recent legislative changes in many states, optometry is now using therapeutic pharmaceuticals to treat ocular disease and performing primary care examinations once solely under the purview of the ophthalmologist.

Ophthalmologists continue in their role as surgeons who diagnose and treat ocular pathology with surgery and medications as well as performing primary care examinations. In treating strabismus, ophthalmologists may perform surgery to correct the eye deviation. Ophthalmologists have also used *orthoptics*, a type of visual therapy, to treat strabismus.

Optometry has always diagnosed pathology but traditionally did not treat it, focusing instead on the diagnosis and correction of problems of vision that related to acuity, binocular fusion, comfort, and efficiency. Both optometry and ophthalmology dealt with spectacles and contact lenses, with optometry being more apt to be involved on a clinical level than ophthalmology. Overall, optometry as a profession was functionally based whereas ophthalmology was medically based.

Opticians were previously integral to the equation as ophthalmology was not a dispensing profession. Hence, opticians fit and sold glasses from ophthalmologists' and some optometrists' prescriptions.

Now all that has changed. The lines differentiating ophthalmology and optometry are often blurred because most states have passed legislation certifying optometrists to both diagnose and treat ocular pathology with therapeutic pharmaceuticals. In an increasing number of states, optometrists have been certified to treat glaucoma as well. With the advent of therapeutic certification, optometry has moved into a primary care role within the managed care model.

The shift in optometry's role has resulted from the schools and colleges of optometry changing their focus to medical primary care with a resultant downgrading of functionally based core material. Private opticianry has also been caught in this change in patient care delivery as many ophthalmologists now dispense glasses from their adjoining dispensaries.

Behavioral Optometry

Behavioral optometry as a branch of organized optometry has roots dating back to the late 1920s when A. M. Skeffington, OD, began probing the mysteries of vision beyond the mere determination of refractive error. Armed with his insights, a new philosophy of optometry was formed—that the process of vision involves learned skills and is as complex a process as learning to speak, with its origins intimately related to a whole mind and body system.

The foundations of behavioral optometry are closely associated with the original Yale University Clinic of Child Development and the contributions of individuals such as Arnold Gesell, MD, who referred to the "whole human action system" being governed by "the input and output arrangement of the eye and brain," and Darrel Boyd Harmon, OD, who argued that a purely optical theory of vision was inadequate as it failed to include the role of the brain in integrating experience nor did it explain the phenomenon of brain–eye–hand–body coordination, which involves a constant process of instruction, feedback, and modified instruction.

Optometrists interested in this specialty area (known as behavioral, functional, or developmental optometry) chiefly pursue their knowledge base through the College of Vision Development (COVD) (described in chapter 4) and the Optometric Extension Program. Additionally, individuals who desire the services of a behavioral optometrist can contact the COVD for a listing of optometrists certified through the COVD in their area. Maintaining certification in the COVD requires completing a specified number of continuing education hours on the part of the optometrist.

In addition to performing a primary care examination, behavioral optometrists examine the visual system in regard to its relationship to dynamic functions. A behavioral vision analysis, for example, would assess the underlying causes of binocular dysfunction, such as a mismatch between an individual's focusing and convergence. It also probes the relationship of vision to the other senses, especially gross motor function, eye–hand coordination, and visual–auditory perception. A behavioral optometrist might also analyze the developmental history of the patient to determine periods of developmental lags such as delayed self-lateralization and established hand dominance.

In addition to the prescription of corrective eyewear and pharmaceuticals, behavioral optometrists may use vision therapy to treat visual skill dysfunctions. Therapy involving visual skills concerns itself with the flexibility and tonic state of the oculomotor act as well as the learned integration of sensory information. It is *not* extraocular muscles strengthening. The extraocular muscles as well as the ciliary body have unlimited strength. Their dysfunctional behavior results from inappropriate neural control, and tonicity problems; muscle strengthening is *not* a consideration.

In addition to the three Os, some developmental and behavioral optometrists have therapists working in their offices who perform therapy with patients. The optometrists supervise treatment and advise the therapists. Certified Optometric Vision Therapy Technicians, or COVTTs, must be sponsored by a Fellow member of the College of Optometrists in vision development and must take a written and oral exam. They must re-certify each year by attending continuing educational seminars on vision therapy.

Neuro-Optometry

Like behavioral optometry, neuro-optometry is a subspecialty of optometry. Neuro-optometrists perform diagnostic testing to determine specific acquired visual dysfunctions or deficits that are a direct result of physical disability, traumatic brain injury, or other neurological insults, such as cerebral palsy, multiple sclerosis, and so forth. Neuro-optometrists may prescribe lenses and prisms as well as in- and out-of-office visual therapy with and without occlusion.

Collaboration

Occupational therapy and behavioral optometry are in the process of joining forces in sharing professional concepts, especially in the areas of vision's relationship to man's *total action system* and man's total action system's relationship to vision. This partnership has the potential for a long and fruitful collaborative union because the origins of both disciplines are deeply rooted in *function*. Steven Cool, a noted health-care educator, has written on the subject of collaboration between the occupational therapy and functional optometry communities noting these similarities. He states that "these two health professions adopted a whole person, integrated, functional approach to treatment long before it was even vaguely fashionable" (1987).

In addition to having an emphasis on function in common, both professions share commonalities in an understanding of the processes of development and integration. The area of integration is steeped in the contributions of occupational therapy and this is the perfect place to begin rapport between the two functional Os: optometry and occupational therapy. On the one hand, occupational therapy has honed techniques for creating "movement" as regards behavioral integration. Behavioral optometry, on the other hand, has honed and developed skills in the use of lenses and prisms for creating "movement" both within the visual system and the body's related motor systems. In chapters 2, 3, and 4, the significant contributions that occupational therapy brings to this collaboration are described. In addition, chapter 4 references several optometrist and occupational therapy teams who have written about their experiences in collaboration. It is my hope that this book will help to move the collaboration between the two professions further along its evolutionary journey.

REFERENCES

Carpenter, M. B. (1991). *Core text of neuroanatomy*. Philadelphia, PA: Williams and Wilkins.

Cool, S. (1987, September). Occupational therapy and functional optometry: An interaction whose time has come? *Sensory Integration Special Interest Section Newsletter, 10*(3).

Gesell, A. G. (1952). *Infant development*. Westport, CT: Greenwood Press.

Gesell, A., Ilg, F., & Ames, L. (1946). *Growth: The child from five to ten* (rev. ed.). New York: Harper and Row.

Gesell, A. (1979). In A. Hoopes, & T. Hoopes. *Eye power*. New York: Alfred Knopf.

Streff, J. (1962). Preliminary observations of a non-malingering syndrome. *Optometric Weekly, 53*(12).

Streff, J. (1971). Lecture Notes, Southern College of Optometry.

Appendix A
Anatomy and Function of the Eye

Steven Schiff, OD

The following is intended to serve as a reference for health care professionals who encounter patients with ocular conditions. The information contained herein will provide the anatomical basis for an overall understanding for such conditions. Emphasis will be placed on those structures that play the most important role in the visual sense.

As light enters the eye, it travels through various media, and the rays are bent, or refracted. Refraction of light rays make it possible for light from a large area to focus on a small surface, the *retina*.

The Eyelids

As the eyelids are the most anterior structure, they serve a protective function. They protect the eye in several ways: when closed, they shield the eye from foreign objects; when open, the eyelashes catch and filter fine airborne particles. In addition, the many glands found on the edge of the eyelids produce the tear film. The tears moisten and hence lubricate the cornea and contain antibodies to destroy pathogenic bacteria that may be present in airborne particles.

Several neurologic disorders will cause the eyelids to either droop, which is known as *ptosis*, or to retract, causing the eyeball to seem larger on the affected side. Should a patient present with ptosis or lid retraction without previous history, immediate referral to the appropriate specialist is in order.

The Cornea

The *cornea* is the main refracting element of the eye due to its steep curvature. It is primarily the curvature of the cornea that determines the presence and extent of myopia (nearsightedness), hyperopia (farsightedness), and astigmatism. It is excessive curvature that produces myopia, insufficient curvature that produces hyperopia, and unequal curvature or "warpage" of the cornea that produces stigmatism.

The cornea is composed of three basic layers. The *epithelium* is the outermost layer and is therefore most vulnerable to damage by foreign objects. If there is a history of "foreign body" removal in the past, there may be a visible scar, with subjective complaints of glare, possibly worse in dark environments.

The *stroma* is the middle layer and comprises 90% of the corneal thickness. Here is where the corneal nerves are found, and as the cornea is richly supplied with sensory nerves, it is one of the most sensitive tissues of the body.

The *endothelium* is the single layer of cells that separate the cornea from the anterior chamber, the next structure in the eye. Biochemical reactions between this layer and the aqueous humor maintain proper osmotic balance of the cornea.

In its normal state, the cornea is transparent, which is essential for proper image formation on the retina. Microscopic anatomy of the cornea makes it an ideal optical instrument—the smoothness and uniformity of the epithelial cell layer allows for uninterrupted transmission of light rays. In addition, the corneal cells have no pigmentation and blood vessels to interfere with light transmission.

The Sclera

The *sclera*, or "white of the eye," is the tough external layer that surrounds the eyeball everywhere except at the cornea (which may be considered the forward extension of the sclera). It is composed of numerous layers of connective tissue that give it its strength, and it is opaque, allowing no light to enter the eye, which reduces light scatter and glare.

The Aqueous Humor

The *aqueous humor* is the watery fluid that fills the anterior chamber, which comprises the area behind the cornea but anterior to the lens. In most of the major ocular structures, there are no blood vessels. The aqueous humor is the source of nutrients to these structures; it also functions as the vehicle for disposal of metabolites of cellular processes. It is derived from the bloodstream and is manufactured by the ciliary body.

By way of steady aqueous formation and drainage, the pressure within the eyeball is maintained at a fairly constant level. Excessive amounts of aqueous occur when there is too much production or impaired drainage. This causes an increase in intraocular pressure, which is known as *glaucoma*.

The ciliary body is found in the anterior chamber. It is responsible for production of aqueous humor. In addition, the ciliary body contains the ciliary muscle, which is responsible for altering the shape of the lens during the process of accommodation.

The *iris* is the colored part of the eye. It is a circular structure, with a hole in the center which is the pupil. The size of the pupil is regulated by the musculature of the iris. The iris contains two muscles: the sphincter and the dilator. When contracted, the sphincter decreases pupil size, thereby reducing the amount of light entering the eye. The dilator muscles radiate away from the pupil and serve to increase the size of it, and therefore the amount of light entering it. The size of the pupil is quite variable, ranging from 1 mm when fully contracted to more than 9 mm when dilated. Pupils are reflexive, responding to light stimuli on the retina. This is known as the light reflex. It is linked to accommodative function (near reflex).

Pupil size can also be affected by neurological, cardiac or central nervous system conditions, or by drug use. Unequal size and/or reactivity can signal neurological problems such as a stroke. Dilated, unresponsive pupils are often seen in cardiac arrest, unconscious patients, or those on amphetamines. Constricted pupils may indicate central nervous system disorders or narcotic use.

Hippus is the term used to describe pupils that are constantly changing in size. This is a normal phenomenon, often seen in young people, and is not indicative of pathology of any kind. *Anisocoria* is by definition an unequal pupil size in one eye as compared to the other. About 25–30% of the general population have this condition, with no associated pathology.

The Lens

The crystalline *lens* is found immediately behind the iris and is a secondary refractive element of the eye. It accounts for approximately 25% of the eye's refractive power. At distances of 20 feet or more, light rays that enter the eye are for all purposes parallel. Within this distance, the ciliary muscle acts upon the lens in varying degrees to provide accommodation. This enables the eye to focus on objects at various distances. The lens is normally transparent, elastic, and very flexible. It is avascular and obtains its nutrients from the aqueous.

With aging, the lens undergoes a loss of its elasticity, and the accommodative function decreases at a steady rate. This makes it difficult to focus clearly on near objects. Patients over age 40 generally require spectacles for reading to compensate for this condition, which is known as *presbyopia*.

The lens also becomes increasingly "sclerosed" (accumulation of yellowish pigment) with aging. This may be partially due to absorption of ultraviolet radiation in sunlight. When this pigment begins to decrease light reaching the retina, visual acuity becomes worse. This is known as a *cataract* and is treated via surgical removal of the lens, which is replaced with an artificial lens, known as an *implant*. Implants have been used for the past decade or so. Prior to this, high powered contact lenses or spectacles were required to compensate for the refractive power that the lens originally provided.

The vitreous is the jelly-like substance that fills the posterior chamber, the largest chamber of the eyeball. It fills the entire space between the lens and the retina. The vitreous keeps the eyeball firm and round and physically supports the retinal layers by keeping them under constant pressure against the sclera. Dead red blood cells within the vitreous are seen as "floaters," or objects perceived by the patient to be present in their visual field.

The retina can be thought of as "the film" where the image develops. It is transparent, and contains 10 different layers of nerve cells. It is actually an extension of brain tissue. Here we find the photoreceptors, the *rods*, which are more concentrated in the periphery, are sensitive to low light and red light. They are primarily responsible for night vision. Incidently, this is why most instrument panels are shades of red; the rod photoreceptors are better able to respond to this color. The *cones* are more centrally located, and they provide fine object detail and color vision. They function best in bright light. During dark adaptation, the rods gradually take over visual function.

The photoreceptors function by way of pigments that are light sensitive. Production of these pigments depends on vitamin A. Color blindness is caused by deficiency or absence of one or more cone types. Red Green color blindness is most common; this is an inherited condition seen in 10% of all males but rarely seen in females.

The Macula

The highest concentration of cones is found at the fovea/macula: The macular region is the central retina, about 5 mm in size. This is the area of the retina responsible for high visual resolution and color vision. Here we find the highest concentration of cones and the best visual acuity. The fovea is a small 1.5 mm depression in the center of the macula, and the cones found here have the finest diameters and provide the best visual acuity. When an object is viewed, the person reflexively moves the eyeball so that the most important part of the image falls on the fovea. This is known as *central fixation*. The several common conditions associated with the macula include macular degeneration, macular edema, and macular hole.

The Optic Nerve

The *optic nerve* carries visual information generated by the rods and the cones and transmits the visual sensory messages to the brain for processing. It is the only area on the retina where vision is absent; this is known as the "blind spot." Optic nerves leave the back of each eye and meet at the chiasm.

The Extraocular Muscles

The extraocular muscles attach from the skull bones to the sclera. They control the movements of the eyeball within its orbital socket. There are six muscles per eye, and they can be divided into two groups, based on their position and resultant effect on movement: The *recti muscles*, of which there are four, are responsible for the basic up-down and left-right movements; and the two *oblique muscles*, which give the eye the ability to perform diagonal movements (see Figure 1).

The superior rectus muscle is named for its attachment to the top of the globe, and it is responsible for upgaze. The inferior rectus attaches at the bottom of the globe and pulls the eyeball downwards, for downgaze, such as required in reading. The medial and lateral recti muscles are used to direct the eyeball in a sideways (lateral) direction.

The superior oblique muscle, when innervated, primarily causes the eyeball to turn inward (adduction) and downward. The inferior oblique

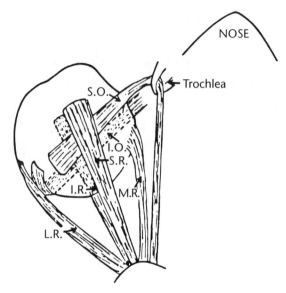

Figure 1. The extraocular muscles, viewed from above. From *Ophthalmology Made Ridiculously Simple* by S. Goldberg. Copyright 1966 by MedMaster, Inc. Reprinted with permission.

has the opposite effect, causing the eyeball to turn out (abduction) and down.

The extraocular muscles are among the most rapidly acting and precisely controlled skeletal muscles in the body. Cranial nerves 3, 4, and 6 innervate these muscles. They are yoked, meaning each muscle is paired with muscles in the opposite eye; this allows the eyes to move in the same direction at the same time. Conjugate movements of the two eyes are known as "*versions*," compared to "*ductions*," which refers to the movements of a single eye in its various fields of gaze. When the eyes move in opposite directions, the term *vergence* is used. Movement of the eyes toward each other, or nasally, is known as *convergence*, and the movement of the eyes outward is known as *divergence*. The medial and lateral recti muscles are primarily responsible for vergence movements, and improper coordination of these muscles causes the binocular deficits.

Appendix B

Table 1. Overview of ocular diseases and disorders*

Condition	Affected Area	Cause	Visual Effects	Mode of Detection	Treatment	Prognosis
Achromatopsia (total color blindness)	Retina (cone malformation	Hereditary	Decreased visual acuity to 20/200, extreme photophobia, and nystagmus. Visual fields are normal	Color vision screening test and electrodiagnostic tests, especially using the electroretinogram (ERG)	Optical aids, sunglasses, and dim illumination.	Nonprogressive; nystagmus and photophobia reduce with age.
Albinism (total or partial lack of pigment)	Macula (underdeveloped)	Hereditary	Decreased visual acuity (20/200 to 20/70), nystagmus, photophobia, high refractive effor, and astigmatism. Visual fields variable and color vision is normal.	Family history and ocular examination.	Painted or pinhole contact lenses, absorptive lenses, optical aids, and dim illumination.	Nonprogressive.
Aniridia	Iris (underdeveloped)	Hereditary	Decreased visual acuity, photophobia, possible nystagmus, cataracts, displaced lens, and underdeveloped retina. Visual fields are normal. Secondary complication: glaucoma, with accompanying constriction of the visual fields, squint, and lens opacification.	Clinical observation of missing iris tissue	Pinhole contact lenses, sunglasses, optical aids, and dim illumination.	Milder forms develop slow, progressive cataracts; severe forms develop glaucoma and corneal opacification.

* Source: R.T. Jose (Ed.). (1983). *Understanding Low Vision*. NY: American Foundation for the Blind. Reproduced with permission.

Table 1. Continued

Condition	Affected Area	Cause	Visual Effects	Mode of Detection	Treatment	Prognosis
Cataracts (congenital)	Lens (opacity)	Hereditary, congenital anomalies (rubella, Marfan's syndrome, Down's syndrome), infection or drugs during pregnancy, and severe malnutrition during pregnancy.	Decreased visual acuity, blurred vision, nystagmus, squint, photophobia, slight constriction in the peripheral visual fields is possible, but visual fields are normal.	Ophthalmoscopy and slit-lamp biomicroscope.	Surgery as early as possible, cases of visual impairment.	After surgery, inability to accommodate; problems with glare, which are corrected with spectacles or contact lenses. Complications from surgery: glaucoma, retinal detachment, hemorrhage of the vitreous or retina.
Cataracts (senile)	Lens (opacity)	Age	Progressively blurred vision; near vision is better than distance vision.	Same are for congenital cataracts.	Surgery, with resultant cataract spectacles, contact lenses, lens implant, (IOL, intraocular lens).	Same are for congenital cataracts. Complications from surgery: glaucoma, retinal detachment, hemorrhage of the vitreous, infection, Better candidate for intraocular lens (IOL) implants.
Cataracts (traumatic)	Lens (opacity)	Head injury or metallic foreign body in the eye.	Blurred vision, redness and inflammation of the eye, and decreased visual acuity. Complications: infection, uveitis, retinal detachment, and glaucoma.	Same as for congenital and senile cataracts.	Surgery after inflammation subsides.	Same as for congenital and senile cataracts.
Coloboma	Various parts of the eye may have been deformed, severity depending on when deformity occurred during development.	Hereditary	Decreased visual acuity, nystagmus, strabismus, photophobia, and loss of visual and superior fields. Secondary			

48

Table 1. *Continued*

Condition	Affected Area	Cause	Visual Effects	Mode of Detection	Treatment	Prognosis
Coloboma (*continued*)			complication: cataracts. Associated conditions: microphthalmia, polydactyly, and mental retardation.	Fundus examination	Cosmetic contact lenses, sunglasses, and optical aids.	Usually fairly stable.
Diabetes Mellitus	Retina	Hereditary	Diplopia, inability to accommodate, fluctuating vision, loss of color vision or visual field refractive error, decreased visual acuity, hemorrhaging of blood vessels in the retina, retinal detachment. Secondary complications: glaucoma and cataracts. Associated conditions: cardiovascular problems, skin problems, and kidney problems.	Ophthalmoscopy; reports of fluctuating vision	Insulin injections, dietary controls, spectacles, and laser-beam surgery. Various illumination control aids.	Variation in acuity common.
Degenerative Myopia (nearsightedness)	Elongation of the eye; stretching of the posterior of the eye.	Hereditary	Decreased visual acuity in the distance, vitreous floaters, metamorphopsia. Normal visual field unless retina is detached. Secondary complications: retinal detachment and swelling or hemorrhaging of the macula.	Fundus examination	Prescription correction, preferably contact lenses; optical aids, and high illumination.	Unpredictable rate of progression.

* Source: R.T. Jose (Ed.). (1983). *Understanding Low Vision*. NY: American Foundation for the Blind. Reproduced with permission.

Table 1. Continued

Condition	Affected Area	Cause	Visual Effects	Mode of Detection	Treatment	Prognosis
Down's Syndrome (mongolism)	Various parts of the eye.	Hereditary; extra No.21 chromosome.	Decrease of visual acuity, squint, nystagmus, severe myopia, Brushfield spots, congenital cataracts, and keratoconus. Color vision and visual fields are normal. Associated conditions: mental retardation, cardiac abnormalities, hypotonia, saddle-shaped nose, large protruding tongue, and a short, squat stature.	Physical appearance. Complete medical workup.	Depending on patient's intellectual level, optical aids, prescription correction.	Medical problems more severe than usual. Good prognosis.
Glaucoma (congenital)	Tissues of the eye damaged from increased intraocular pressure.	Hereditary	Excessive tearing, photophobia, opacity or haze on lens, buphthalmos, poor visual acuity, and constricted visual fields.	Tonometry, study of the visual fields, and ophthalmoscopy.	Eye drops; surgery as soon as possible to prevent extensive damage.	With treatment, depends on the innate resistance of the structures of the eye. Blindness if not treated.
Glaucoma (adult)	Same as for congenital glaucoma.	Hereditary of the result of changes in the eye after surgery.	Headaches in the front portion of the head, especially in the morning; seeing halos around lights; decreased visual acuity, loss of visual fields, photophobia, and constricted peripheral fields in severe cases.	Same as for congenital glaucoma.	Eye drops, optical aids, sunglasses.	Same as for congenital glaucoma.
Glaucoma (acute attack)	Same as for congenital and adult glaucoma.	Inability of the aqueous to drain.	Nausea, severe redness of the eye, headache, and severe pain.	Same as for congenital and adult glaucoma.	Emergency surgery.	Without surgery, permanent damage to the ocular tissues and loss of visual acuity and in peripheral vision.

Table 1. *Continued*

Condition	Affected Area	Cause	Visual Effects	Mode of Detection	Treatment	Prognosis
Histoplasmosis	Macula or periphery (scattered lesions)	Fungus transmitted by spores found in dried excrement of animals.	In the macula: decreased visual acuity, central scotoma, and deficient color vision. In the periphery: scotoma corresponding to the area of lesions.	Ophthalmoscopy	Optical aids for visual problems; steroids for physical condition.	Can be life-threatening if not treated.
Keratoconus	Cornea (stretched to a cone shape)	Hereditary. Manifests in second decade	Increased distortion of entire visual field; progressive decrease in visual acuity, especially in the distance. Associated conditions: retinitus pigmentosa, aniridia, Down's syndrome, and Marfan's syndrome.	Ophthalmoscopy, retinoscopy, keratometry, and slit-lamp biomicroscope.	Hard contact lenses in the early stages; keratoplasty (corneal transplant) as needed.	Without keratoplasty, progressive degenerative thinning of cornea until cornea ruptures and blindness ensues.
Marfan's Syndrome (disease of the connective tissues of the body)	Various parts of the eye.	Hereditary	Dislocation of the lens, decreased visual acuity, severe myopia, dislocated or multiple pupil, retinal detachment with accompanying field loss, different-colored eyes, squint, nystagmus, and bluish sclera. Associated conditions: skeletal abnormalities, long, thin fingers and toes, cardiovascular problems, and muscular underdevelopment.	Medical examination and evaluation.	Optical aids. Surgical or optical management of the dislocated lens.	Vision problems stable; medical problems are more significant.

* Source: R.T. Jose (Ed.). (1983). *Understanding Low Vision*. NY: American Foundation for the Blind. Reproduced with permission.

Table 1. *Continued*

Condition	Affected Area	Cause	Visual Effects	Mode of Detection	Treatment	Prognosis
Retinal Detachment	Retina (portions detach from supporting structure and atrophy)	Numerous, including diabetes, diabetic retinopathy, degenerative myopia, and a blow to the head.	Appearance of flashing lights; sharp stabbing pain in the eye; visual field loss; micropsia, color defects, and decreased visual acuity if the macula is affected.	Ophthalmoscopy and an internal eye examination.	Laser-beam surgery and cryosurgery, depending on the type and cause of the detachment; optical aids; and usually high illumination.	Guarded.
Retinitis Pigmentosa	Retina (degenerative pigmentary condition)	Hereditary	Decreased visual acuity, photophobia, constriction of the visual fields, (loss in the peripheral field), and night blindness. Usher's syndrome, Laurence-Moon-Biedel's syndrome, and Leber's syndrome are associated with R.P.	Electrodiagnostic testing, especially ERG, and ophthalmoscopy.	Optical aids, prisms. No known medical cure; genetic counseling is essential.	Slow, progressive loss in the visual fields that may lead to blindness.
Retrolental Fibroplasia	Retina (growth of blood vessels) and vitreous.	High levels of oxygen administered to premature infants; occasionally found in full-term infants.	Decreased visual acuity, severe myopia, scarring, and retinal detachment, with resultant visual field loss and possible blindness. Secondary complications: glaucoma and uveitis.	Ophthalmoscopy.	Optical aids and illumination control devices.	Poor, in severe cases, where further detachments can be expected in third decade.

Table 1. *Continued*

Condition	Affected Area	Cause	Visual Effects	Mode of Detection	Treatment	Prognosis
Rubella	Various parts of the eye.	Virus transmitted to the fetus by the mother during pregnancy.	Congenital glaucoma, congenital cataracts, microphthalmia, decreased visual acuity, and constriction of the visual fields. Associated conditions: heart defects, ear defects, and mental deficiency.	Ophthalmoscopy, slit-lamp biomicroscope, tonometry, and family history.	Surgery for glaucoma and cataracts, optical aids, establishment of appropriate educational goals.	Poor; post-surgical inflammation.
Toxoplasmosis	Retina, especially macula (lesions)	Intraocular infection caused by *Toxoplasma gondii.* In congenital type, fetus exposed to organism; in acquired type, through contact with infected animals or ingested.	Loss in visual fields corresponding to location of lesion, squint, decreased visual acuity if macula is affected, severe brain damage if congenital.	Ophthalmoscopy.	Optical aids — usually good responses to magnification.	Nonprogressive, although new lesions may develop.

* Source: R.T. Jose (Ed.). (1983). *Understanding Low Vision.* NY: American Foundation for the Blind. Reproduced with permission.

2 Neuromotor Prerequisites of Functional Vision

Renee Okoye, MS, OTR, BCPOT

Introduction

In order for vision to become functional, neurons located throughout every level of the central nervous system (CNS) must first become accustomed to responding to the body's demand for (a) postural support to position the head and neck so that the eyes can take in visual information, (b) movement synergies to coordinate positioning of body parts in order to contact or avoid targets in the environment, and (c) integration of neural circuits to coordinate movement of the eyes with movement of the trunk and body parts in space. Without this postural basis of support, functional vision would be a moot point, and the individual would be unable to interact with his or her environment. It is only after the motor prerequisites have been met that the upper portions of the brain can begin their work of decoding, analyzing, and associating visual data with other incoming stimuli.

Unfortunately, because functional vision tends to be thought of as a highly cortical task, it is easy to forget the postural components of the process. It seems that only when challenged by the patient who is unable to perform on the cortical level and progress is painfully slow, that the memory is jogged just enough to remember the need to get back to those basic elements of preparing the body as a whole in order to engage the eyes in the processes of functional vision.

Recent discoveries in the neurosciences, particularly in the area of the development of visual perception, provide validation of the intimate link between the development of movement in the body as a whole and the development of vision as a perceptual process.

The purpose of this chapter is to review foundational aspects of neuro-motor development that affect the development of functional vision behavior (see Figure 2.1).

General Organization of Neuromaturational Processes

The following discussion is intended to be a brief survey of how the structures and functions of the CNS relate to maturation of cognitive, motor, and sensorimotor skills inherent to the development of functional vision.

Neuromaturation Progressions

The general organization of structures within the CNS reflects a dynamic interplay between both vertical and horizontal hierarchies of function. The interplay among these hierarchies results in neuromaturation (processes surrounding emergence and development of the functional support mechanisms that link central structures with the sensorimotor events that fall within their sphere of influence) unfolds in clearly identifiable strands of repetitive progressions. The overall structure, shape, and definition of the neuromaturational progression is repeated throughout each level of the CNS within structures of the brain and spinal cord. The repetition is analogous to the leaves of a maple tree, which conform in overall shape and veinal pattern. Regardless of its location on the maple tree, or where on the branch a leaf is found, one can identify the leaf

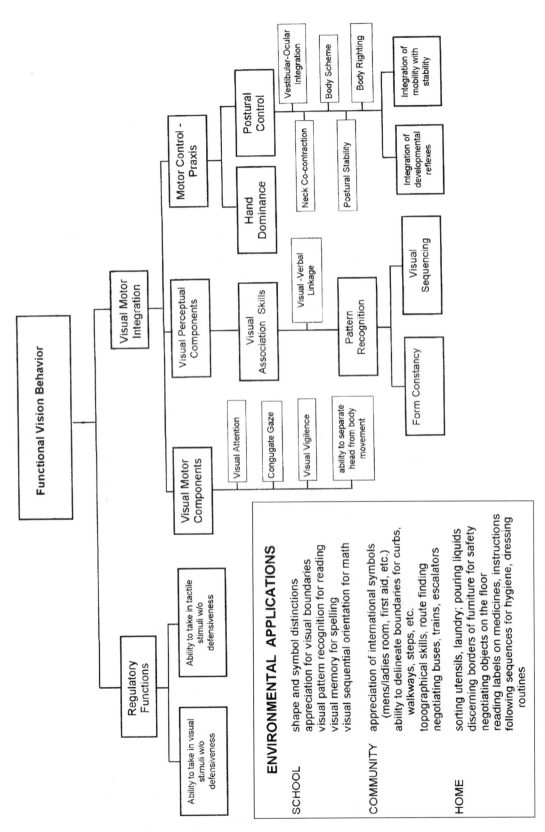

Figure 2.1 Neurodevelopmental task: Acquisition of functional vision behavior.

because each bears a recognizable pattern. Neuromaturational processes also conform to recognizable patterns that are repeated at every level of the CNS and tend to be organized according to basic developmental progressions.

The Phylogenetic Progression

The clinical significance of the phylogenetic progression is quite broad and affects treatment outcomes in almost every rehabilitative service. This progression reflects the neurobiologic observation that phylogenetically primitive functions, rather than those specific to the human species, will emerge earlier in neuroma are species specific. For example, development of phylogenetically older, neurobiologically protective motor responses, such as the blink of an eye or gross grasp of the hand, will precede development of phylogenetically newer, exploratory motor responses, such as conjugate gaze or superior pinch.

Clinical Application. For example, if sustained visual regard were selected as the treatment objective during a particular phase of treatment, then within a phylogenetic progression, introduction of a strong-smelling food item or a visually interesting blow toy would be preferable to introduction of a picture to stimulate visual attending behaviors. From the perspective of the phylogenetic progression, pairing a primitive approach behavior, such as an orienting response to something that smells interesting or an oral motor activity with visual output, would be preferable to pairing a language response with visual output. The behavioral response to olfaction and oral motor activity is a phylogenetically older behavior than that of a cognitive response to symbolic language. Particularly when treating patients whose attending behaviors fluctuate, adjusting the level of CNS state (lowering the level of arousal if it is too high or raising the level of arousal if it is too low) is a necessary first step in treatment.

When the phylogenetic progression is used as a consideration in treatment, it is usually sequenced into the early stages of treatment by (a) selecting an appropriate developmental continuum within which the target behavior (or short-term treatment objective) may be demonstrated or achieved, (b) having the patient rehearse a phylogenetically older response pattern within that developmental continuum as a prerequisite activity, and then (c) moving toward production of the target behavior later in treatment. From the perspective of this progression, stimulating primitive centers within the brainstem early in treatment results in the involvement of a wider network of neural support for the target behavior. When the target behavior is finally facilitated, a more thoroughly integrated motor response may be affected. Current neurobiological theory supports the notion that the resulting sensory motor output would then have greater amplitude (projecting further through the neuraxis) and last longer because of the influence of reverberating neural networks (Faber, 1982). Clinically, one would expect that arousal and sustained attention to task would result.

The Cephalocaudal Progression

The cephalocaudal progression embodies the concept that development proceeds in a head-to-tail fashion. This is a foundational concept that demonstrates a vertical hierarchy in the emergence of sensorimotor skills. The cephalocaudal progression is demonstrated by the emergence of sensorimotor patterns that involve cephalic regions (muscles of the head, face, and neck) developing the ability to control sensory motor events before more caudal regions (the trunk or legs). This pattern of neuromaturation may be seen when an infant begins to develop mobility in the prone position and neck extension emerges before scapular stabilization and shoulder extension. Within a treatment context, therefore, cephalocaudal progressions of motor output would be facilitated early within a therapeutic sequence designed to improve eye–hand coordination, since the face, neck, and upper trunk are physically closer to the head. Direct involvement of the hand as a tool or means of output would be introduced later since the hand is physically located more caudally.

Clinical Application. Direct application of the cephalocaudal progression is seen clinically during the planning stage of treatment as the clinician carefully selects therapeutic sequences that proceed in a head-to-tail fashion to optimize results. For example, in planning treatment sequences to improve integration of functional vision behavior with reciprocal upper extremity movement, sequences to improve reciprocal interaction of the eyes and mouth (such as use of a blow toy or whistle) would be presented before sequences to improve eye–hand coordination. Because of the cephalocaudal progression of neuromaturation, treatment sequences should involve body segments that are closer to the head first and incorporate involvement of the more caudal body segments later. This plan will result in recruitment of supportive neuromotor activity and produce more semiautomatic motor responses.

The Proximal-Distal Progression

The proximal-distal progression describes a horizontal hierarchy of neuromaturation that begins within the midline or proximal regions of neural structures and body segments and flows toward the periphery or distal regions. The proximal-distal progression may be observed in cranial structures such as the cerebellum where neuromaturation begins in the central zone or vermis, which controls movements of the trunk, and spreads to more distal, paracentral regions that control movements of the limbs. On a functional yet microscopic level, the proximal-distal progression may be observed in the major lobes of the cortex, such as in the occipital lobe where neuromaturation begins in the central zone of the occipital lobe (area 17), which only responds to signals from the retina and is responsible for primary reception of visual data. From area 17, neuromaturation of the occipital lobe spreads toward its association regions in the peripheral regions of the occipital lobe (areas 18 and 19) where the neurons respond to signals arising from other structures and are responsible for interpreting or associating visual data with movement, language, and other sensory motor codes. The organizational structure supporting this progression may be seen in motor maps throughout the central nervous system. A classic example of this is the observation of the organization of the central gray matter within each segment of the spinal cord. Neurons responsible for innervating the midline regions of the limbs are located proximally, or in the center most portions of the central gray matter, while those responsible for innervating the distal regions of the limbs are located in peripheral regions of the central gray matter (DeGroot & Chusid, 1988).

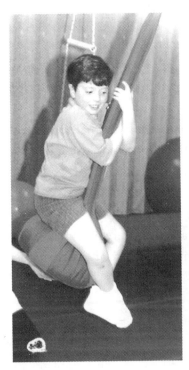 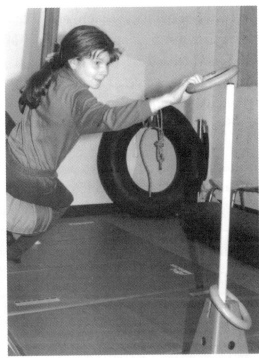

Figures 2.2A and 2.2B. The moon swing is being used as an exercise to stimulate and strengthen proximal stabilizers of the trunk. When the proximal stabilizers of the trunk contract with sufficient strength, their coordinated action serves to stabilize the trunk while the body moves through space. When the proximal stabilizers perform their work, the more distal segments of the body (the arms and legs) are free to engage in the skill component of activities. The flexion component of proximal stabilization is weak (left). This boy's lack of chin tuck indicates that his neck flexors are weak. His extended, rather than flexed, trunk indicates that his abdominals and other trunk flexors are not responding with sufficient strength to stabilize his trunk for this activity. The youngster is unable to free the distal segments of his arms to reach for a target because they are engaged in helping his weak proximal stabilizers to hold on. The dynamic rotation of the girl's trunk (right) shows synergistic action of her trunk stabilizers. Because her proximal muscles are contracting with sufficient strength to stabilize the trunk for this activity, her distal body segments (eyes, forearms, and hands) are free to engage in the skill component of this task, and she is able to place the ring onto the rod. Courtesy of Picturesque Photography. Reprinted with permission.

Clinical Application. Proximal motor functions tend to contribute stabilizing (holding or tonic) components to motor activities. When the proximal muscles contract, they tend to preposition the midline segments of the body in steady holding patterns that provide postural support for the movements that are to come. This means that when proximal motor patterns (such as neck flexion) are facilitated before distal motor patterns (such as visual fixation), the very act of moving the neck into flexion tends to prepare for the movement to come, in this instance, visual fixation upon a target. The proximal-distal progression is reinforced on a neurokinesiological basis, in that movement of proximal synergists facilitates action of more distal motor patterns. The proximal-distal progression is generally touted as the foundational basis for strengthening postural control in children with poor eye–hand coordination before attempting to develop oculomotor or in-hand manipulation skills. By strengthening the proximal muscles of the neck, back, and upper body first, the child will be able to demonstrate the prerequisite postural stability. Fine motor skills may then be superimposed on a stable base (see Figures 2.2A and 2.2B).

The Gross-to-Fine Progression

The interaction of structures and functions of the CNS are organized so that neuromaturation proceeds from the ability to coordinate gross-motor patterns, involving large muscle groups first, to the ability to coordinate fine-motor patterns, involving groups of small muscles working together. This means that gross-motor patterns, such as the ability to control the upper body and neck to allow for early monocular fixation upon the hand, will mature long before the fine-motor skills that allow for smooth visual pursuit of a moving target. The gross-to-fine progression also shapes the development of control of upper-body stability for sitting erect long before control of the digits for handwriting.

Clinical Application. The clinical significance of the gross-to-fine progression is such an essential feature of neuromaturation processes that entire programs of therapeutic exercise have been based on this progression. For example, neurokinesiological approaches to treatment that emphasize the use of movement to facilitate CNS response patterns, such as neuro-development therapy (Bobath), proprioceptive neuromuscular facilitation (PNF) (Voss, Ionta, & Myers, 1985; Brunnstrom 1970), all stress that the approaches to patient treatment be organized in this fashion. For example, one technique of PNF is to apply proper pressure to the shoulder girdle to activate the muscles of the rotator cuff before giving the command to "look at your hand." This is done in preparation for an exercise designed to facilitate coordinated movement patterns in the upper extremity. Similarly, one NDT technique used to prepare a patient with spastic hemiplegia for exercise is to shake out or normalize tone in the spastic shoulder before attempting to gain opening of a tightly fisted, spastic hand.

The General-to-Discriminative Progression

The final progression, in which neuromaturation proceeds from general (or nonspecific) sensorimotor functions to increasingly discriminative skills, has been a popular theme of most neurobiological treatment approaches (e.g., Ayres; Fisher & Murray, 1991; Rood; Stockmeyer, 1967). Clinically speaking, general sensorimotor skills, such as the ability to localize a sound source and visually fixate on it, will tend to be available to a child long before discriminative skills, such as the ability to pair relationships between sound and sight necessary for phonics.

Treatment techniques based on the hierarchical principles of neuromaturation progressions (phylogenic, cephalocaudal, proximal-distal, gross-fine) are called developmental approaches because they tend to facilitate emergence of skills in a manner consistent with a general developmental continuum of neurobiological processes.

The Role of the Brainstem in the Development of Functional Vision

Both myelination and neuromaturation begin at the pontomedullary junction in the brainstem (Aoki & Siekevitz, 1988). From this point, neuromaturation proceeds upward and downward in a vertical orientation, as well as forward in a horizontal orientation to activate the cranial nuclei, and reticular and olivary complexes. Fibers entering the neuraxis at this point bifurcate to project both downward to the spinal cord to activate muscles of the neck and upper back, upward to the oculomotor nuclei and the diencephalon, and from there to the cortex.

Reflexes and sensorimotor reactions that are integrated by structures housed within the brainstem are of clinical significance to neurorehabilitation therapists because these reflexes and sensorimotor reactions provide a background of postural support without which normal movement and functional vision is not possible. Most of the structures of the brainstem subserve neurobiologically primitive functions by integrating their input with the more sophisticated directives from the cortex (Gilfoyle, Grady, & Moore, 1990). This integration is accomplished as the neurobiological sum of the inputs change thresholds at terminals of neural pathways whose interconnections are located in the brainstem. For the most part, sensorimotor functions of the brainstem tend to involve phylogenetically older rather than newer movement patterns. This means that the phylogenetically older movement patterns provide for primarily cephalic movements of the head, neck, and upper body more than for the more caudal movements of the lower body, movement patterns of proximal rather than distal musculature, and movements that are gross rather than fine.

The tonic labyrinthine reactions and the tonic neck reactions, sustained postural reactions that are stimulated by vestibulo-proprioceptive input that is modulated in the medulla, are typical of brainstem-level reaction patterns. These mass movement patterns distribute additional postural tone to the trunk and extremities depending on the combined stimulation from the proprioceptors in the neck and the vestibular organs in the middle ear. For neurorehabilitation clinicians who treat patients with deficits of functional vision, successful formulation of treatment sequences hinges in large measure on an appreciation of how motor patterns at the level of the brainstem affect visual motor and other adaptive skills. Because all levels of the neuraxis are intricately interwoven, the central core of these patients' deficits does not rest in any one part of the whole. That is to say, it is not the eyes alone nor the vestibular system alone nor the reticular attending system alone, but the sum total of their interactions, albeit played out at the level of the brainstem, which is at the central core of the problem. Patients who sustain injury to these primitive centers tend to have disorders of postural tone and other regulatory functions that have a profound affect on their ability to maintain a consistent level of arousal and to perform smoothly coordinated movements. These types of disorders affect ocular motility, visual perceptual skills, postural stability, eye-hand and eye-foot coordination skills, and balance (see Figure 2.3).

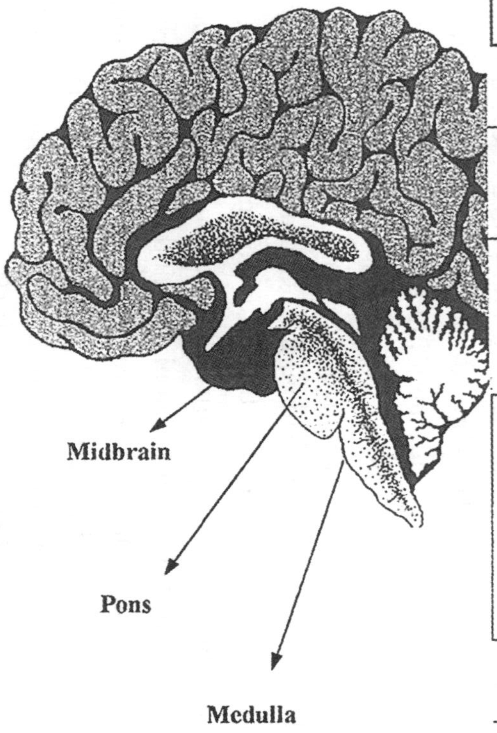

POSTURAL REACTIONS SUPPORTING FUNCTIONAL VISION

Level of Integration	Reaction Patterns	Receptors	Stimulus	Response Pattern
Spinal cord	Stretch Reflex 1) Stretch Reflex 2) Crossed Extension 3) Reciprocal Innervation 4) Reciprocal Inhibition	Proprioceptors Muscle spindles	Stretch	1) contraction of muscle 2) contralateral extension 3) facilitation of synergists 4) inhibition of antagonists
Medulla	Tonic Labyrinthine Reflexes 1) supine 2) prone 3) sidelying	Otoliths	Positioning of the head relative to gravity	1) increased extensor tone 2) increased flexor tone 3) increased flexor tone in topmost extremities; increased extensor tone in bottom most extremities
Medulla	Tonic Neck Reflexes 1) Symmetrical 2) Asymmetrical	Neck proprioceptors	Turning the head 1) up 2) down 3) to the side	1) increased extensor tone in the arms and increased flexor tone in the legs 2) increased flexor tone in the arms and increased extensor tone in the legs 3) increased extensor tone in the nasal extremities and increased flexor tone in the occipital extremities
Midbrain	Labyrinthine righting reactions	Otoliths	Gravity	Head rights to the head vertical, mouth horizontal position
	Body righting reactions	Proprioceptors about the axial skeleton	Stretch	Body rights to align itself with the head
	Neck Righting reactions	Proprioceptors in the neck	Stretch	The body rights to align itself with the neck
Cortex	Optical Righting reactions	Eyes	Visual cues	The body rights to align itself with the field of vision
	Equilibrial reactions	Otoliths	Gravity	Counterbalancing in the trunk and protective extensor tone in the extremities

Midbrain

Pons

Medulla

Figure 2.3 Postural reactions supporting functional vision.

The brainstem consists of three primary structures known as the me-dulla, the pons, and the midbrain. The organization and structure of the brainstem reflects a hierarchy of functions. The interaction of vertical and horizontal zones of function within the CNS is apparent in both the macroscopic and microscopic columnar arrangement of structures throughout the brainstem. On a macroscopic level, central structures are arranged longitudinally. On a microscopic level, the nuclei for the cranial nerves are arranged in seven longitudinal columns (Nieuwenhuys, 1992). Each of these columns is specifically related to somatic, motor, or vis-ceral functions.

The Medulla

The medulla is located at the base of the brainstem. It is a phylogenetically old structure and houses nuclear complexes that perform vital functions essential to growth and development of the individual. Structures within the medulla that have been shown to impact neuromaturation processes involved with functional vision include the vestibular nuclear complex, the olivary nuclear complex, and the medullary reticulospinal tract. The interaction of vestibular and oculomotor complexes allows for normal development of body scheme and temporal-spatial orientation, or visual perceptual skills that allow the individual to estimate distances and negoti-ate skillfully among objects while moving through space.

The vestibular nuclear complex contains four paired nuclei that have an extensive network of relays throughout the neuraxis that project downward to the spinal cord and upward to the cortex. The individual nuclei within the vestibular nuclear complex have direct connections with the extensor motoneurons within the gray matter of the spinal cord, the cerebellum, the reticular formation, the oculomotor complex, and the thalamic relay nuclei. Their functional components affect cognitive skills as well as motor and sensorimotor skills. These structures contribute in a powerful way to the labyrinthine, tonic labyrinthine, and equilibrium reaction patterns that signal normal development of neuromaturational processes within the CNS. The combined effect of these reaction patterns provides additional extensor tone for postural muscles during antigravity activities and postural stability for balance (Molina-Negro, 1980).

The olivary nuclear complex is involved in almost every resistive exercise regimen used in neurorehabilitation. One function of this nuclear complex is to awaken the parasympathetic division of the nervous system to the need for additional physiological support as sustained muscular activity begins to drain local reserves. The blushing of the skin and additional turgidity of muscle tissues that accompany sustained effort is one of the outcomes of the function of the olivary nuclear complex.

The medullary reticulospinal tract affects neurorehabilitation functions by inhibiting antigravity extensor muscles while providing some degree of facilitation to the flexors. This action serves to counterbalance the extensor tone generated by the combined output of the vestibular and pontine reticular systems and allows for smoother transition of movements during activities that require alternate reciprocal motor patterns.

The Pons

The pons is located in the middle of the brainstem. Structures within the pons that have been shown to impact neuromaturation of functional vision include the phylogenetically older portions of the reticular formation and the nuclei of the trigeminal, abducens, facial, and vestibulocochlear cranial nerves. Phylogenetically more recent structures of the pons directly involved in development of neuromaturation processes include the medial longitudinal fasciculus and the pontine nuclei.

The reticular formation is more expansive in the pons than elsewhere in the brainstem. These reticular nuclei give rise to the reticulospinal tract, a descending tract that conveys excitatory impulses to extensor motoneurons throughout the length of the spinal cord. Pontine reticular nuclei interact with ascending fibers that project to the thalamic nuclei and interact with descending fibers that project to the inferior olivary complex. Because of the early maturation of this communicative network that conveys attending and orienting behaviors between the eyes and ears, muscles of the face, and spine via the medial longitudinal fasciculus, treatment modalities that awaken the pontine reticular formation can be used clinically to facilitate anticipatory readiness for sensorimotor and perceptual skills. Clinically speaking, this network is responsible for much of the increased level of arousal, focused attention, and increased visual regard that results from use of sucking, chewing, blow toys, and other forms of oral motor stimulation.

Cranial nerve V, the nuclei for the trigeminal nerve, is located in the pons. This cranial nerve contains both sensory and motor fibers and communicates directly with almost all of the other cranial nerves. Again, because this is a phylogenetically older structure, its pathways are developed early during neuromaturation. Sensory modalities applied to trigeminal areas of sensory innervation on the face can be used to stimulate this cranial nerve and enhance primitive sensorimotor functions of the eyes and mouth. Neurophysiological treatment approaches emphasized stimulation of the trigeminal nerve as a preliminary stage of treatment for persons with CNS dysfunction (Stockmeyer, 1967). Tactile stimulation to the face and use of sour balls and ice pops can be used to stimulate the trigeminal nerve.

Cranial nerve VI, the nuclei for the abducens nerve, is located in the pons. It is a motor nerve that innervates the lateral rectus muscle of the eye and serves to abduct the eye. Although fibers of the abducens nerve communicate with the other cranial nerves within the oculomotor complex, the function of the abducens nerve is integrated early during neuromaturation because of the location of the nuclei within the more primitive part of the brainstem and synergistic action with the extensors of the neck and upper back.

Clinically speaking, it is significant that abduction is a synergistic function of extension. The ability to abduct the eyes emerges early, along with reflexive maturation of extensor patterns in the neck, trunk, and upper extremities. Development of coordinated patterns of extension in the neck and upper trunk paired with abduction of the eyes will, therefore, emerge as a functional motor synergy early in the development of the infant because the structures that affect these patterns lie in phylogenetically older portions of the brainstem. Skilled patterns of trunk flexion are paired with eye adduction. Because the structures that subserve these movement patterns lie in phylogenetically more recent areas of the brainstem, eye adduction and skilled use of flexor patterns represent developmentally newer skills and are more difficult to acquire.

The nuclei for cranial nerve VII, the facial nerve, is located in the pons. It innervates muscles of facial expression (the buccinators, the orbicularis oculi, and the stapedius) as well as the platysma, a muscle that superficially acts to flex the head upon the neck. These muscles can also be stimulated by use of oral-motor activities, whistles, and blowing or sucking toys. Because of the way in which the neural circuits are integrated in the brainstem, blowing tends to reinforce postural extension including neck extension and eye abduction. Sucking tends to reinforce postural flexion including neck flexion and eye adduction.

The Midbrain

The midbrain is located at the top of the brainstem. Structures within the midbrain that have been shown to affect neuromaturation of functional vision include the inferior and superior colliculi, and the oculomotor nuclear complex.

Integration of sensorimotor signaling between auditory, visual, and motor output occurs at the level of the midbrain. Sensorimotor relays through the midbrain constitute a major thoroughfare for visual and auditory orienting responses as the body responds to incoming sensory signals from its distance receptors by righting or aligning its parts. This is the first developmental level of the CNS that provides mechanisms that allow the body to take in information from its external environment and to pair that input with a motor response.

The inferior colliculi in the midbrain receive information from many sources within the brainstem including the cochlear nuclei, which are located in the pons. The sum of the auditory information from this level is then relayed upward to the thalamus where the information is then projected to the auditory cortex of the cerebrum. As paired structures, the inferior colliculi also relay information to each other for spatial comparison. Some fibers from the inferior colliculi branch to the superior colliculi where their signals are paired with incoming visual information. Finally, signals from the inferior colliculi provide for motor response through collateral discharge to the tectospinal tract and the medial longitudinal fasciculus. These fibers terminate in the cervical regions of the spinal cord and facilitate turning or orienting the head in the direction of a sound source. This positions the head so that the eyes may begin to investigate the sound source.

The superior colliculi in the midbrain receive information from the retina, cerebral cortex, oculomotor nuclei, vestibular nuclei, and the spinal cord. The superior colliculi are paired and information is relayed back and forth between them for spatial registration purposes. Although the superficial layers of each colliculus are functionally related to vision, and the deeper layers are functionally related to eye and head movements, both layers are intimately linked for spatial registration (Carpenter, 1991). The superior colliculi relay visual information upward to the thalamus where the information is then projected to the visual cortex. Other fibers from the superior colliculi project to the oculomotor nuclei and downward to the inferior colliculi where reverberating circuits can provide comparator information. Other fibers from the superior colliculi project to the tectospinal tract. Some of these projection fibers travel via the medial longitudinal fasciculus to terminate in the cerebellum. Other fibers course through the medial longitudinal fasciculus to terminate in upper segments of the spinal cord to facilitate head turning or orienting the head in the direction of the visual stimulus. Integration of visual, vestibular, and motor inputs at the collicular level allow for involvement of the superior colliculi in coding the location of an object in the visual field relative to the fovea and in eliciting saccadic eye movements that produce foveal acquisition of the object (Ornitz, Kaplan, & Westlake, 1985).

The oculomotor nuclear complex is a collection of cell columns and discrete nuclei that innervates the inferior oblique and the superior, medial, and inferior recti muscles of the eyes; innervates the levator palpebrae muscle; and provides visceral support between the ciliary ganglion and lower brainstem (Kernhuber & Frederickson, 1970). The visceral nuclei are involved with oculomotor reflexes that produce nystagmus, saccadic eye movements, and the queasy stomach associated with too much nystagmus.

Fibers from the oculomotor nuclear complex project downward to the vestibular nuclei, where they terminate in each of the four vestibular nuclei. The oculomotor complex is the only structure that provides direct afferent fibers to the vestibular nuclei from higher levels of the neuraxis (Moore). Visual information has a profound impact upon vestibular processing within the CNS. Development of relays between oculomotor and vestibular complexes, referred to as *vestibulo-ocular integration* (VOI), is an essential ingredient in the development of dynamic balance and functional vision.

Clinically speaking, VOI allows for the grading of movements as the person nears an object in the environment such as when walking up or down steps, crossing thresholds, or moving from a narrow corridor into a wide-open vestibule. The relays used to compare visual with vestibular information as the body moves in space toward a target serve to continually compute distance and point of contact. This servomechanism provides a framework for spatial orientation that is projected cortically and incorporated into skills that require serial ordering (see Figures 2.4A, 2.4B, and 2.4C).

Adaptive behaviors, motor planning, and motor sequencing skills, such as the ability to negotiate space without bumping into objects, to negotiate curbs and escalators, to find a route and orient to topography, to dress and perform hygiene routines, and even to understand time and number concepts, emerge from information derived from VOI. Although our focus in this text is primarily on the affect of VOI on visual parameters, it is clinically significant to note that secondary social and emotional issues arise when VOI fails to mature properly. Some of the social and emotional maladaptive behaviors observed in persons with poorly developed VOI include apprehension and avoidance of new environments and new people, difficulty transitioning from one activity to another, avoidance of eye contact, visual hypersensitivity, visual defensive behavior, and shutdown when presented with visually complex images. These maladaptive behaviors affect quality of life in social and academic contexts and signal the need for sensory integrative approaches to treatment to facilitate development of VOI before visual training or eye–hand coordination exercises per se can be effective.

Neural transmission from the vestibular nuclei facilitates transmission from the oculomotor nuclei. The reverse is also true. In order for development of vestibulo-ocular relays to occur, concomitant factors of sufficient

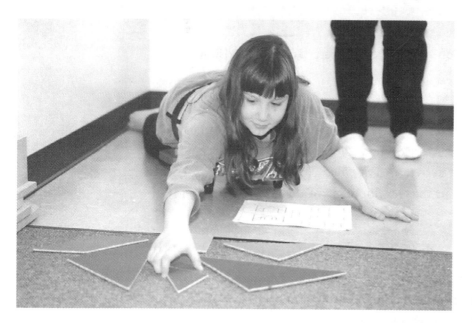

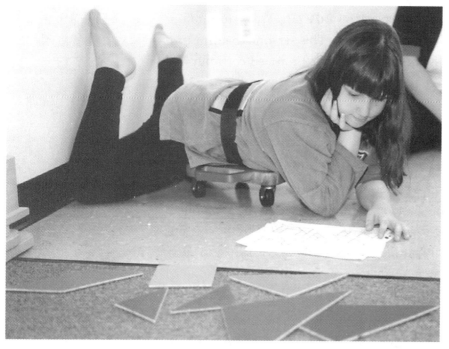

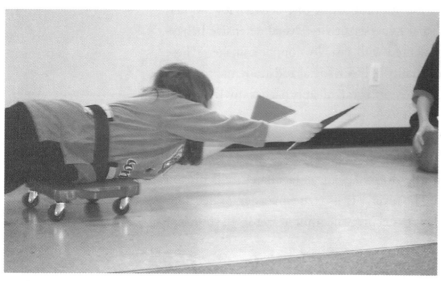

Figures 2.4A, 2.4B, and 2.4C. These pictures demonstrate how VOI is used in daily living skills. In Figure 2.4A, the oversized manipulatives are being handled so that tactile sensation may reinforce the visual image and form constancy of each shape. Use of another sensory channel to compare and verify visual input helps to code each piece in preparation for mental manipulation. In Figure 2.4B, a sequential plan is formulated and the girl begins to plan how each puzzle piece is to be oriented in space. In Figure 2.4C, the plan is executed, using input from both the vestibular and oculomotor systems to (a) guide the girl's movements accurately through space within the boundaries of the tiled runway, (b) grade the timing of her motor output as she nears the target, and (c) maintain her spatial orientation so that she can position each piece correctly. Courtesy of Picturesque Photography. Reprinted with permission.

signal strength and adequate neurotransmitter levels must be present. Unfortunately, these relays are highly susceptible to toxins early in pregnancy, before the mother may know that she is pregnant (De Benabib & Nelson). When significant levels of toxins are introduced to these rapidly developing structures early in embryonic development, movement disorders result and VOI fails to develop properly. The result is low-normal postural tone, impaired dynamic balance, poor ability to shift from peripheral to central vision, postural-ocular dyspraxia, and poor fine-motor skills. Secondary social and emotional maladaptive behaviors also may be noted.

The availability of postural righting mechanisms on a subcortical level is central to the ability to move about safely and independently in space. Postural righting mechanisms integrated at the midbrain level that support development of functional vision include the labyrinthine righting reflexes, body righting reactions, and neck righting reactions. These postural righting mechanisms serve to provide postural alignment and head and neck orientation on a semiautomatic basis, so that attention and visual vigilance may be directed toward learning tasks and problem solving. When these postural mechanisms fail to develop properly, cortical attention must be reallocated to supporting posture and visual functions, and less attention is available for other tasks.

Developmental postures may be used to assess integration of postural control and availability of cortical attention for cognitive tasks by having the patient perform simple cognitive tasks while in an antigravity developmental posture (e.g., the Sensorimotor Performance Analysis). If postural righting mechanisms have been integrated properly, the patient will be able to maintain postural control on a semiautomatic basis while performing the cognitive task (see Figure 2.5).

If postural righting mechanisms have not been properly integrated, the posture of the head, neck, and arms will quickly become compromised, and the patient will not be able to perform both activities at the same time. This means that this patient is not likely to be able to perform challenging eye–hand, visual discrimination, or oculomotor tasks smoothly until the body has first been supported in a sedentary position. The clinician is then left to consider which goals in treatment should be

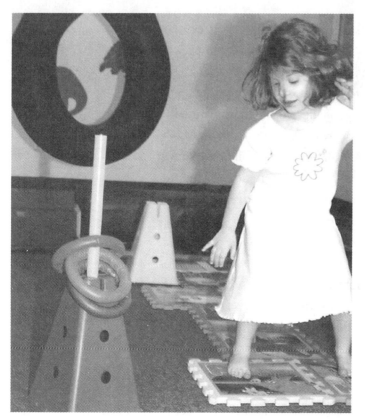

Figure 2.5 The girl demonstrates how traditional childhood games depend on the ability to subordinate postural control so that cortical attention may be allocated to specific skills. The ability to play hopscotch requires a background repertoire of postural adaptations, such as the ability to alternate leg movements, so that visual attention can be directed to counting out number or letter sequences. Courtesy of Picturesque Photography. Reprinted with permission.

addressed first. Should this patient be propped up to perform visual training activities, or should treatment address faulty postural mechanisms? Which approach will result in improvement of functional vision skills for this patient?

When the patterns of background postural adjustments and motor skills are analyzed for the patient with deficits of functional vision, often vestiges of poorly integrated developmental reflexes may be seen. Failure to integrate developmental reflexes or reaction patterns into coordinate patterns of movement is considered to be a soft sign of neurological involvement. That is to say, one of the primary tasks of neuro-maturational processes is to integrate primitive reflexes and reaction patterns with successively higher levels of motor control as development progresses. When this process fails to develop normally, acquisition of fine-motor skills, such as eye-hand coordination and ocular motility, fail to develop normally and acquisition of functional vision is delayed. Another way of saying this is that the failure to integrate basic reflexive patterns of movement beyond infancy may block development of functional vision (Barnes, Crutchfield, & Heriza).

The Role of Developmental Reflexes in the Emergence of Functional Vision

The emergence of functional vision is codependent on the presence of primitive developmental reflexes that are present prior to or at birth and the development of postural reaction patterns that appear during infancy. These patterns, working together with visual influences, become integrated into functional patterns of motor coordination during early childhood. Primitive reflexes and postural reactions involved with the develop-

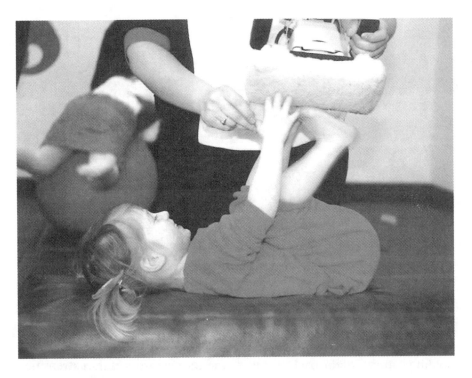

Figure 2.6 The ability to rehearse the tonic flexion pattern with synergistic recruitment of trunk, neck, eyes, arms, and legs in a variety of positions is typical of normal neuromaturation. The position of this toddler is sometimes referred to as the inverted tonic labyrinthine prone position. It is characterized by tonic holding of proximal flexors of the neck, trunk, arms, and legs with adduction and fixation of the eyes in near to midpoint. Courtesy of Picturesque Photography. Reprinted with permission.

ment of functional vision tend to be whole-body patterns of movement that serve to integrate postural tone with basic patterns of coordination. The reaction patterns provide for integration of movements of the head and the body by integrating local neurophysiological reflexes at the spinal level with the supraspinal relays of the brainstem. Developmental postural reactions that are involved in the emergence of functional vision tend to be responsive to vestibular-proprioceptive and vestibulo-ocular influences. This response tends to facilitate development of tonic stabilizing or holding patterns about the midline while pairing the response with vision to provide for rotation and organization of motor patterns in three-dimensional space.

Developmental reflexes that divide the midline of the body along the frontal plane (e.g., the tonic labyrinthine prone reflex) affect tonic holding patterns of either the flexors or extensors. When the abdominals and flexors of the extremities located on the front of the body are innervated, because these are flexors, their synergistic action helps to recruit adduction of the eyes (see Figure 2.6).

The contrasting pattern of the developmental reflexes affects tonic

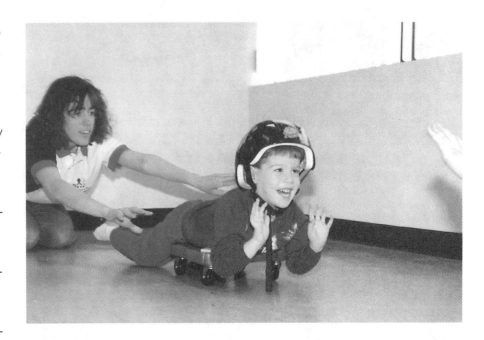

Figure 2.7 The ability to rehearse the tonic extension pattern with synergistic recruitment of trunk, neck, eyes, arms, and legs in an antigravity position is being demonstrated by this preschooler as he practices an exercise in tonic stability. This position is often referred to as pivot prone and also prone extension. It is characterized by neck, upper back, and shoulder extension with hips, knees, and ankles extended as well. The position promotes abduction of the eyes with visual fixation in far range. Courtesy of Picturesque Photography. Reprinted with permission.

holding patterns of the back extensors and the extensors of the extremities located on the back of the body (e.g., the tonic labyrinthine supine reflex). Because these are extensors, their synergistic action helps to recruit abduction of the eyes (see Figure 2.7).

Developmental reflexes that divide the midline of the body along the horizontal plane (top half and bottom half) affect holding patterns of the neck, upper body, and arms. Their contrasting pattern affects tonic holding patterns of the legs and lower body (e.g., the symmetrical tonic neck reflex) (see Figure 2.8). These movement patterns are sometimes referred to as being *homologous*, since they tend to provide for simultaneous contrasting patterns. When the neck is extended, the upper extremities are also extended, and the lower extremities are flexed. Alternatively, when the neck is flexed, the upper extremities are also flexed, and the lower extremities are extended.

Developmental reflexes that divide the midline of the body along the sagittal plane (right and left sides of the body) affect ipsilateral or holding and stabilizing patterns on the same side and mobilizing patterns on the opposite side (e.g., the asymmetrical tonic neck reflex) (see Figure 2.9).

Developmental reactions that serve to help organize patterns of rotation

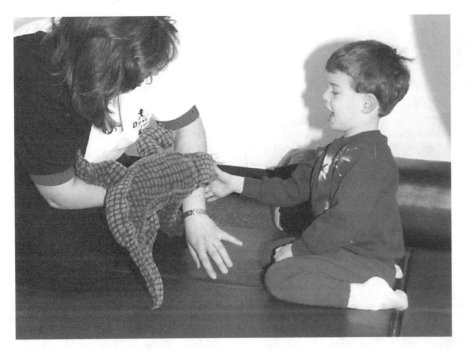

Figure 2.8 The need to "W" sit with his lower extremities flexed, adducted, and internally rotated to provide him with a stable base in the low back while he actively extends is arm and neck shows that this boy has not yet integrated the symmetrical tonic neck reflex. The neck extension provides the impetus for extension of the arms but at the cost of imposed lower extremity flexion. Courtesy of Picturesque Photography. Reprinted with permission.

about the midline are referred to collectively as *body righting reactions* (see Figure 2.10). These reactions function collectively to realign the person so that the head or the body face the same direction, following rotation of one of the body's segments.

Primitive reflexes and developmental reactions may be observed most clearly in the neonate when the influences of more sophisticated motor patterns are not yet available. The neonate is delivered into a sensory environment that has only been vaguely experienced in utero. After birth, while the CNS adapts and begins to ascribe causal relationships to sensory experiences, gravitational, vestibular-proprioceptive, and visual influences begin to interrelate to form organized patterns of movement.

Neonatal Neck Righting and Neonatal Body Righting Reflexes

One of the earliest of these whole body, organized patterns of movement that influence the emergence of functional vision are the neonatal neck righting and neonatal body righting reflexes. This early form of neck righting and body righting has been described as localized stretch reflexes (Padula, 1988). (The stretch reflex is one of several reflexes of a normally

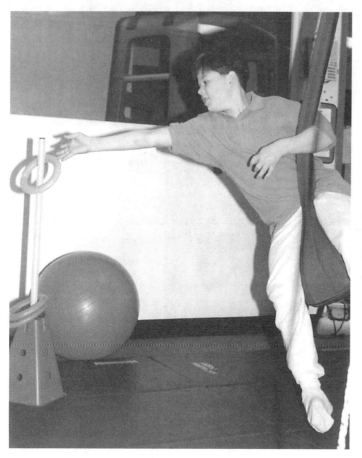

Figure 2.9 The action of the asymmetrical tonic neck reflex along the sagittal plane divides movements on the nasal side of the body into extension and movements on the occipital side of the body into flexion. This primitive motor pattern becomes integrated during the first year of life but may be seen throughout the lifespan during times of stress or motor challenge. Courtesy of Picturesque Photography. Reprinted with permission.

active spinal cord. The stretch reflex is stimulated by proprioceptors lying within muscle tissues. When these proprioceptors are stimulated, they send a neural impulse to their corresponding segment of the spinal cord, which results in contraction of the muscles in which they lie). The neonatal neck righting reflex is a pattern that serves to realign the body with the spatial orientation of the head in the newborn, after the head and the neck have been rotated. Rotating the head of a newborn either to the left or the right and holding the head in the rotated position usually will provide adequate stimulus to initiate the neonatal neck righting reflex. If the newborn is less than 4 months old and postural tone is normal, the entire body of the neonate will usually rotate in the same direction as the head was rotated, so that the body will be realigned with the new position of the head and its fields of vision.

The neonatal body on body righting reflex is a pattern that serves to realign major body segments once they have been rotated. Rotating a major body segment, such as the shoulder girdle or the pelvic girdle, away from midline and holding the segment in the rotated position usually will provide adequate stimulus to initiate the neonatal body on body righting reflex. The infant usually will respond by rotating the body as a whole unit so that the head and its field of vision will be aligned with the body as a whole.

One function of the neonatal neck righting and neonatal body righting reflexes as they relate to functional vision is the maintenance of alignment of the head and fields of vision with the body to develop organized responses to proprioceptive input as the neonate rotates in space. Another function of the neck and body righting reflexes is to aid early processing of visual information. From a neurobiological point of view, body righting serves to position the neonate to investigate, avoid, or simply wait as the nervous system processes the visual information brought into focus by the rotary movements. These reflexes help maintain the distance receptors, the eyes and the ears, aligned with the mobilizers of the body. This may be viewed as a precursor to early survival responses that allow the neonate to prepare for movement by rolling and visually orienting in response to environmental demands.

The positioning of body parts in response to emerging visual, visuomotor, sensory integrative, and cognitive processing is an initial phase of motor sequencing. As such, these reflexes represent a rudimentary form of organized motor behavior for the neonate. These neonatal reflexes link the motor neurons of the spinal cord with sensory receptors lying within the muscles, joints, and connective tissues into patterns of sensorimotor interaction. Although the neonate moves slowly into this response as the pattern is learned, motor patterns that become integrated at the spinal level do not require cortical direction and are available for rapid deployment. Having the pattern readily available at the spinal level is necessary for both survival and fluidity of postural adaptation mechanisms.

The neonatal neck righting and neonatal body on body righting reactions assist the development of functional vision by facilitating early motor responses that pair movement of the head and neck with response to body rotation. Rotary influences occur about the midline of the body constantly during the course of daily activities. Not only do these reaction patterns bring the body's effectors into alignment with what is viewed in the visual field, but they also provide the neural bias to activate synergistic muscle patterns that will assist eye–hand and eye–foot teaming. These early reaction patterns help to prepare the individual to interact with objects within the visual field and serve to establish neurokinesiological motor patterns at the spinal level that will subserve practical eye–hand and eye–foot patterns of coordination later in life.

Clinically speaking, a key point to note is that although the neonate

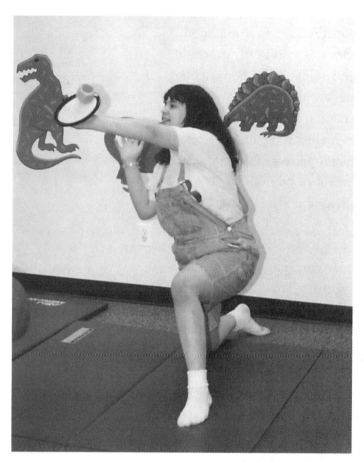

Figure 2.10 Body righting reactions provide for alignment and repositioning of body segments as they rotate around the midline. The body righting reactions coordinate movement patterns between the neck and body segments as each rotates around the midline of the body. The girl demonstrates body righting of her head and neck with her shoulder girdle and upper body as she first turns her head to keep her eyes on the ball and then reaches out to cross her midline in order to catch it. Courtesy of Picturesque Photography. Reprinted with permission.

responds to rotational influences by righting the body in whole segments as the nervous system matures, it is essential that this primitive beginning becomes integrated into more discrete patterns of movement. Patients who move the entire upper quarter of the body during handwriting or use ambulatory aids demonstrate that they are dependent on this primitive reflexive pattern to team eye–hand movements. Neither their eyes nor their hands are truly free to perform independently (see Figures 2.11A and 2.11B).

Tonic Labyrinthine Reflexes

The tonic labyrinthine reflexes provide additional facilitation for development of postural tone about the frontal plane of movement. Tonic flexion and tonic extension, short-leveraged holding patterns centered in the midranges of the trunk, form proximal stabilizing bases from which skilled motor patterns can emerge. (For example, without the steady holding patterns of neck cocontraction, the head is not held still, and visual fixation is faulty. Without the steady holding of the shoulder girdle, the arms are not held still, and prehension is faulty). The tonic labyrinthine prone reflex serves to facilitate organization of flexor tone when the neonate is placed in a prone position. The stimulus for the reflex is the prone position, per se, and the sensory receptors responsible for the reaction are the otolithic organs in the inner ear and the proprioceptors located in the skin and muscles of the body segments that are in contact with the supporting surface. When these sensory receptors are stimulated as the neonate is placed in the prone position, their response pattern stimulates muscle action of the postural flexors of the body. The pattern stimulates the neck and trunk flexors along with the flexors of the extremities. Activation of the deep-lying flexors of the neck with synergistic flexion of the trunk

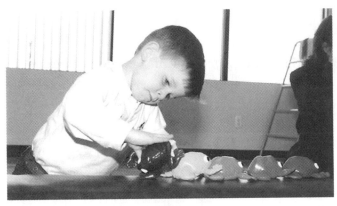

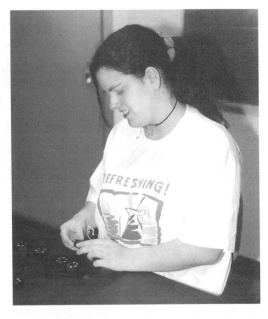

Figures 2.11A and 2.11B The preschooler in Figure 2.11A demonstrates a primitive pattern of eye–hand teaming as his entire shoulder girdle, arm, and head are recruited to perform a simple hand-turning maneuver. As long as sustained visual engagement is needed to direct every hand and finger movement, this boy's eyes are not free to take in simultaneously other relevant information (such as awareness of where his body is in relation to other objects and people in the environment). The head tilt coupled with the asymmetrical positioning of the arms in Figure 2.11B indicates that this young adult is dependent on vision rather than tactile and proprioceptive stimuli to manipulate the small pieces of her game. Until her tactile processing skills are improved, functional vision will be delayed as her eyes, rather than her hands, direct manipulation of small objects. Courtesy of Picturesque Photography. Reprinted with permission.

and upper extremities brings the head with eyes adducted into near contact with the hands on a reflexive basis. The motor pattern is one that will be used later in life as a subset of eye–hand coordination.

The tonic labyrinthine supine reflex serves to facilitate organization of extensor tone when the neonate is placed in the supine position. The stimulus for the reflex is the supine position, per se, and the sensory receptors responsible for the reaction are the otolithic organs in the inner ear and the proprioceptors located in the skin and muscles of the body segments that are in contact with the supporting surface. When these sensory receptors are stimulated as the neonate is reclined in the supine position, their response pattern stimulates muscle action of the postural extensors of the body. The pattern activates the neck and trunk extensors along with the extensors of the extremities. Activating the deep-lying extensors of the neck with synergistic extension of the trunk and upper extremities stimulates relays that reflexively abduct the eyes when extensor tone predominates in the neck and trunk.

The steadying influence resulting from tonic labyrinthine coactivation of the proximal musculature results in a dynamic tension about the midline of the body. Activity of the more distal mobilizers can then be initiated from a steady springboard of movement, rather than from a wobbly base. Skilled patterns of movement in the peripheral regions of the body can then emerge smoothly.

The stability derived from this position coupled with synergistic motor and oculomotor patterns are rehearsed throughout developmental motor activities, such as prone on elbows or quadruped creeping, as the infant learns to recruit tonic extension and far vision to explore the environment. However helpful the primitive tonic labyrinthine reflexes may be, failure to integrate their powerful tonic stabilizing influence with developmentally higher mobilizing rotary and vestibular influences results in rigid and fixed movement patterns. When the tonic labyrinthine reflexes predominate, poor ability to alternate between flexor and extensor patterns in the extremities is correlated with poor ability to alternate between adduction and abduction of the eyes. In these instances, both flexor and extensor movement patterns will be characterized by too much tone with little control over body rotation; functional vision will be characterized by little control over the midranges of ocular motility.

Tonic Neck Reflexes

Motor patterns of the tonic neck reflexes affect development of functional vision as the neonate uses these primitive patterns of mobility about the horizontal and sagittal planes. Primitive fixation on the hand occurs when the neonate uses the tonic neck reflexes to mobilize the arms, legs, and eyes into reciprocal alternating patterns (Corelle & Henderson, 1979).

The symmetrical tonic neck reflex provides alternating patterns of stability and mobility about the horizontal plane. The reflex is activated when the infant flexes the neck. The sensory receptors involved in this reflex are the proprioceptors in the neck; they produce one of two different motor patterns, depending on which muscles are contracted. When the infant flexes the neck by contracting the neck flexors while reciprocally relaxing the neck extensors, this action serves to signal the nervous system in such a way that the upper extremities flex, while the lower extremities simultaneously extend. This position also results in adduction of the eyes because of synergistic action. When the eyes are adducted and the arms are flexed, the upper extremities are automatically brought into near visual range, and the infant fixes on the hands. The pattern of flexing the neck to look at objects within the hand is a primitive response programmed very early in the neuromaturation of the infant. An alternate motor pattern results when the infant extends the neck by contracting the neck extensors while reciprocally relaxing the neck flexors. This action serves to signal the nervous system in such a way that the upper extremities extend, while the lower extremities simultaneously flex. This action results in abduction of the eyes. While the neck is extended and the upper body is propped up off the supporting surface on extended arms, the eyes are positioned to engage the distant environment. Many developmental activities of the infant, such as crawling, pulling up into standing, and even heel sitting for play, incorporate use of these motor patterns. Vestiges of the symmetrical tonic neck pattern remain available throughout life and may be seen even in the adult, particularly when resistive activity is required.

The asymmetrical tonic neck reflex provides alternating patterns of stability and mobility about the sagittal plane (see Figure 2.12). The reflex is activated when the infant rotates the neck and head. Reciprocal stimulation of the neck proprioceptors and the semicircular canals produces different motor patterns on the right and left side of the body. When the infant rotates the neck, the side toward which the nose is pointing (or the nasal side) tends to move into extension, while the side toward the back of the head (the occipital side) simultaneously moves into flexion. The action involves both the arms and the legs in reciprocal patterns of stability in the extremities on the nasal side with mobility in the extremities on the occipital side of the body. Visual fixation occurs on the nasal side (Ottenbacher, 1979) and offers the neonate an opportunity to examine the hand while in a stable position.

The asymmetrical tonic neck reflex positions the body in what is sometimes referred to as the *fencing position*. Although the reflex allows the neonate to briefly regard the hand, it is a motor pattern that tends to block development of feeding, dressing, and similar self-care activities.

Figure 2.12 As the girl rolls toward her right, she not only shows the typical asymmetrical tonic neck reflex pattern of movements in the sagittal plane, but she also demonstrates the visual fixation of her extended hand that is afforded by the reflexive pattern of movement. As her head rotates, postural tone in the extensors on her nasal side increased and the extremities on this side tend to move into extension. Meanwhile, postural tone in the flexors on her occipital side increased and those extremities then move into flexion. While the neck is stabilized, it provides the opportunity for fixed visual regard on the extended hand. Courtesy of Picturesque Photography. Reprinted with permission.

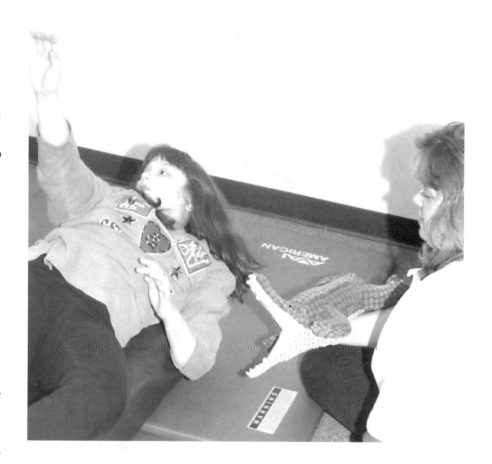

Clinically speaking, the tonic reflexes produce sustained holding postural tone. While the tone is helpful to the neonate and prepares the proximal regions of the body (head and neck, trunk and central girdles) for the sustained holding muscular activity needed for normal development, disorders of tone signal dysmaturation of the brainstem and pose a major problem. Because the brainstem is a key structure in relaying sensorimotor data between the proprioceptors and vestibular and oculomotor complexes, damage to this area invariably results in disorders of tone, vestibular processing, and ocular motility. When patients present disorders of tone in the clinic, the therapist should look to see if comorbid disorders are present in vestibular and oculomotor skills as well.

The implications for clinical practice are far-reaching for therapists who hope to ameliorate disorders of functional vision, either through the means of developmental optometry, occupational therapy, educational therapy, or other means of developing fine-motor skills. Acquisition of functional vision is inexorably wed to development of postural mechanisms. This would suggest that treatment of disorders of functional vision should of necessity address postural issues in some measure. Studies in the past have shown that when postural issues are addressed in treatment along with functional vision, the results are positive (Forstrom & von Hofsten, 1982).

REFERENCES

Aoki, C., & Siekevitz, P. (1988, December). Plasticity in brain development. *Scientific American.*

Barnes, M.R., Crutchfield, C.A., & Heriza, C.B. *The neurophysiological basis of patient treatment* (vol. 12), Morgantown, WV: Stokesville Publishing.

Carpenter, M. (1991). *Core text of neuroanatomy* (4th ed.). Baltimore, MD: Williams and Wilkens.

Cohen, H. (Ed.). (1993). *Neuroscience for rehabilitation.* Philadelphia, PA: J. B. Lippincott.

Corelle, J., & Henderson, A. (1979). Role of the asymmetrical tonic reflex in hand visualization in normal infants. *American Journal of Occupational Therapy 33.*

DeBenabib, R.M., & Nelson, C.A. Efficiency in visual skills and postural control: A dynamic interaction.

DeGroot, J., & Chusid, J. G. (1988). *Correlative neuroanatomy* (12th ed.). East Norwich, CT: Appelton & Lange.

de Quiros, J., & Schrager, O. (1979). *Neuropsychological fundamentals in learning disabilities* (rev. ed.). Novato, CA: Academic Therapy.

Faber, S. (1982). *Neurorehabilitation: A multisensory approach.* Philadelphia, PA: W. B. Saunders.

Forstrom, A., & von Hofsten, C. (1982). Visually directed reaching of children with motor impairments. *Develop. Med. Child Neurol 24,* 653–661.

Gilfoyle, E.M., Grady, A.P., & Moore, J.C. (1990). *Children adapt.* Thorofare, NJ: Slack.

Kernhuber, H.H., & Frederickson, J.M. (1970). Recent clinical and experimental results concerning vestibular and oculomotor mechanisms. *International Journal of Neurology 8,* 23–24.

Molina-Negro, P., et. al. (1980). The role of the vestibular system in relation to muscle tone and postural reflexes in man. *ACTA Otolaryngol 89,* 524,533.

Moore, J. Current concepts in the neurosciences. AOTF Mini-Course handouts and personal notes.

Nieuwenhuys, R., Voogd, J., & van Huijzen, C. (1992). *The human central nervous system.* NY: Springer-Verlag.

Ornitz, E.M., Kaplan, A.R., & Westlake, Jr. (1985). Development of the vestibulo-ocular reflex from infancy to adulthood. *ACTA Otolaryngol 100,* 180–193.

Ottenbacher, K., et. al. (1979). Nystagmus and occular fixation difficulties in learning disabled children. *American Journal of Occupational Therapy 33.*

Padula, W. (1988). *A behavioral vision approach for persons with physical disabilities.* Optometric Extension Program. Santa Ana, CA: Optometric Extension Program.

Semans, S. (1967). The Bobath concept in treatment of neurological disorders. *American Journal of Physical Medicine, 46,* 732–985.

Stockmeyer, S. (1967). An interpretation of the approach of Rood to the treatment of neuromuscular dysfunction. *American Journal of Physical Medicine 46,* 900–957.

Voss, D., Ionta, M., & Myers, B. (1985). *Proprioceptive neuromuscular facilitation.* NY: Harper and Row.

3 Sensory Integration and Visual Functions

Jeannetta D. Burpee, MEd, OTR/L

A Developmental Hierarchy of Sensory Systems Supporting Awareness of Body-Self and Surroundings

Sensory integration is an operation intrinsic to everyone's life. It enables functioning, relating to our world, being who we are, and understanding who and what is occurring around us. It is this very basic sensory process that allows visual functions to work for us. Without it, we might see, but what we see would mean nothing to us and we would probably have little or no control over how we use the oculomotor system. In my clinical work it has been extremely important for me to continue to work at recognizing how and where the visual-motor, visual-spatial, and visual-relational components fit into the overall sensory-integrative developmental process in order to evaluate patients and to treat them with any reasonable effectiveness. I do not consider myself in any way an expert in the area of visual function per se, but I do have some insights into where, how, and why visual function fits into the context of a larger sensory motor developmental process. I would like to share these insights and caution people to consider the larger sensory integrative developmental process within the context of visual sensory-motor function before coming to conclusions about any presumably specific visual dysfunction.

Sensory integration is a fundamental process that enables the body to take all the sensory input (tactile, proprioceptive, vestibular, visual, auditory, gustatory, olfactory) we receive from our own bodies and from the external environment and to then process it. Our central nervous systems organize, synthesize, and analyze the input as a sort of database for possible functional use. This assimilated input is integrated and used by each body to formulate a type of sensorimotor scheme and eventually to create a cognitive map of itself. We become a body-self and we have a presence. With this physical presence we begin simple interactions and form relationships with our surroundings. By having a reasonably accurate sense of our own body and its physical form within space, we are able to then project from this base an elementary understanding of that which is external to us. We experience within ourselves the sensory-perceptual constructs of movement in space (e.g., speed, distance, direction [forward, side-to-side, backward, up, down, etc.]) and of physical form (e.g., our weight, height, width, the contours of our form, the distance of reach, the texture and density of our tissue). We experience sensory-emotional reactions and feelings associated with our own body and with interactive experiences while relating to objects and others (pain, pleasure, fear, anticipation, sadness and separation, anger and frustration, etc.). These immediate and primitive sensory-perceptual and sensory-emotional experiences eventually become cognitive constructs used to project a basic but essential judgment about how things and people beyond us also function. Further interaction and feedback correct and revise these initial perceptual presumptions. We develop a sensorimotor map of our body-self and use it to do the same with those around us and with the environment.

One important feature of this map is that it is not static. Sensory integration is an ongoing process. It occurs from moment to moment and throughout our lives. In any one moment or series of moments, sensory integration allows us to have an idea of what is happening and enables us to formulate a plan or a sequence of actions in order to execute an intention or carry an idea to fruition. This process is called *praxis*, or motor planning. It is a highly cognitive sensory-integrative process that is necessary for us to do what we need to do, from reaching for a specific toy behind or under several others to maneuvering a pen through each letter of each word of each sentence we write. Without sensory integration and without learning the basics of organization through praxis (motor planning), I would be unable to organize a sequenced plan of ideas to pull the words and sentences of this chapter together. Sensory integration very simply and initially gives us a body-self with which we can proceed to relate effectively and efficiently (adaptively) with others and our environment. In a word, it allows for and facilitates the organization of *relationship* and everything thath spins off from that.

To engage our sense of body, to develop a dynamic sensorimotor map, we need three sensory systems functioning with relative integrity: the tactile, proprioceptive, and vestibular. These three systems give us a body-self. It is what we might call a body-body operation. The body focuses its work on gathering input and assimilating stimuli fairly intensively to get to know itself. This occurs approximately between birth and 3 to 4 months of developmental age.

The visual and auditory sensory systems, which are also important to sensory integration and to organizing relationship, are most effective once the body-self awareness is in a process of healthy development. Their function is secondary to basic body awareness developmentally and functionally. These two phylogenetically newer systems essentially take a person beyond his or her own body and out into the expanse of space beyond the self. They extend a person's awareness so that information can be acquired without the need to be in immediate physical proximity to what is happening. The visual and auditory systems bring the beyond to a person or take a person to the beyond without the need for direct physical involvement. This is a major step toward efficiency and also adds a significant safety margin by allowing a person to look and listen before approaching with direct physical contact and engagement.

When assessing a person for visual function, inclusive of oculomotor and visual-motor attention, and visual-perceptual integrity, it is necessary to have some sense of a person's more basic sensory-integrative process. If there are problems with basic body awareness—the "body-on-body" assimilative process utilizing tactile/proprioceptive/vestibular input—it is not at all uncommon to have problems that at first may seem primarily visual in nature but in fact are not. The following example of how our visual perceptions can be compromised by an inadequately developed body awareness is instructive:

Sharon was a 29-year-old woman of average intelligence who was referred to us by her psychologist for an evaluation and possible therapy. She was diagnosed as an agoraphobic, fearful of leaving her home, and extremely anxious. She could not climb steps unless they were completely enclosed. She panicked if she could look down and see herself at a height. She could not take escalators, walk across bridges, or stand on any platform where she could see herself to be above ground level. She was also frightened of walking down her street because she could not figure out how to handle a speed bump—how to go around it or over it. Potholes were major obstacles: she could not figure out how to get around or over them either. When we first met, I asked Sharon to draw a picture of a person for me. The result was telling. She drew a head without a neck or trunk. The legs were attached to the head, and the arms protruded from the legs close to the head. The drawing was simplistic and primitive. Sharon did not seem in any way concerned with the discrepancy between what she drew and what her eyes must have looked at every time she saw an individual in front of her or herself in a mirror. Sharon's only comment was that she was not much of an artist. There was no problem with her intelligence and nothing wrong with her eyesight. There was, however, something significantly wrong with her body awareness and sensory processing, particularly the tactile-proprioceptive systems. Sharon had great difficulty feeling even firm touch pressure on her body. I took a hair brush and applied enough pressure to bend the bristles against the soles of her feet (normally a very sensitive part of the body). She simply could not feel it. I then took a vibrator at full speed and also placed it on the soles of her feet. She only momentarily noticed. This scenario was replayed over the full surface of her body. She could not feel her body, except vaguely. She could not project or draw an accurate representation of it on paper. Her picture of a person was a reflection of her limited body awareness, and this was secondary to a tactile, proprio-ceptive, and vestibular processing disorder. The visual discrepancies between what she saw on paper in her picture of a person and what she saw when she stood in front of a mirror were neither substantive enough nor in enough conflict to enable resolution or correction. What she could not feel, she could not draw. Because she could not feel her feet against the stair or platform surface, she panicked when she looked down and saw she was high off the ground. She could climb only the stairway that was enclosed, and this was only because she could not see anything except her walking surface. Her lack of body awareness, even while visually perceiving herself as high off the ground and without anything more than vision to place herself at this higher point, was overwhelming and left her feeling out of control and at risk. She could not secure her body on a platform above the ground without the necessary concrete sense of body in contact with that platform surface. Her 20/20 vision was inadequate to the task of securing her on the ground because she was only vaguely aware of being in her body.

Sharon's inability to maneuver over or around the speed bumps or the potholes in the street was not the result of any visual system or visual processing disorders. We might assume vision could have guided her over or around the obstacles without a complete understanding of sensory integration and sensory integration dysfunction. These struggles were instead the result of poorly developed body awareness, secondary to a somatosensory (tactile and proprioceptive systems = somatosensory) and vestibular processing deficit, and subsequent dyspraxia, a motor planning deficit. She could not feel her body adequately, had an extremely limited sense of how her body was put together (remember the picture she drew of a person), and as a result developed a poor sense of space, how objects fit in it, and how her body related to it all. Without a solid sense of body, sorting out the external world had little basis, no context, and no means for organization. Agoraphobia had developed, and reasonably so.

Sharon is a very good teaching example of why body awareness must be developed first, how visual perception and representation and function are inadequate to do the job without the integrity of body awareness having been established or in the process of being established.

Visual Motor Attention, Relationship, and Self-Stimulation

Visual Attention, a Developmental Function

As the body-self is establishing itself, an individual becomes aware of himself or herself as a physical presence in action. Primitive movement patterns (extremities moving about, head movement, trunk flexion, and extension, etc.) expand and help to satisfy the continued need for input. With an increasing ability to control basic motor coordination (reaching to grasp, pushing up against gravity, turning the head and eyes side to side, etc.) simple interactions with objects occur. Objects are visually observed and eventually reached for and grasped, mouthed, banged, or scratched. They are used by the body to accumulate more stimulative input and to serve the body's purpose in its continued need for more information about itself. This is a body object operation. Shoes are mouthed, keys are banged, and so forth. Even though the primary focus is still body centered, there is a secondary learning process occurring. By default, sensory information about the objects is also gathered. The information, however, is not so much to define object function but rather to accommodate the body's stimulative needs. Shoes are therefore mouthed, found to be nonedible and hard, but are not recognized as footwear for the developmental moment.

Visual clarity, perceptual functions, and oculomotor control clearly are not the operations that give a shoe its footwear identity. Until the person has fairly resolved his or her own body stimulative needs and as a result has developed reasonably good basic coordinative control and good basic sensory discriminative awareness, he or she will not be able or ready to explore objects outside his or her own body with a focus on anything but his or her own bodycentric needs. Likewise, visual attention will pursue an individual's primary needs. When a person's visual attention focuses on an object that bangs the loudest or spins the fastest and inattentively drifts away from playing catch with a Nerf® ball or scribbling with a crayon and paper, consider that body needs may not have been met yet. Visual inattention may not be what it seems. The visual focal set may be drawn toward body-centered needs and not toward any other activity, no matter that others think it would be more appropriate.

When a person sees objects, for example a series of nesting cups, and dives in all hands and feet without any attempt to visually sort out size before grabbing three at once, it often suggests body awareness needs, not so much irreverent impulsiveness or a primary visual-perceptual deficit. To recognize variations in object size and to differentiate and sequence size in series presumes that a person has already internalized and fine-tuned his or her own measure of body size and uses this to base and match kinesthetic object explorations with visual-perceptual memories of that internalized body awareness. Any delay in either of these processes will hinder visual-perceptual reflective thinking and lead a person to immediately seek physical trial-and-error object interactions. When in doubt, always step back and look at earlier developmental function. When a person is able to visually determine the smaller from the larger nesting cup, I can assume that he or she has a solid background of body awareness that is being used to interact with and develop good object/environmental awareness. Much of this is accomplished initially through trial-and-error manipulations. Visual-perceptual reflective thought begins to emerge at a developmental age of 15 to 18 months.

Visual Attention and Relationship

Avoidance versus Approach, Gaze Aversion versus Eye Contact

Eye contact is one of our first indicators that a person's attention has been gained. We receive a simple stimulus when we enter into or are introduced to a situation. We orient to it and register information that allows us to determine its use to us, its newness, and its safety or irrelevance. Visual attention occurs immediately following an orienting reflex and is an indication that the body/person is ready to give this input/situation meaning, perhaps to make an approach and investigate. If, however, a stimulus is presented and the body finds it threatening, a defensive reflex is activated instead of an orienting reflex. When a defensive reflex is elicited (as when a person who is tactually hypersensitive is touched) the response is apt to be acknowledged with gaze aversion, turning the head away, closing the eyes, even total shutdown and falling asleep rather than direct visual attention and other preparatory reactions leading to approach.

Eye contact is very much a type of contact, albeit across a distance. When an individual avoids eye contact it may reflect some of the dynamics or means of coping with relationship, rather than be a sign of visual-motor or visual-perceptual dysfunction or both, or even an indication of poor visual attentiveness. It is, of course, important to check out visual acuity, visual-motor control, and visual-perceptual functions as much as is possible. Along with this, we need to assess the person's ability to physically make an approach, engage in, and to then maintain interpersonal interactions. We need to evaluate the person's ability to trust primary caregivers and whether he or she enjoys being with and communicating with others (verbally or otherwise). The person who is withdrawn, hesitant to make eye contact or to physically approach and engage others, who is perhaps shy of communicating and withholds affection, who is perhaps irritable, unhappy, unsure, and frustrated, likely has some serious emotional/relational issues precluding eye contact as well as other relational gestures.

Eye contact, like other means of contact and interaction, tends to encourage people to approach and engage each other. If people are in any way threatened by interaction with others, eye contact will be one of the first responses they will drop from their repertoire altogether or diminish significantly. This gaze aversion is a defensive response, quite natural and appropriate for anyone to use when uncomfortable or fearful of what a situation with another might bring.

People who are shy of interaction may use peripheral vision to keep tabs on the activities of others. They may also turn their heads and briefly and occasionally watch an activity or situation out of the corner of their eyes so that their faces are not directed at the targeted situation but their eyes can sneak up, scan, and quickly leave in an attempt to remain surreptitious. With emotional or relational intervention and attention to those issues that are at the root of their feelings of fear toward relationship, which is may be sensory integrative in nature, avoidance of eye contact will usually spontaneously resolve itself.

Optokinetic Self-Stimulation: Other Considerations

In dealing with those diagnosed with autistic and pervasive developmental disorders (PDD), emotional or relational withdrawal is often evident.

Another behavioral sign is apt to be self-stimulation. This is sometimes sought out specifically through optokinetic stimulative input, for example, watching a spinning object while the body remains essentially stationary. Nystagmus occurs as the eyes attempt to track the movement of the object through slow phase eye movements with fast phase eye movements following in the opposite direction. To an observer, this simply looks like the eyes are repeatedly moving sideways, quickly returning, and then moving sideways again and again. This input stimulates the vestibular nuclei and central vestibular processing mechanism in a way similar to actual physical rotation or spinning in a swing. I have found that individuals who crave vestibular input but who are also fearful of body movement per se (often due to postural instability leading to postural insecurity) will avoid actually spinning their own body or moving their body in other ways to achieve movement input. Instead they choose to find objects they can spin (a ball, a spinning top, anything dangling from the end of a string) and proceed to quietly sit, spin the object, and intently focus on the movement external to their own body.

Another effect of optokinetic stimulation is its support in assisting an individual's avoidance of expanded interaction with the surrounding world of people and objects. Bruno Bettleheim (1967) described the use of a dream screen by individuals diagnosed with autism. His example is the use of waving fingers and moving hands in front of the eyes. To focus on one's hands moving at close range in front of the eyes helps to diffuse the poignancy of any environmental input. The person more easily stays focused on himself or herself and his or her own inner world of self.

Evaluation and Treatment Processes

Just a word to reiterate that an evaluation of individuals with visual functional deficits who are also dealing with developmental or sensory-integrative dysfunction or both, or with sensorimotor deficits, needs to consider possible causal factors outside the visual system (both peripheral and central processing).

Intervention clearly needs to address root issues when identifiable, and although behavioral intervention or specific visual intervention techniques can be helpful, if the root issue is not specifically visual and/or behavioral in nature, the results are apt to be short-lived.

Oculomotor Control, a Total Body Sensorimotor Developmental Process

Any consideration of an individual's oculomotor control, when dealing with those who have developmental disabilities and particularly concomitant sensory-integrative and sensorimotor deficits, needs to look carefully at total body responses and needs, the reason being (in my experience) that the integrity of many oculomotor functions is dependent on earlier, more central and proximal foundation functions of both a sensory processing and motor control nature. Those that seem to be the most common are mentioned below. For more in-depth theoretical, evaluative, and treatment information, specific reading material (see references listed at the end of the chapter) and courses dealing with these issues are recommended.

There are three primary levels of muscle coordinative tone: phasic, tonic, and cocontraction. The latter two are most relevant to this discussion, but an awareness of the progression starting with phasic tone helps clarify the impact on function. *Phasic tone* is tone that is initially used by the infant and developmentally young to allow for generalized movement of the extremities, head, and trunk. This movement is nonsupportive. The muscles do not bear weight or hold a position. The individual using this level of tone is often apedal and incapable of holding an erect posture against gravity. It allows movement for the sake of movement, creating stimulative input and feedback to the body about itself as it moves against itself.

Tonic tone is the next level of coordinative tone and the first indication that the body is capable of holding a position by contracting either the flexors or the extensors in a unitary and essentially total body pattern. Asymmetrical or symmetrical tonic neck reflexes are examples of this tone being elicited reflexively. Total body flexion or extension patterns against gravity are also examples of tonic tone in action. This tonic tonal pattern is essential because it enables the body and all of its muscles to learn to sustain or hold a contraction of one muscle group (either the flexors *or* the extensors) for an extended period. It is, if you will, a precursor to the strength of muscle contraction in any future stabilizing movement.

The third level of coordinative tone is cocontraction. *Cocontraction* (or coactivation of muscles around a joint) builds on tonic tone and enables the body to move with fluidity and smoothness. Tonic tone does not permit flexibility because either the flexors *or* the extensors are at work. There is no movement, only the assumption of a posture/position and the pursuit of holding this same position. If a person tries to use tonic tone in the process of moving the body, the movement is jerky and rigid. If a person, however, has developed cocontraction, the movement allows for cooperative interaction between the flexors and extensors. This is also called coactivation of muscle groups around a joint.

Cocontraction is essential for smooth control of movement and muscle use in both gross and fine motor coordinative activities. Without adequate development of cocontraction, movement control is limited, usually jerky and inept, and often described as clumsy.

One further note of importance has to do with the need for specific input to support each level of muscle coordinative tone development. Very simply, the tactile system is primary (though not exclusive) in its support of phasic tone development, the proprioceptive for tonic tone, and the vestibular for cocontraction. These sensory systems provide only primary support for each level of muscle tone. They are only a focus, not the exclusive requisites. All input, especially from these three sensory systems, is used at each level.

The impact that all this has on oculomotor development is hierarchical. Oculomotor control is certainly a type of fine motor control, even very fine motor control. Eye movement control depends on the ability of the head and neck to stabilize themselves against the movements of the trunk. Of course, the trunk needs to find its stability against the point of contact with the ground, as do the hips and pelvis of someone seated in a chair with both feet on the ground. All of this relies on holding or controlling a steady posture either while still or while moving about. This further depends on the development of muscle cocontraction, and this from well-developed tonic tone flexors and extensors, from phasic tone, and from ongoing specific sensory-stimulative touch support and the body awareness that comes from sensory-discriminative support.

An example of an oculomotor control deficit that can be related to possible problems in the development of coordinative muscle tone is difficulty crossing the midline with the eyes and difficulty separating eye movements from movements of the head and neck. If there is a predominance of tonic tone, it may be reflected in a rigid postural set with excessive use of either the flexors or the extensors such that when the person wants to move his or her body, he or she is often able to move only as one unit and with the inflexibility that comes from relying on more extensors than flexor tone (or the reverse). People with a predominance of extensor tone may walk on their toes and show lordotic tendencies, shoulder girdle retraction, and perhaps head and neck hyper-extension. Following the rest of the body, the eyes also tend to have difficulty moving with fluidity; show more tonic tone response; and move to end range, lock into a position, and stay put. In other words, if cocontraction has not yet developed in the rest of the body, it cannot be expected to do so in the eyes. Also, if the rest of the body is struggling to stabilize itself, then there is no firm base from which oculomotor control can project any finely tuned movements.

Crossing the midline requires good cocontraction, fluidity of move-ment, and a good cooperative interaction between the flexors and the extensors. Efficient oculomotor control also requires an automatic disso-ciation or separation of the eye movements from movements of the head and neck, shoulder girdle and upper trunk, and lower trunk, hips, and pelvis. This likewise requires efficient cocontraction. Tonic tone tends to elicit more of a total body response of primary flexion or extension. Good cocontraction develops when and only when good strong tonic tone extensions are balanced with equally good strong sustained contraction of the flexors. With the strength of tone in these antagonistic muscles, a person can then work to develop dynamic balanced interplay between the two, such that total body rotation develops and with it a simple dissociation of one body part from another.

When you observe an individual having difficulty keeping his or her eyes focused on the object and activity placed in front of him or her, perhaps tying a shoe or buttoning buttons, it probably would be wise to assess overall muscle tone before addressing the visual problem. If the person is using heightened tonic extensor tone in the trunk to sit upright, then perhaps having the person flex the head and neck while simultaneously asking the eyes to move freely in their orbit, expecting the person not only to separate the movement of the eyes from that of the head and neck but also to smoothly follow a targeted activity, is asking for too much.

When a person does not seem to be able to scan the tabletop or the floor for missing pieces of a puzzle, and always misses items beyond the immediate frontal visual field, question whether the eyes are able to separate these movements from those of the head and neck, and so forth. If the person cannot, then question whether adequately balanced tonic tone flexors and extensors are available. If not, then cocontraction is also in all likelihood inadequate, causing the body to move rigidly as a unit and disallowing dissociation of body parts for efficient movement.

When a person cannot move his or her eyes back and forth from a book to writing paper on the desk, to the blackboard, and to the teacher without becoming lost in the shuffle, consider and assess for this same problem, ditto for missing one's place in the text while reading, skipping letters or words, miscounting objects, and so forth. The more finely tuned the demand for oculomotor proficiency, the more finesse a person needs to have achieved in the development of cocontraction and the dissociation of body parts, leading to dissociation of the eyes. The need is also great with these demanding oculomotor tasks for a good solid postural base of support off of which the eyes can move. The eyes need no interference from a wobbly head on a wobbly trunk to do needlepoint work, for example. If a child is struggling with reading, parents will often ask when I think it appropriate for their child to receive visual training from the developmental optometrist. My answer comes from experience. Those who have developed cocontraction, such that there is dissociation of eyes from the head and neck, necessitating also dissociation through the rest of the body, generally benefit more from oculomotor training than those who have not. An overall evaluation for visual function is appropriate at any point, and I would never object to people trying intervention with developmental optometry before cocontraction is reasonably established, but it seems to influence the results positively when overall body cocontraction is accomplished first.

An assessment of antigravity total-body supine flexion and also prone extension will show you whether or not an individual has developed adequate tonic tone strength to sustain contraction of these muscle groups such that muscle cocontraction can develop. If both antigravity postures are weak, both need to be developed. If one is weaker than the other, the weaker needs to be developed. Sustained strength of both the flexors and the extensors needs to be available if we expect muscle stability and postural stability through cocontraction to develop. Remember that the development of tonic muscle tone proceeds in a cephalocaudal and proximal-distal fashion. Often we tend to overlook the head and neck musculature and then become frustrated in our attempts to elicit oculo-motor proficiency. A bobbing head, or even slight head lag when a person is tipped backwards in supine, or a neck that gets sore during desk work, or a head that needs to be propped up on an arm all suggest inadequate development of head and neck tonic flexion and tonic extension or both. Emphasize the development of head and neck tonic tone control and proceed caudally, while also working from the trunk out toward the extremities. Remember that muscle-coordinative tonal deficits are often the result or partial result of sensory-integrative processing deficits, and intervention needs to be specific concomitantly to both sensory processing and muscle-coordinative tonal deficits. With these preliminaries in place, oculomotor control often follows quickly and easily.

Visuo-Vestibular-Proprioception Triad and Visual Perception

Some aspects of visual perception stem directly from a three-way sensory collaboration. The visual system, in concert with discriminative awareness from the vestibular and proprioceptive systems, enables each of us to grasp how we and the rest of our world fits together in space in such a beautifully organized or frustratingly disorganized fashion, as the case may be in normal or abnormal sensory-integrative function of these three sensory systems. At least two basic components evolve as a result of these three systems sharing, analyzing, and synthesizing information in such a way that we can make sense of the forms within space and the form (if you will) of space itself.

Vestibular-Proprioceptive Impact on Visual-Spatial Percepts

The ability to organize visual space so that we can be aware of and understand where things are and their position in relation to each other, thus allowing us to order things correctly (writing the alphabet left to right, drawing things right side up, stacking blocks vertically to make a tower, holding a plate top side up to accept food, etc.) comes from a more basic and primitive awareness of how our body orients and organizes itself in space. For us to know up from down, to feel linear direction (side-to-side or front-to-back), to recognize rotation and its perceptual derivations (circles and curves), we need a sense of gravity. We perceive this thanks to vestibular system functions. In concert with this, our proprioceptive system gives us information about our body's movements against itself and against the ground or other surfaces that we push, pull, and move against. These two systems, the vestibular and proprioceptive, give us our own experience of the movement patterns of our body. With these experiences and with the use of the visual system, we can master our sense of going down, down, down to the bottom of the slide and up, up, up to the top of the jungle gym and then to project this awareness onto a piece of paper and eventually label its top and its bottom. We do the same with side-to-side linear or horizontal movements.

So many times we meet people who confuse their right and left sides and then, of course, the right and left sides of objects. Chances are they never thoroughly physically and sensorily felt the difference between their right and left body sides. It would be a mistake to assume a person can visually see front from back, right from left, and so forth without having experienced discriminative body awareness (which comes from somatosensory awareness) and body awareness during movement through space (which comes from vestibular-proprioceptive awareness).

Visual Form and Space Concepts

Seeing size and discriminating object position and placement is, of course, based on body awareness and a sense of the body in space as just described. Sharon, the woman mentioned earlier who was diagnosed with agoraphobia, had a very poor sense of her body, and an even more limited sense of how her body fit into space. Fearful of standing on any platform and looking down, such as from a stairway or escalator, unable to sort out how to maneuver around a pothole or over a speed bump, she had never found her own position in space or on the ground, and thus had not figured out how her body related to other objects in the environment.

Ryan could not figure out how to make a creative block tower (a tower with any design more complex than simply one block on top of another) or a road of blocks, or how to draw lines on paper going from the top to the bottom or keep the lines of letters within the lines on the page, until his sense of body and then his sense of body in space (vestibular-proprioceptive awareness) became more discriminative. Until he could make clear sense of his own body in space, he had no accurate basis for comparison and no grounded sense of what other objects or designs would or could do in space.

Ian had a very poor sense of where and how letters should be sized and spaced on a line in relation to each other and how words should be placed next to each other. John, an adult, could not figure out where things fit on or in his desk at work, or how to organize the space in his car and apartment (after having been evicted from three apartments because of the clutter and mess he would create). Map reading was a struggle for John, as was organizing time and schedules. His life was a seriously disorganized mess, not from a root visual-perceptual problem, but because he had major body-awareness and organizational problems. He had been diagnosed as seriously dyspraxic.

Treating such issues is not the intent of this particular book. Recognizing the foundation functions that lead to certain visual functions is. Sensory integration is a primary area for assessment, along with developmental optometric and ophthalmological evaluations when we find visual function deficits in people who clearly have developmental disorders, learning disabilities, attention deficit disorder, and so forth.

SUGGESTED READINGS

Ayres, A. J. (1975). *Sensory integration and learning disorders.* Los Angeles: Western Psychological Services.

Ayres, A. J. (1979). *Sensory integration and the child.* Los Angeles: Western Psychological Services.

Bettleheim, B. (1967). *The empty fortress, infantile autism and the birth of the self.* New York: The Free Press.

Borello-France, D. F., Whitney, S. L., & Herdman, S. J. (1994). *Assessment of vestibular hypofunction.* In S. J. Herdman (Ed.), *Vestibular rehabilitation.* Philadelphia: F. A. Davis.

Cermak, S. A. (1991). Somatodyspraxia. In A. J. Fisher, et al. (Eds.), *Sensory integration theory and practice.* Philadelphia: F. A. Davis.

DeGangi, G. A. (1991). Assessment of sensory, emotional, and attentional problems in regulatory disordered infants. *Infants Young Child, 3*(1).

DeGangi, G. A., Goodin, M. M., & Wietlisbach, S. (1994). Treatment of vestibular deficits in children with developmental disorders. In S. J. Herdman (Ed.), *Vestibular rehabilitation.* Philadelphia: F. A. Davis.

Fisher, A. G., Murray, E. A., & Bundy, A. C. (1991). *Sensory integration, theory and practice.* Philadelphia: F. A. Davis.

Fraiberg, S. (1977). *Insights from the blind.* New York: Basic Books.

Gellhorn, E. (1964). Motion and emotion—The role of the proprioception in the physiology and pathology of the emotions. *Psychology Review, 71,* 357–372.

Gilfoyle, E. M., & Grady, A. P. (1971). Cognitive-perceptual-motor behavior. In H. S. Willard & C. S. Spackman (Ed.), *Occupational therapy.* Philadelphia: J. B. Lippincott.

Gilfoyle, E. M., & Grady, A. P. (1981). *Children adapt.* Thorofare, NJ: Slack.

Ginsburg, H., & Opper, S. (1969). *Piaget's theory of intellectual development.* New York: Prentice-Hall.

Gruber, H. E., & Voneche, J. J. (1977). *The essential Piaget.* New York: Basic Books.

Heack, L., Short-DeGraff, M., & Hanzlik, J. R. (1993). Relationship of oculomotor skills to vestibular-related clinical observations. *Physical and Occupational Therapy in Pediatrics, 13,* 113.

Honrubia, V. (1994). Quantitative vestibular function tests and the clinical examination. In S. J. Herdman (Ed.), *Vestibular rehabilitation*. Philadelphia: F. A. Davis.

Kantner, R. M., Clark, D. L., Allen, L. C., & Chase, M. F. (1976). Effects of vestibular stimulation on nystagmus response and motor performance in the developmentally delayed infant. *Physical Therapy, 56,* 414–421.

Leigh, R. J., & Zec, D. S. (1991). *The neurology of eye movements* (edition Z). Philadelphia: F. A. Davis.

Masterton, B. A., & Biederman, G. B. (1983). Proprioceptive versus visual control in autistic children. *Journal of Autism and Developmental Disorders, 13,* 141–152.

Montague, A. (1978). *Touching.* New York: Harper & Row.

Ohwaki, S., & Brahlek, J. A. (1973). Preference for vibratory and visual stimulation in mentally retarded children. *American Journal of Mental Deficiency, 77*(6), 733–736.

Ohwaki, S., & Strayton, S. E. (1976). Preference by the retarded for vibratory and visual stimulation as function of mental age and psychotic reaction. *Journal of Abnormal Psychology, 85,* 516–522.

Ornitz, E. M. (1969). Disorders of perception common to early infantile autism and schizophrenia. *Comprehensive Psychiatry, 10.*

Ornitz, E. M., & Ritvo, E. R. (1968). Perceptual inconstancy in early infantile autism. *Archives of General Psychiatry, 18*(5), 76–98.

Piaget, J. (1954). *The construction of reality in the child.* New York: Ballentine Books.

Posner, M. I., & Peterson, S. E. (1990). The attention system of the human brain. *Annual Review of Neuroscience, 13,* 25–42.

Resman, M. (1984). Effect of sensory stimulation on eye contact in a profoundly retarded adult. *American Journal of Occupational Therapy, 38*(8).

Ritvo, E. R., Ornitz, E. M., Eviatar, A., Markham, C. H., Brown, M. D., & Mason, A. (1969). Decreased postrotary nystagmus in early infantile autism. *Neurology, 19,* 653–658.

Ross, R. G., Radant, A. D., et al. (1994). Saccadic eye movements in normal children from 815 years of age: A developmental study of visuospatial attention. *Journal of Autism and Developmental Disorders, 24,* 413–431.

Silver, L. B. (1992). *Attention deficit hyperactivity disorder: A clinical guide to diagnosis and treatment.* Washington, D.C.: American Psychiatric Press.

Stern, D. N. (1985). *The interpersonal world of the infant.* New York: Basic Books.

Watson, P. J., Ottenbacher, K., et al. (1982). Visual motor difficulties in emotionally disturbed children with hyporesponsive nystagmus. *Physical and Occupational Therapy in Pediatrics, 2*(2/3), 67–72.

4

Functional Visual Skills

Laurie Efferson Chaikin, MS, OTR, OD, and
Shannon Downing-Baum, MS, OTR

Vision Therapy: Optometry and Occupational Therapy Collaboration

Vision therapy has traditionally been within the realm of ophthalmology and optometry. Initially, it was referred to as *orthoptics,* and therapists interested in providing this service could attend an orthoptic training course. A few of these programs are still in existence on the East Coast of the United States and in Canada and England. Orthoptists would generally work with ophthalmologists on patients with strabismus, particularly after surgery. Their training consisted primarily of work in vision instruments such as an amblyoscope. Currently, many ophthalmologists do not offer vision training, which has become more the purview of optometry. Optometrists either train patients themselves or educate the therapist in his or her office. However, more formalized training programs are in existence. One such program is offered by the College of Optometrists in Vision Development, or COVD. The COVD is an organization of optometrists interested in formally associating with other optometrists who practice developmental optometry. The COVD offers recognition of the successful completion of a written and oral examination for vision therapists by conferring the title of Certified Optometric Vision Therapy Technician (COVTT). In order to sit for the exam, applicants must have completed a specified number of hours working in an optometrist's office and must be sponsored by a fellow of the COVD (FCOVD). In order to maintain COVTT status, COVTTs must continue to work in an optometrist's office, maintain sponsorship by an FCOVD, and complete continuing education approved by COVD.

Many individuals study and collaborate with optometrists and ophthalmologists to legitimately obtain skills in vision function remediation, including occupational therapists, physical therapists, speech and language pathologists, and professionals with nursing and education backgrounds. Some of these individuals may also call themselves "vision therapists," although their knowledge and skill base varies widely. Educational criteria are not well established. Future study by all interested parties is recommended to establish a more standardized role for the vision therapist.

One large contribution that optometry has made to the practice of vision therapy is the use of free space training for generalization of the visual skills to the environment. Instruments are still used, but in addition visual activities are employed that allow feedback about how the eyes are being used in real space as opposed to optical space, which is illusory space created by the optics in an instrument. In addition, some optometrists, called *behavioral* or *developmental optometrists*, look at the importance of posture, muscle tone, and the vestibular system's interaction with visual function.

These are areas in which occupational therapists both contribute knowledge to and collaborate with optometry. Occupational therapists working with individuals who have neurological deficits, and with the pediatric population, began to interact with optometrists. Optometrists started to appreciate the developmental and neurological knowledge base that occupational therapists had, as well as their functional orientation. A number of collaborative conferences have been hosted between occupational therapists and optometrists, as well as articles written about what they have to offer each other (Cool, 1990; Downing-Baum & Maino, 1996; Gianutsos, Ramsey, & Perlin, 1988; Hellerstein & Fischman, 1990;

Kalb & Warshowsky, 1991; Suchoff, 1995). Occupational therapists are also writing articles about integrating vision therapy into occupational therapy services (Arnsten, 1994; Downing-Baum 1995; Schnell, 1992). A new model of interaction appears to be developing where the optometrist is more involved in the early diagnosis of visual problems in pediatrics, stroke, and head injury (Gianutsos & Ramsey, 1987; Padula, 1988). The early correction of refractive errors, and the initiation of visual training, patching, or use of prisms can certainly affect the outcome of fine and gross motor, and speech and language treatment when one considers the primacy of the visual sense in functional abilities.

Optometry–occupational therapy interaction may take place in the hospital setting if the doctor has hospital privileges, in the outpatient clinic if the doctor has a contract, or in the doctor's office. Referrals to optometrists for vision evaluation often come from therapists involved with patients with vision dysfunction. Vision therapy may be prescribed by the optometrist and implemented by the trained therapist in the hospital, clinic, or school. Communication between the optometrist and therapist should be ongoing when performing vision rehabilitation to determine progression of treatment and when further evaluation is warranted. After discharge from occupational therapy, the patient may be followed in therapy in the optometrist's office. Occupational therapists may simply wish to become more aware of therapy performed for clients by vision therapists in optometrists' offices, and not perform vision rehabilitation themselves (as the agenda for the occupational therapy session may already be quite full). Occupational therapists may add to a vision therapy regimen for a client by performing neurodevelopmental treatment, sensory integration, and other occupational therapy modalities with some modification to include vision therapy principles, as prescribed by the optometrist.

When prescribing vision therapy to the clients, families, teachers, and other medical personnel, occupational therapists should be cognizant of potential controversy. A potential conflict may occur between optometrists and allied health professionals. Some optometrists are of the opinion that "vision therapy" should be performed only in their offices. Terminology such as functional vision training, retraining, and rehabilitation may be preferentially used by allied health professionals to describe these services. The authors have generally found that if the controversial issues are openly discussed with clients and colleagues, understanding and resolution of conflicts can be obtained.

The efficacy of vision therapy has been well researched by Cohen (1988). However, significant conflict exists between ophthalmology and optometry regarding efficacy. Some of the arguments involve only turf issues. The literature is replete with well-documented scientific research as well as anecdotal evidence, both in pediatrics and in rehabilitation cases (Aksionoff & Falk, 1992; Andrezejewska & Baranowska, 1969; Cohen, 1992; Krobel, Simon, & Barrows, 1986; Padula, 1988; Soden & Cohen, 1993; Stanworth, 1974).

Functional visual skills are based on certain physiological norms. Generally speaking, they are developed within the first year of life, paralleling reflex integration. In this chapter the various visual skills will be defined, symptoms of dysfunction will be described, and both therapist screening techniques and optometric evaluation will be discussed. Each section will include considerations for how limitations in this skill area could affect function and suggestions for remediation. The visual skills include accommodation, vergence, oculomotilities, stereopsis, and central and peripheral awareness. Developing functional visual skills is an educational as well as physiological process. Dysfunction may be influenced by developmental anomalies affecting muscle tone, vestibular dysfunction, refractive errors, and eye turns. It is essential that therapists interested in this area seek continuing education and work closely with an eye care professional before addressing visual issues.

A full description of the options available in vision therapy is beyond the scope of this chapter. Training is available in a variety of skill areas, but in none of these areas does the occupational therapist work in isolation. Communication between the optometrist and the occupational therapist should be ongoing when vision rehabilitation is performed with patients with vision dysfunction. This is necessary to determine the progress of treatment and when further evaluation is warranted.

Disorders of Accommodation: Definition, Evaluation, and Treatment

Accommodation is the ability to bring near objects into clear focus automatically and without strain. Relaxation of accommodation allows distant objects to come in clearly. The primary action is that of the ciliary muscles acting on the lens controlled by sympathetic and parasympathetic nervous system components (Moses & Hart, 1987). Problems in accommodation can be caused by uncorrected refractive error, such as hyperopia or fatigue caused by prolonged or excessive use of the focusing system (e.g., hours of computer use, video games, or reading).

Symptoms

A patient with accommodative dysfunction generally has problems with clarity for near activities. Symptoms include near-point blur, intermittent near-point blur, a feeling of eye strain or headache after sustained near work, and reduced concentration and comprehension. One may observe the patient moving his or her head or reading material closer or further; he or she may squint or avoid near activities. Patients may complain about their glasses not working well. These symptoms could be caused by accommodative infacility or insufficiency, but accommodative problems are not the only diagnosis possible. Other possibilities include presbyopia, hyperopia, or astigmatism. Accommodative infacility involves difficulty in rapid shifts of focus from near to far, as when, for example, one looks from the chalkboard to the desk in a copying task. Accommodative insufficiency is reduced accommodative ability compared to what is expected for that patient's age; it is *not* a result of aging.

It is possible to have accommodative spasm, in which the patient looks across the room at a distant object like a clock or a calendar and the object does not become immediately clear. In this case, the ciliary muscles are not allowing the lens to return to its flatter curvature, creating the symptom of distance blur. Distance blur, however, could also be a symptom of myopia or astigmatism.

Evaluation

The need for optometric referral would be indicated with 20/40 or worse on a near visual acuity test, or with the above symptoms, or both. Paying attention to patient complaints can be a more sensitive indicator of accommodative problems than results from near acuity test.

Optometric evaluation includes monocular measures of near-point accommodation expressed in diopters. A diopter is the reciprocal or inverse of meters. For example, if a small target is viewed as blurry at 0.8 meter, 1/0.8 equals 1.25 diopters. The expected amount of accommodative ability changes with age, and certain formulas are applied to determine if an individual's accommodation is at or below age expectations.

Other optometric measures may be binocular in combination with convergence ability. Additionally, lenses may be used to determine accommodative ranges. Sometimes rapidly changing lenses (flipper bars) are used to determine the patient's ability to sustain near focus over time and can indicate accommodative infacility.

Therapeutic considerations are to

- instruct the patient that if reading glasses have been prescribed, they should be used for all near-point tasks
- encourage the patient to take frequent breaks, looking off into the distance to relax accommodation
- increase direct lighting of the task; this will reduce the pupil size and increase the depth of focus.

Vision Rehabilitation Techniques

Many fine and gross motor skill improvement activities already being performed by therapists may be slightly modified to improve visual accommodation. The additional principle that must be incorporated is to alternate the patient's visual regard between close and distant visual targets (anywhere from a few inches from the eyes to infinity). Key elements of this principle include the speed of visual adjustment between close and distant targets and the ability to clearly focus on the targets.

When therapy with a patient who has an accommodative disorder begins, the targets could be larger and the involvement of gross motor skills, particularly use of the upper extremities and muscles of the neck and back, should be incorporated to improve success with the task. Much discussion by optometrists and therapists has revolved around using the upper extremities and neck and back musculature to enhance visual skills. It is a generally recognized principle used by both professions in daily practice but is in need of further research justification. Examples of exercises employing large targets include throwing a ball at close and distant targets or operating a "going game"—propelling a large oblong bead along a pair of strings between two players.

As the patient progresses, smaller targets may be added to challenge the patient and to provide feedback regarding the patient's ability to clearly focus on the targets. The therapist could ask the patient to concentrate on clarity of focus. For nonverbal patients and young children this communication would need to be adapted. Providing opportunities for discrimination among targets may assist in these cases. For example, one such technique is to ask that the patient shine a flashlight beam on a nearby small detailed design, such as one might find on a decorative sticker, then use the flashlight to select a matching design from a group of designs several feet away.

An example of an accommodation exercise for school-age children and adults is near-far letter charts (Griffin, 1976). Patients hold a typed series of letters at a comfortable viewing distance from their eyes (12–16 in.) and alternate reading these letters and those from a chart that has been affixed at eye level on a wall at a distance of 10 ft. The distance between the near hand-held chart and the wall chart is graded to increase the visual challenge.

Very few activities exist that exercise accommodation without also requiring vergence (unless the activity is monocular). An example of maintaining vergence demand while varying accommodation is reading while using plus-minus flipper lenses (McGraw, 1988)—reading a line using the plus lenses and then flipping the lens set over to read the next line with the minus lenses.

Therapists should bear in mind that activities with movement components and visual targets generally use accommodation function. An example would be swinging on a trapeze traverse swing while looking for differences among a group of stationary pictures.

Vergence Disorders: Definition, Evaluation, and Treatment

Vergence ability includes convergence and divergence. Convergence is the ability to smoothly and automatically bring the eyes together along the midline axis in order to observe near objects singly. Conversely, as the eyes move outward to keep a distant object single, divergence is employed. Vergence is a reflex related to accommodation, convergence with accommodation, and divergence with relaxation of accommodation. The function of this reflex is to allow objects to be both single and clear at both distance and near.

Problems can occur in vergence ability when the eye movement system is out of coordination with accommodation or when cranial nerves III, IV, or VI have suffered damage. Two basic types of problems, phoria or tropia (strabismus), are known.

Phoria

Phoria is the positioning or aiming of the eyes relative to where the eyes are focused. Phoria in general means that the eyes are being used together; fusion and some degree of depth perception are present. Figure 4.1 graphically describes the relationship between the accommodative point and the convergence point. The dotted line is accommodation; the solid line is the eye aiming system (vergence).

The eye aiming system is controlled by the eye muscles. The focusing system, as noted above, is controlled by the ciliary muscles acting on the lens. Ideally, the eyes are both aimed and focused on the same object. In order for the eyes to maintain their position, a balance must exist between the inward pulling muscles of convergence (medial recti) and the outward pulling muscles of divergence (lateral recti). Think of it as a balance of tone between these two opposing sets of muscles. The average eye position relative to the accommodative point is slightly outward: the eyes are slightly diverged, so that the inner muscles have to exert some force to maintain alignment. This state is called *exophoria*. Most people have a slight exophoria. When the convergence tone is greater than the divergence tone and the eyes have a tendency to pull inward, then divergence must be used to create alignment between the focusing and aiming systems. This is called *esophoria*. Established optometric norms help to determine when a large amount of exophoria or esophoria may be contributing to a patient's symptoms of reduced visual efficiency.

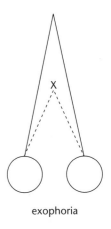

exophoria

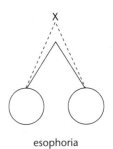

esophoria

Figure 4.1

Symptoms occur when the amount of compensatory vergence is great enough to cause the individual fatigue by the effort to sustain focus at a certain point. Symptoms are usually task specific and occur, for example, when reading, using the computer, doing near-point activities, or driving. It is the sustained effort involved that becomes difficult. Symptoms include eye strain, fatigue, headaches (temporal or frontal), difficulty concentrating, reduced comprehension of reading matter, sleepiness after reading, and eye burning or stinging after reading printed matter or the computer screen.

Phorias are measured in units called prism diopters. This is the size of the prism needed to measure the eye position in or out from the straight-ahead position (Fannin & Grosvenor, 1987).

Evaluation

A subjective screening tool that can be used by therapists is the Modified Thorington card, or eye alignment card, which uses a Maddox rod and a point source of light (Griffin, 1976). The distance between the dots on the scale on the card is equal to 1 prism diopter of eye turn as long as the card is held at 16 in. (40 cm). The patient holds the card at 16 in. while the therapist touches the penlight to the back of the card aiming the light through the small hole. The Maddox rod is held over the right eye with the lines horizontal. This creates a vertical red streak that will pass through the horizontal scale on the patient's card. If the line falls 5 prism diopters to the right of the light (5 esophoria) or 10 prism diopters to the left (10 exophoria), this would be outside the normal range. To test vertical eye alignment problems, the paddle is turned so that the lines are vertical. This creates a horizontal red streak that crosses the vertical scale on the card. If the red line is more than 2 prism diopters above or below the light, this is considered outside the normal range. A referral is indicated when there are also symptoms or signs of a dysfunction in this area.

The optometrist would evaluate using the cover test (see *Strabismus* later in this chapter) along with prisms for objective results, the Modified Thorington card, or prism dissociation technique to separate the two eyes. If symptoms or signs are observed, the patient may benefit from visual retraining. The alternate cover test may be used as a screening tool, but it requires additional training.

Treatment

Optometric lens treatment may include the use of lenses or prisms to help the vergence problem. Sometimes a minus lens is used to stimulate accommodation that then stimulates more convergence. This treatment would be used for someone who had a convergence insufficiency. A plus lens may be used to relax accommodation, thereby reducing overconvergence. Prisms may be used to reduce the amount of over- or underconvergence, effort, and fatigue effects.

Vision Rehabilitation Techniques

Patients with high degrees of exophoria, or other causes of poor convergence, may benefit from exercises aimed at improving visual convergence skills. Many fine motor tasks that are usually performed within a range of 12–16 in. from the eyes may be moved closer as a convergence exercise.

Because positioning is critical in this type of exercise, therapists may want to have their patients assume a supine position for these activities.

In this position, gravity will help bring hand-held objects closer to the patient's eyes while also helping to hold the patient's head in a stable position. Small bilateral tasks, such as stringing beads, assembling pop-beads, and using lace-cards made of note card-sized cardboard, typically make good convergence exercises for young children. Prone or prone-on-elbows positioning promotes neck musculature co-contraction of extensors and flexors, which may in turn facilitate visual skills.

Convergence tasks may also be performed with patients in a sitting position. In this case, it is not unusual for patients to assume a hunched-shoulder, kyphotic posture. In such cases, upright posture should be emphasized and a firm high-back chair used as reinforcement.

In cases in which only one eye is having difficulty converging, occlusion (patching) of the dominant eye may be useful. Patching regimens should be prescribed by an eye care specialist. Often the patient is not aware that one eye is not involved in the convergence skill. An activity could be performed with occlusion, followed immediately with binocular performance of the activity to reinforce the sensory awareness that is learned when the deficient eye is stimulated.

As the patient's convergence skills improve, increased challenge may be provided by having the patient stand or by adding a movement component, such as sitting in a swing. After midline convergence skills are improved, the visual targets may be moved to different positions (up, down, left, right, or diagonally, often referred to by optometrists as positions of gaze). (See Figure 4.2.)

An example of a convergence activity for older children and adults is the Brock string (Brock & Folsom, 1962). The Brock string may also be used to check for visual suppression. Using one string, the patient is asked to focus on one bead. If the patient's eyes are both "turned on," meaning that the patient is employing binocular vision, the patient should see two string images leading up to the bead, one coming from the left and one from the right, and two string images leading away from the bead. These string images should appear to form an X with the bead at the center. If one or more of these string images is missing, neurological visual suppression may be indicated.

Convergence Fusion

The principle of converging in front of the plane of focus requires cognitive abstraction and is generally not useful to young children or those patients with cognitive impairment. However, many free space fusion activities may be done with school-age children and adults to improve their convergence abilities. An example is the penny card fusion activity, which may easily be constructed and used at home (McGraw, 1988).

Two pennies of similar appearance (same year of issue) are affixed to an index card, 1½ in. apart, head side up. The patient should hold the penny card in one hand about 16 in. from the face at eye level while holding a pen in the other hand about 10 in. from the face. The pen should be held to appear at midpoint between the two pennies with the pen tip just below the penny level. The patient should then focus his or her eyes on the tip of the pen (not on the pennies) and notice a third image of a penny appearing at midpoint just above the pen tip. This image may be blurry at first and may disappear quickly. The patient's eyes may feel uncomfortable because they are "crossing" because of the convergence demand. The patient should work at intervals to increase the time the third, middle image of the penny can be maintained, and should eventually stop using the pen as a prop. Accommodative and convergence flexibility is increased in this activity as the patient learns separate control between these two skills. The patient should try to clearly focus the fused image of the pennies to discern the small details of the face, date, and words. Later, motion of the patient or the card may be added as an additional challenge.

Divergence Fusion

Patients with a high degree of esophoria may need to work on exercises that require divergence fusion. The most common example of this exercise is the stereogram, now popularly known as Magic Eye pictures (N. E. Thing Enterprises, 1995). To view these pictures as three-dimensional images, the patient's eyes must assume a divergence posture, focusing on an image beyond the plane of the picture, and relax accommodation. If successful, the stereo image implanted within the picture will appear to float out in three-dimensional space.

Several other convergence and divergence activities are available commercially through various sources, including the Optometric Extension Program. Examples of available activities include vectograms, tranaglyphs, Keystone stereoscope (Keystone View), and the aperture rule trainer. Use of these activities requires specialized training that is beyond the scope of this chapter.

Strabismus (Tropias)

Strabismus may occur either when a muscle imbalance or weakness exists, a cranial nerve has been damaged, or when the phoria becomes excessive and binocularity breaks down. In strabismus, no fusion and no depth perception are present. The eye may be seen to wander inward, outward, upward, or downward. The condition may be constant, intermittent, or alternating from one eye to the other.

Generally, symptoms are less task specific, except in the case of an intermittent strabismus. Symptoms include double vision, or if patients have had the strabismus during their developmental years, up to about age 7, their brains may have learned to neurologically suppress or turn off the nondominant image. In time an amblyopia may develop, although an amblyopia can exist without strabismus. The patient may have an obvious inability to judge distances, may be seen to close or cover one eye, or to turn or tilt the head. The patient may be confused or disoriented and be unable to describe the double vision.

Some of the more common types of strabismus are *esotropia* (one eye turns in), *exotropia* one eye turns outward, and *hypertropia* (one eye turns up relative to the other eye). With *intermittent strabismus*, the individual with an exophoria or an esophoria that is outside the optometric norms may be able to function fairly well for some period of time. When the task demand increases and fatigue sets in, however, the individual may not be able to compensate for the high phoria. At this point, the tentative binocular system breaks down and the patient experiences double vision, becoming at that moment strabismic. In *alternating strabismus*, the person switches the deviating eye, and in *constant strabismus*, no fusion is present. With comitant strabismus, the angle of the eye turn is the same regardless of which direction the eyes turn. However, when one particular nerve or muscle is affected, the magnitude of the eye turn may change as the eye moves more or less into the area of action of the involved muscle. This is a noncomitant strabismus. This is more common in acquired strabismus.

Evaluation

The presence of strabismus is best screened using the cover test (Griffin, 1976). An occluder and a distant and near target (such as a tracking pencil) are needed. The patient should wear his or her glasses if usually worn for the distance tested.

The therapist should ask the patient to look at the distant target. Cover the patient's right eye and observe the left eye for horizontal, vertical, or diagonal movement. Remove the occluder and repeat, covering the right eye until the therapist is sure about what has been seen: no movement, inward, outward, downward, or upward movement of the uncovered eye. When uncovering the eye, wait about a second to allow the eyes to recover fusion between trials. Repeat by covering the left eye and observing for any movement of the right eye. Repeat the test at near. Ask the patient to keep the close target clear.

If either eye moved when covered, then one eye was not looking directly at the target and thus is strabismic. This indicates the need for referral to an eye doctor.

Optometric evaluation will include the cover test, with a measurement of the angle of the deviation in prism diopters. The doctor will indicate what type of strabismus is present (constant, comitant, alternating, developmental), which eye muscle is involved in the deviation, and what the prognosis is for recovery of function.

Vision Rehabilitation Technique

The optometrist may recommend patching one eye or a portion of one eye's visual field to eliminate the confusion caused by double vision. If the two images are fairly close together, the patient should have the opportunity to make fusional responses. The stimulus to fusing two images together is double vision. If the patient is constantly patched, the eyes will not have that opportunity. Partially occluding one lens is a good alternative to complete patching. Sometimes, as in the case of acquired strabismus, just one zone of space exists where the double vision is seen. A partial patch, such as one made by partially occluding the lens of one or both eyes with "magic tape," can allow ambient light and peripheral vision in the deviating eye. This is an alternative to a black eyepatch, which completely eliminates all vision in the occluded eye. "Cling patch," another type of partially clear occlusion material available from Bernell, has variable amounts of transparencies and is easily removed.

In the developmental case, where the pathological suppression of one of the double images exists, antisuppression techniques, such as using red/green and polarized lenses, may be employed. (See Use of Red and Green Filters and Polarized Lenses.) Clinical use of these techniques must be closely supervised by the optometrist.

Prisms may be used in the treatment of strabismus, either the temporary (Fresnell) press-on prism or ground-in. The object is to bring the lines of sight closer together to help achieve fusion. The prism may be reduced over the course of therapy as improvement occurs.

Therapeutic considerations need to be made. The therapist should realize that fatigue affects visual performance leading to strabismus and symptoms such as double vision, eye strain, headaches, excessive blinking, rubbing eyes, and loss of concentration. In cases of *diplopia* (double vision), the following suggestions should be prescribed by an optometrist:

- For a constant and large angle of strabismus, a slightly translucent occluder can be used on the patient's glasses such as magic tape or alternating eye patch. The doctor would recheck the angle periodically to determine if the condition changes.
- For a constant but small angle strabismus, the patient is encouraged to experience double vision, as this will encourage fusional responses. Remember that diplopia is the stimulus for fusion. Taping (e.g., binasal) or periodic patching may be done when frustration, confusion, or balance issues are present.
- For occasional diplopia, no patching is required. The patient should be encouraged to take a break or do eye relaxation exercise such as palming: while seated at a table, place cupped hands over eyes without putting any pressure directly on the eyes. Allow the weight of the hands to rest on the palms, with the elbows resting on a table. Take a few deep breaths, and rotate palms in a slow circular massaging motion.

The referring doctor can be asked if certain positions are better particularly for noncomitant strabismic. Vision therapy may be appropriate in specific cases.

The subject of vision rehabilitation for strabismus is replete with controversy, particularly as related to the appropriate level of therapist involvement. However, occupational therapists, physical therapists, and speech and language pathologists are often faced with the dilemma of how to respond to patients' inquiries about possible vision rehabilitation for strabismus problems, especially following surgery or injury. Patients may have both ophthalmologists and optometrists involved in their cases. Open communication between therapist and doctor is always the best policy. Without additional training, therapists should be cautious about using vision rehabilitation techniques for patients with strabismus. Even if a therapist may not feel comfortable enough to employ vision rehabilitation techniques, increased awareness of techniques used by others may enable the therapist to recommend alternate pathways for a patient to consider.

Occlusion is often used by doctors as a treatment technique for strabismus. Therapists may communicate with doctors and patients about enhancing the occlusion regimen to include directed, structured activities performed by the therapist with the patient and by the patient on his or her own. Understanding the type of strabismus involved is crucial to planning these activities. For example, if the patient has been diagnosed with esotropia of the left eye and is wearing a patch on the right eye, activities may be used to encourage the patient to "stretch" the left eye from a nasal midline position toward the temple of his or her head. One such activity consists of asking the patient to hold the head at midline and look at a ball that is suspended by a string (Marsden ball), held by a therapist at the far left of the patient's visual field. The therapist then releases the ball and the patient tries to hit it back when the ball reaches his or her midline. For younger patients, supine positioning would, again, be helpful in maintaining the head at midline while the therapist positions a visually attractive item in the patient's left visual field.

Use of Red and Green Filters and Polarized Lenses

With some patients, difficulties may arise when they are asked to move beyond monocular functioning. In cases of constant unilateral strabismus occurring during the developmental period (under age 7), the dominant use of the nondeviating or fixating eye may override using the deviating eye, thereby causing suppression of the deviating eye's visual function. The patient is often unaware of this suppression while it is happening. Various devices may be used to increase the patient's awareness of this suppression, thereby helping the patient to learn to use binocular vision. One such device is a set of red and green filters (Griffin, 1976). For example, the patient with left eye esotropia described above would wear a special pair of eyeglasses consisting of frames with the green filter over the right eye and the red filter over the left eye. The patient would then watch a red suspended ball with black letters on it and try to touch the letters as they are called out by the therapist. If only the right eye is being used to view the ball, the patient will not see the letters because the green filter will cancel out the black letters. Only if the left eye is functioning will the patient be able to see the letters. Such suppression monitoring is more difficult to do with young children and nonverbal patients, because it requires more abstract reasoning and communication skills. Another example of a suppression check activity uses polarized filters. The patient wears a pair of polarized filters while looking into a mirror

(Griffin, 1976). If binocular vision is being used, the patient will be able to see both eyes reflected in the mirror through the filters. If one eye is being suppressed, that eye will appear black in the mirror.

Amblyopia: Definition, Evaluation, and Treatment

Amblyopia is reduced visual acuity that cannot be improved by optical means. Amblyopia is developmental in nature. Normal visual development does not occur because of abnormal visual stimulation. Examples are congenital cataracts that are not removed during the critical period of development (by 1 year of age at least), traumatic cataract, uncorrected refractive error (especially one very farsighted eye), or strabismus. In general, the earlier these conditions are identified and treated, the better the acuity will be.

Evaluation

The therapist screening consists of a visual acuity measurement: if the patient has corrective lenses on and a difference of two lines of letters is observed, then an amblyopia may be present. For the school-age child, a regular Snellen type acuity chart should be used to elicit the "crowding phenomenon" present in amblyopia—where a reduction in acuity results from the presence of surrounding letters. Single-letter acuity is always better. In younger children, however, the rotating E card may be used or the Broken Wheel Test available from Bernell Corporation.

In the optometric evaluation, the optometrist identifies the amblyopia by complete correction of the refractive error. If a difference in refraction exists between the eyes or an eye turn, then an amblyopia can be identified.

Visual Rehabilitation Technique

Amblyopia affecting one eye often results in neurological suppression of the affected eye. The blurry images observed using the amblyopic eye are canceled out in favor of the clearer images obtained through the nonamblyopic eye. As a result, the patient loses the efficiency and advantages of binocular vision. Monocular exercising of the amblyopic eye, achieved by occluding or patching the nonamblyopic eye, is the first step in remediation. Initially, verbal patients will express an inability to see anything at all with the amblyopic eye. Young children will often cry or be intolerant of the patching procedure. Beginning remediation may consist of having the patient perform easy tasks such as throwing a ball at a wall, walking on a dark, broad line on a lightly colored floor, or, especially for young children, playing with modeling dough. The motor component of these tasks serves to divert the patient's attention from the patching procedure while stimulating an adaptive visual response that may surprise the patient. As the patient becomes more comfortable using the amblyopic eye, more difficult tasks may be attempted, such as throwing balls at targets, walking on a path made of dots on the floor, or stacking blocks while sorting them by color. Progressive treatment leads to more challenging fine motor tasks, such as hammering nails into a design or placing pegs into a pegboard. Using high-contrast materials and increased illumination assists performance of these activities. Filling in Os in a line of print or looking for details or hidden pictures in a drawing are examples of more challenging tasks (McGraw, 1988). Patients may then proceed to biocular activities (see Visual Rehabilitation Techniques), where both eyes are being used but each eye is looking at a different target and they cannot be fused together. The binocular activity, by contrast, uses similar images presented to each eye, thereby allowing fusion to occur. Generally, the biocular and binocular phase is not begun until the acuities are at least only one acuity line different.

Binocular amblyopia is generally referred to as *low vision*. In terms of remediation, a large body of knowledge on this subject is beyond the scope of this chapter. However, the monocular procedures described above can be used to improve functional vision in either or both eyes.

Oculomotor Disorders: Definition, Evaluation, and Treatment

Oculomotor disorders include dysfunction in both the smooth pursuit skills and rapid saccadic skills. *Pursuits* are the smooth, coordinated movement of all the eye muscles together, allowing accurate tracking of objects through space. Perception is continuous during pursuit movements. *Saccades* are rapid shifts of the eyes from object to object, allowing quick localization of movements in the periphery. This would include any object immediately outside of the 1° to 2° of central vision. Once an object attracts interest, the ballistic-like eye movement swings the foveas around, placing the image directly on the fovea for identification. Perception occurs during moments of fixation. Saccades are the eye movements used for reading.

Peripheral vision is a critical part of the efficient execution of eye movements. While the peripheral system has very poor acuity, it is exquisitely sensitive to detecting small movements. As an unidentified motion is sensed to the side, the eyes are swung around so the central vision can view the source of the movement. The finer central acuity can then identify the source and a decision can be made. Thus, peripheral vision is extremely important in the efficient functioning of the oculomotor system (Moses & Hart, 1987).

The vestibular system plays a central role. The vestibular ocular reflex is intimately involved in oculomotor function by providing a stable platform for vision, contributing to the smoothness of the eye movement, and allowing a differentiation between movement of the object and movement of the eye. Scientific research has demonstrated that improvement in vestibular function also leads to an improvement in saccadic function (Chaikin, 1983).

Problems in pursuits and saccades can be the result of an injury or dysfunction of a muscle or nerve supplying a muscle or group of muscles, a vestibular dysfunction, an optical problem, or a generalized head injury, certain disease processes such as multiple sclerosis, or thyroid disease. Field loss can affect localizing ability.

Symptoms of oculomotor disorders include difficulty reading where a loss of place, skipping lines, or rereading lines occurs. In such cases, the words may appear to jump around on the page and letter order confusion exists in reading words. The patient may have poor ball skills and poor eye-hand coordination. Signs could include incomplete ocular range of motion, saccadic intrusions during a pursuit (e.g., a smooth pursuit is interrupted by a series of jerky, jumping movements), nystagmus, or a series of saccades instead of one direct movement. The eyes may overshoot or undershoot fixation on a target during fine motor tasks. For evaluation, optometric and therapist screenings are essentially the same.

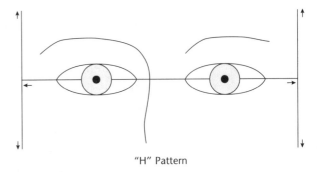

"H" Pattern

Figure 4.2

Pursuits. Ask the patient to follow a small object such as a map pin stuck into an eraser. For younger patients, use a "smiley" face sticker affixed to a popsicle stick. The patient should hold his or her head still or, if unable, have it held still. Move the target along the midline and out to all positions of gaze. The H pattern can be used, or a sidelying figure eight (see Figure 4.2). Standardized tests are available through Bernell Corporation, which include the King-Devick Saccadic Eye Movement Test and the Developmental Eye Movement Test (DEM). Both tests are good for evaluating eye movements in patients where word or number recognition or speech deficits are not problems. Note the smoothness of movement, completeness of range of motion, jerkiness, or jumping eye movements. Generally, such testing should be done monocularly in the case of acquired injury.

Saccades. Hold two pencils with map pins of different colors in them about shoulder width apart. Ask the patient to hold his or her head still and to look at one colored pin when told to. While the patient is fixating on one pin, move the other up or down. Then ask the patient to look at the other pin. Keep repeating the peripheral movement and then calling out the opposite colored pin until you can observe the patient's pattern. Ninety percent of the time the patient should be able to wait until you call the color. Observe for accuracy, under- or overshooting, nystagmus movements, searching movements, ability to isolate the eyes from the head movement, and shifting into all fields of gaze.

Visual Rehabilitation Techniques

Children may sometimes exhibit pursuit disorders complicated by attention deficits. Therapists will be challenged to find activities that will stimulate improved visual tracking skills for these children while retaining their attention. Involving both gross and fine motor skills may encourage patient participation in visual tracking exercises. Supine positioning provides stability for the patient's head and encourages isolation of eye movements from head movement (a beanbag chair can help provide additional head stability). An example of beginning pursuits activity is using a string to suspend a ball, which may be struck using a rod or directly with one's hands. Once the patient has demonstrated tracking improvement, pursuits training may be conducted from sitting and standing positions. Initially, the patient may have greater success with tracking if occlusion is used alternately with each eye prior to attempting binocular pursuit coordination. For more advanced pursuits training, a young child could watch a marble while rolling it inside a box lid or a pie pan (Richards, 1988). Older children and adults may be able to employ more advanced coordination skills to perform pursuit activities such as balancing a small ball on a supporting rod while moving the rod in various directions.

Complaints of losing the place on the page while reading or writing are common among children and some adults. This problem may be a combination of pursuit and saccade skill deficits. Problems with awareness of direction and position in space may be involved. Reading in Western countries requires a learned response of a left-to-right, top-to-bottom scanning orientation. Consideration must be given to cultural differences in reading. For example, Japanese and Hebrew require right-to-left scanning orientations. Remediation of difficulties tracking words on the page can begin with practicing visual jumps to fixed targets in space, gradually progressing to smaller targets on a page. One such fixation activity, especially useful with younger children, is having the patient place shapes onto matching outlines on the left side of a page and then match placement of the shape on the right side of the page. This saccadic activity may be modified to be more appropriate for older children and adults by having them alternately call out letters typed on the right and left sides of the page while clapping hands to a steady rhythm.

Patients are often less intimidated by practicing tracking across a page using material other than words. Using symbols or searching for sequenced letters of the alphabet among a letter jumble are examples of alternatives (Ann Arbor Tracking Pages from the Optometric Extension Program Foundation). Patients with binocular vision difficulties because of pursuit problems often exhibit symptoms of headaches after prolonged reading or writing. Working on endurance through therapy can help patients to extend their periods of tolerance for such activities.

Patients with oculomotor skills impairment may also fall under the category of dyslexia or be considered slow or cognitively impaired. In our present society with its emphasis on information technology, efficiency in visual skills is continually required for success in academics and careers. Oculomotor skills impairment will affect processing skills in other sensory areas and affect perception and fine and gross motor skills (Belgau, 1971; Getman, Kane, Halgren, & McKee, 1968; Locher & Worms, 1977). Patients with a diagnosis of dyslexia, attention deficit disorder, attention deficit hyperactivity disorder, cerebral palsy, and mental retardation may, in addition, have functional visual skills impairment (Duckman, 1980; Greenstein, 1976; Hoffman, 1980; Johnson & Zaba, 1994; Wold, 1978). Such patients may benefit from intervention as described in this chapter.

Nystagmus

Nystagmus is another type of neurological oculomotor disorder with rhythmic oscillating eye movements. It may be either congenital or acquired. The direction of the eye movement may be horizontal, vertical, or torsional (rotating around its own axis). It may be pendular, where the movement is equal in each direction, or jerk, where there is a fast and a slow phase. Many different types of nystagmus have been identified. Acquired types result from brainstem, cerebellar, thalamic, or vestibular dysfunction (Glaser, 1990).

Individuals with congenital nystagmus have reduced acuity but generally have no sensation of *oscillopsia* (the world moving). These individuals sometimes develop a null point, which is frequently achieved by overconverging the eyes. The null point causes significant dampening of the amplitude of the nystagmus, with a resultant increase in the functional acuity. In acquired nystagmus, reduced visual acuity may be accompanied by oscillopsia, dizziness, or nausea. Visual acuity may vary as the amplitude varies.

Evaluation

The therapist may note the presence of nystagmus by observation. It is helpful to note its presence in straight-ahead gaze, worsening of the amplitude of nystagmus in right or left gaze, and whether the movements appear equal or unequal in both directions. The optometrist may use a +20 diopter lens (which prevents fixation and magnifies the image) and observation under the biomicroscope.

Visual Rehabilitation Techniques

Treatment methods are limited. Some success has been found in using rigid gas-permeable (RGP) contact lenses for acquired nystagmus. The mechanism for the reduction in amplitude is not known but may be a type of feedback mechanism. This author has tried RGPs on two cases. In one case of brainstem-related damage with horizontal jerk nystagmus, the acuity improved from 20/60 to 20/40. In the second case, the nystagmus was torsional and no improvement was seen.

Summary

This brief overview of functional visual disorders and their remediation is meant to provide basic background information. The purpose of doing screening of visual conditions is to decide on referral to a vision specialist. If no visual problems are apparent, a referral is probably not necessary. If the therapist has questions regarding the patient's visual status, a referral to an optometrist or ophthalmologist should be made. Therapists may not, by law, diagnose visual conditions; they should not treat any visual conditions without a diagnosis. Therapists are encouraged to develop referral relationships with vision specialists for the good of their patients as well as to help further the therapist's education. Ongoing progress evaluations with the specialist can help to monitor progress and modify therapy programs.

REFERENCES

Aksionoff, E., & Falk, N. (1992). Optometric therapy for the left brain injured patient. *Journal of the American Optometric Association, 63*(8), 564–568.

Andrezejewska, W., & Baranowska, G. (1969). Accommodative disorders after head injury and cerebral concussion. *Clin Oczna, 7-39*(3), 431–435.

Arnsten, S. (1994). Vision therapy within occupational therapy. *OT Forum.*

Belgau, F. (1971). *A perceptual, motor and visual perception handbook of developmental activities for schools, clinics, parents and preschool programs.* Port Angeles, WA: Perception Development Researching Association.

Brock, F. W., & Folsom, W. C. (1962). A clinical measure of fixation disparities. *Journal of the American Optometric Association, 33*(7), 497–502.

Chaikin, L. (1983). *The effect of vestibular stimulation on visual function.* Master's thesis, Department of Occupational Therapy, San Jose State University, San Jose, CA.

Cohen, A. (1988). The efficacy of optometric vision therapy. *Journal of the American Optometric Association, 52*(2), 95–105.

Cohen, A. (1992). Optometric management of binocular disorders secondary to head trauma. *Journal of the American Optometric Association, 63*(8), 569–575.

Cool, S. (1990). Behavioral optometry and occupational therapy, an interaction whose time has come. *Journal of Behavioral Optometry, 1*(2), 31.

Downing-Baum, S. (1995a). OT and vision therapy in pediatrics—Finding pathways. *OT Forum.*

Downing-Baum, S. (1995b). *Pediatric vision therapy. OT Week.*

Downing-Baum, S., & Maino, D. K. (1996). Case studies show success in OT–OD treatment plans. *Advance for Occupational Therapists.*

Duckman, R. H. (1979). Effectiveness of visual training on a population of cerebral palsied children. *Journal of the American Optometric Association, 50,* 1013.

Fannin, T., & Grosvenor, T. (1987). *Clinical optics.* Stoneham, MA: Butterworths.

Getman, G., Kane, E., Halgren, M., & McKee, G. (1968). Developing learning readiness: A visual/motor/tactile skills program. New York: McGraw Hill.

Gianutsos, R., & Ramsey, G. (1987). Enabling survivors of brain injury to receive optometric services. *Journal of Visual Rehabilitation, 2,* 37–58.

Gianutsos, R., Ramsey, G., & Perlin, R. (1988). Rehabilitative optometric services for survivors of acquired brain injury. *Archives of Physical Medicine and Rehabilitation, 69,* 573–577.

Glaser, J. S. (1990). Neuro-ophthalmology (2nd ed.). Philadelphia: J. B. Lippincott.

Greenstein, T. N. (Ed.). (1976). *Identification of children with vision problems that interfere with learning.* Proceedings from American Optometric Association conference on Vision and Learning Disabilities, St. Louis, MO.

Griffin, J. (1976). *Binocular anomalies.* Chicago: Professional Press.

Hellerstein, L., & Fischman, B. (1990). Vision therapy and occupational therapy, an integrated approach. *Journal of Behavioral Optometry, 1*(5), 122.

Hoffman, L. H. (1980). Incidence of vision difficulties in children with learning disabilities. *Journal of the American Optometric Association, 51,* 447–451.

Johnson, R., & Zaba, J. (1994). Examining the link between vision and illiteracy. *Journal of Behavioral Optometry, 5.*

Kalb, L., & Warshowsky, J. (1991). Occupational therapy and optometry: principles of diagnosis and collaborative treatment of learning disabilities in children. In *Occupational therapy practice* (pp. 77–87). Gaithersburg, MD: Aspen.

Krobel, K., Kirsten, R. W., Simon, W., & Barrows, N. A. (1986). Post traumatic convergence insufficiency. *American Ophthalmology, 18*(3), 101–102.

Locher, P. J., & Worms, P. P. (1977). Visual scanning strategies of neurologically impaired, perceptually impaired and normal children viewing the Bender-Gestalt Drawings. *Psychology in the Schools, 14,* 147–157.

McGraw, L. (1988). *Guiding strabismus therapy.* Santa Ana, CA: Optometric Extension Program.

Moses, R. (1987). Accommodation. In R. Moses & W. Hart (Eds.), *Adler's physiology of the eye* (p. 298). St. Louis, MO: Mosby.

N. E. Thing Enterprises. (1995). *Magic Eye stereograms.*

Padula, W. (1988). *Behavioral vision approaches for persons with physical disability.* Santa Ana, CA: Optometric Extension Program.

Richards, R. (1988). *Classroom visual activities.* Novato, CA: Academic Therapy Publications.

Schnell, R. (1992). A vital part of rehabilitation. *OT Week.*

Soden, R., & Cohen, A. (1993). An optometric approach to the treatment of noncomitant deviation. *Journal of the American Optometric Association, 54*(5), 451–454.

Stanworth. (1974). Defects of ocular movement and fusion after head injury. *British Journal of Ophthalmology, 58,* 266–271.

Suchoff, I. (1995). A rationale and clinical model for collaboration between optometry and occupational therapy. *Journal of Behavioral Optometry, 6,* 142.

Wold, R. (1978). *Vision: Its impact on learning.* Seattle, WA: Special Child Publications.

RESOURCES

Bernell Corporation, PO Box 4637, South Bend, IN 46634-4637.

College of Optometrists in Vision Development (COVD), PO Box 285, Chula Vista, CA 91912.

Keystone View, 4673 Aircenter Court, Reno, NV 89502.

Optometric Extension Program Foundation (OEPF), 2912 South Daimler Street, Santa Ana, CA 92705.

5 Visual-Perceptual-Motor Dysfunction

Effects on Eye-Hand Coordination and

Skill Development

Rhoda P. Erhardt, MS, OTR, FAOTA, and
Robert H. Duckman, MA, OD, FAAO

Introduction

The visual function of many children and some adults with developmental and learning disabilities or both is often compromised because of central nervous system damage as well as optic insufficiencies. Terms such as *perceptual-motor* (Barsch, 1968; Roach & Kephart, 1966), *visual-perceptual* (Hung, Fisher, & Cermak, 1987; O'Brien, Cermak, & Murray, 1988), *visual-motor* (Erhardt, 1987; Farrell & Schultz-Krohn, 1990), and *visual perceptual-motor* (Williamson, 1987) have been used to describe certain problems that affect the quality of functional performance in almost all daily activities at home and school and in community environments.

This chapter will discuss those visual-perceptual-motor problems as

133

they affect eye–hand coordination and skill development. The term *visual-perceptual-motor* dysfunction has been selected because *visual* means relating to sight, *perceptual* refers to awareness through the senses, and *motor* is concerned with movement. Each of these components is important for function: the visual input, how it is perceived and processed, and the resultant motor output (gross motor, fine motor, and oculomotor).

The normal sensorimotor system receives and processes visual and tactile input efficiently, resulting in well-executed motor output (Williams, 1983). Sensorimotor system organization and disorganization are discussed in terms of the effects on gross motor, fine motor, and oculomotor function. A person who has developmental delays because of damage to the central nervous system may demonstrate hand dysfunction that is fairly obvious. Visual impairments may also be present, but they are often more subtle and difficult to identify and understand (Erhardt, 1992). Clinical observations and subsequent careful analysis are needed to determine how these developmental processes have been disrupted and how eye–hand mechanisms are affected. Eye–hand coordination and skill development are viewed within the contexts of occupational performance in children, that is, self-help, play, and the role of student, or learner, and how dysfunction affects the learning of these skills.

A literature review provides theoretical frameworks for understanding the relationship of these problems to deficits in general visual-perceptual-motor development, eye–hand coordination, and skill development. An observational approach to assessment and treatment of visual-perceptual-motor dysfunction includes guidelines for intervention. A model using clinical observations to chart the process of skill development in children will be presented.

A case study of a 6-year-old boy with subtle neurologic dysfunction and potential learning disabilities is used to demonstrate visual-perceptual-motor dysfunction that causes problems of eye–hand coordination and skill development. The process of evaluation, consultation to home and school, and reevaluation illustrates the effects of intervention on functional skills. Progress during the home program is documented with activity charts showing achievement of structured tasks, as well as charts recording observations of skill development.

Sensorimotor Organization and Disorganization

Many of the functional problems children have can be traced to disorganized central nervous systems that are unable to process sensory input accurately. If sensory input is inadequate or distorted, the central nervous system cannot interpret that information *veridically* (true to the stimulus), and motor output becomes compromised. Vision is a major part of that sensory information, essential for integrating gross motor, fine motor, and oculomotor control. It has been termed the steering mechanism for the body (Gesell, Ilg, & Bullis, 1949). Vision provides the sensory data upon which a person relies to make all spatial judgments. The general purpose of vision is to convey spatial information about the environment. The function of vision is to establish the foundation of sensory information and experience needed to direct movement through the environment. It is this movement through space, led by vision, and the feedback the system receives, comparing the visual input to the motoric output, which ultimately leads to an ever increasing dependence on visual information. Vision, in normal development, becomes the surrogate of movement.

Gross Motor Components

Gross motor skills are essential for balance not only for activities in physical education classes and playgrounds, but also for postural control in sitting positions to support fine motor dexterity in writing and oculomotor efficiency in reading. Many children with learning disabilities have delayed reflex integration, low muscle tone, compromised joint integrity, limited strength and endurance, and inadequate postural control. Without automatic balance reactions, they expend a great deal of effort just maintaining their posture in the classroom and concentrating on academic tasks. They have difficulty learning new motor patterns as well as executing skills already learned.

Fine Motor Components

Fine motor dexterity and coordination are affected not only by inadequate postural stability, but also by missing components in developmental sequences of approach, grasp, manipulation, and release. Thus, higher level skills requiring in-hand manipulation and tool use for activities of daily living are often impaired, despite normal intelligence and essentially normal neurological examinations. These children with learning disabilities frequently have problems with handwriting that include poor body posture, unstable pencil grip, lines too light or too heavy (poor midrange control), and perceptual deficits such as reversals (laterality, directionality, form perception).

Visual Components

Vision and Learning

Unfortunately, functional problems involving vision are not always identified, even in school. Children may be described as distractible, daydreaming, or noncompliant. They learn early to develop strategies and compensations that may be effective in certain situations, but not all. Again, because so much effort is required for controlling the oculomotor aspects of reading or writing, very little energy may be available for cognitive processing. Vision involves many different sensorimotor components, in both the optical and the neural systems.

Questions that need to be asked and answered include

- How well can the child see? (visual acuity)
- Are the eyes aligned properly? Are eye movements coordinated and accurate? Are eye-focusing skills appropriate and efficient? (oculomotor control)
- Is visual information being processed correctly? (visual perception)

The underlying question is actually, "Is there a visual problem contributing to the child's overall performance?"

Visual Acuity

Visual acuity refers to the eyes' ability to resolve detail, an exceedingly important skill for correctly identifying information about a stimulus in space. Optical insufficiencies, such as refractive error and ocular pathology, can interfere with the ability to make these identifications. All further processing in the visual-perceptual-motor "loop" will thus be affected. Insufficiency or inefficiency of *accommodation* (focusing) can affect the ability to resolve detail of stimuli presented in near space, especially when shifting gaze back and forth from a chalkboard to a book on one's desk. Refractive errors and ocular pathology need to be ruled out before functional vision can be considered.

Children with even a mild degree of central nervous system dysfunction are unable to achieve or maintain focus as well as children with intact systems. In addition, they cannot adapt well to minimal refractive errors. They may perform well during brief office testing but cannot sustain visual function during extended classroom tasks (Suchoff & Petito, 1986). Children are not asked to visually attend for only a minute or two at a time but for much longer periods. Therefore, it is not surprising that some children can perform well during a visual examination but have great difficulty with sustained near-point work. After a period of time, the visual system will fatigue and begin to "break down." It is at this point that functioning well on the basis of vision is no longer possible. Because many eye care specialists do not prescribe prescriptive lenses for these comparatively minor insufficiencies, these children need to use extra effort to function; they fatigue much more quickly and more often than their peers. Even if lenses are prescribed for children who need them only for near work, the use of bifocals, which require precise head adjustments, is contraindicated if head and trunk control are inadequate, as in children with moderate or severe cerebral palsy (Duckman, 1987).

Oculomotor Control

Oculomotor efficiency involves rapid, precise, and accurate control of eye muscles. Many children lose their place when reading and writing, have trouble staying on the line (rereading or skipping lines), and are not sure where one word stops and another starts. The slight differences in spaces between letters and words are a challenge to 5- or 6-year-old eyes, trying to make their first accurate discriminations of those differences. Insufficient and inefficient ocular motor control or both are manifested by poor comprehension of material and the need to read it several times to understand it. Coordination of eye muscles for precise eye movements, however, depends on total postural stability, especially of the head and neck (Duckman, 1987). Since extraocular muscles usually operate similarly to muscles in the rest of the body, inadequate control in some children may be related to low muscle tone and poor grading of movement.

The motor components of vision emerge in clear developmental sequences during the first 6 months of life, and include localization, fixation, ocular pursuit, and gaze shift (Erhardt, 1990). Specific voluntary eye movements and examples of their implications for the school environment include

- *localization:* the ability to quickly and accurately localize a visual target (e.g., to find a certain place on a page in a book)
- *fixation:* the ability to maintain stationary gaze (e.g., long enough to discriminate and comprehend a word, sentence, or paragraph in that book)
- *ocular pursuit:* the ability to smoothly track a moving object (e.g., to follow a volleyball across a net in a gymnasium) and
- *gaze shift:* the ability to quickly and accurately shift gaze, with the eyes moving independently from the head (e.g., to scan a line of letters and words while reading across a page to the right, back to the left, and down to the next line).

Visual Perception

Visual perception is defined as the process of obtaining and interpreting information from the environment. Information entering the eye is always processed against a background of information received by all the other sensory systems, as well as memories of past experiences (Schrock, 1978). Visual perceptual processes include visual discrimination, memory, spatial relationships, form constancy, sequential memory, figure-ground, and closure.

Visual *input* is the information that is processed cortically by the organism. Logically, if the input information is distorted in any way, output will be affected, causing observable problems in school and home environments. Visual information may be distorted by impairments originating in the optical structures (the eye itself) or in neural processing throughout the brain. Although the assumption is often made that visual problems are always related to ocular pathology and deficiency, in fact, many can be traced to the neural or motor components of vision, not only coordination of eye muscles, but also the integration of the visual system with other body systems.

The "garbage in, garbage out" syndrome addresses the child who appears to have visual perceptual motor deficits but really does not. Instead, visual input may be significantly distorted by ocular anomalies that may not have been routinely diagnosed. Unlike *myopia* (nearsightedness), which elicits subjective complaints ("I can't see") or objective symptoms (bringing the eyes very close to the page), certain conditions are missed because the child is able to make ocular adjustments that allow him or her to *see* but not to *perceive* accurately what is seen. These conditions may include

- significant uncorrected *hyperopia* (farsightedness)
- intermittent *exotropia* (outward deviation strabismus), with inability to converge the eyes closer than 12 inches (normal reading distance for many young children). Note: The normal ability to converge as close as 2 inches is an indicator of sufficient fusion reserves for sustained function.
- ocular pathology causing significantly compromised input (e.g., nystagmus).

If optical devices are used to improve the visual input (e.g., prescription lenses to correct hyperopia and prisms to realign an exotropic eye or direct gaze to the null point for nystagmus or both), it is not uncommon for these visual-perceptual problems to disappear.

Visual Problems in the Classroom

Figure 5.1, Visual Problems in the Classroom Checklist, is a form that can be used by classroom teachers. It is organized into groups of objective

Child's Name _____ Grade _____ Age _____ Date _____

Teacher observations during reading and writing

☐ Red or watering eyes

☐ Eyes crossed, turned in or out or not moving together

☐ Excessive blinking or eye-rubbing, especially when changing focus between near and far

☐ Losing place when reading, rereads or skips words or lines, using finger for marker

☐ Omitting, substituting, repeating, or confusing similar words

☐ Difficulty comprehending or remembering what is read

☐ Confusion when interpreting or following written instructions

☐ Writing up or down hill, spacing letters or words irregularly

☐ Inability to finish timed assignments with rest of class

☐ Confusion with left/right directions

☐ Persistent reversals after 2nd grade

☐ Errors copying from chalkboard or from book to notebook

☐ Misaligning horizontal and vertical series of numbers

☐ Difficulty remembering, identifying, and reproducing geometric forms

☐ Poor orientation of drawings on page

☐ Eye-hand coordination problems in tying shoes, buttons, sports

Avoidance behaviors

☐ Short attention span, distractibility, or daydreaming

☐ Dislike of close work

☐ Disruptive behavior, emotional outbursts

Physical adaptations

☐ Placing head close to book or desk when reading or writing (7–8″)

☐ Moving head instead of eyes while reading

☐ Attempting to use one eye only by turning or tilting head, closing or covering one eye

Complaints, especially after doing close work

☐ Burning or itching eyes   ☐ Nausea or dizziness   ☐ Seeing double

☐ Headaches ☐ Fatigue   ☐ Sensitivity to light   ☐ Blurring of print

Adapted from checklists of: The American Optometric Association, 243 N. Lindberg Blvd., St. Louis, MO 63141; Optometric Extension Program, 2912 South Daimler, Santa Ana, CA 9205; College of Optometrists in Vision Development, PO Box 285, Chula Vista, CA 91912

Figure 5.1 Visual problems in the classroom checklist.

teacher observations during academic tasks, avoidance behaviors, postural adaptations, and the child's subjective complaints.

Styles, Differences, and Disabilities

Adult learners as well as children need a variety of teaching methods, because each individual has a different learning style. Some learn best through visual material, some through auditory, some through their tactile and proprioceptive senses. The therapist who considers these individual differences as learning *differences* rather than learning *disabilities* will recognize the wide range of "normal" and will be able to respect the clever compensations that children invent to manage their "atypical" learning styles. However, children who are unable to achieve age-appropriate tasks, particularly in the school setting, will need intervention for specific performance components that are interfering with skill development.

Theoretical Frameworks for Evaluation and Treatment of Visual-Perceptual-Motor Dysfunction

Developmental Approaches

The term *development* has been defined in its broadest sense as a process of evolution, maturation, and learning. In other words, learning is a self-determined process occurring through interaction of genetic and environmental (internal and external) variables. The developmental frame of reference can be very helpful when intervention activities need to be sequenced in preparation for functional tasks. Important features of human development are

- tendency toward increased organizational complexity as each component of development becomes activated and functional
- modification of each activity as a result of ongoing experiences
- craving for purpose and variability.

The role of vision in total development originated in the early work of pioneers such as Arnold Gesell (Gesell et al., 1949), a pediatrician; Newell Kephart (1960), an educator; and Gerald Getman (1962), an optometrist. Their theoretical perspectives provided the foundation for better understanding of children with learning disabilities and mild developmental disabilities.

Gesell's research in child development at Yale University began in the 1930s; by the 1940s he extended his work to vision (Gesell et al., 1949). His involvement with optometrists stimulated their interest in developmental vision therapy and led to one of the first multidisciplinary approaches to vision and learning (Wold, 1978). Barbara Knickerbocker (1980) was one of the first occupational therapists who realized the importance of blending visual function with whole body performance. She presented a holistic approach to *learning disorders,* a term she preferred to perceptual-motor handicaps, widely used in the 1960s, especially by Kephart. Since much of her work was based on that of Dr. A. Jean Ayres, she also used terms such as *sensorimotor*, the equivalent of *sensory integration,* defined as the organization and integration of sensory systems and developmental motor patterns (Ayres, 1972).

Knickerbocker (1980) proposed two basic premises about children with learning disorders. First, that when they encountered new experiences without the necessary developmental prerequisites, they were unable to learn spontaneously, often failed at new skills, and became very frustrated. Second, that their pattern of avoidance following these unsuccessful experiences then interfered with the smooth development of underlying foundational skills for new learning.

Perceptual-Motor Approaches

Kephart (1960) referred to new learning acquired as a separate entity as a *splinter skill*, one that cannot be applied or generalized to other similar but not identical situations. He described the following hierarchy of perceptual-motor development as the foundation for efficient function:

- *Posture*, the maintenance of the body in reference to its center of gravity, is the basis for all movement.
- *Body image* provides a point of reference for all external spatial relationships.
- *Laterality*, awareness of left and right within the body, is necessary for projection of left and right in space.
- *Directionality* then develops, first in the relationship of the child to external objects, and then in the relationship of external objects to each other.

Thus, without an *internal* awareness of left and right or up and down, the child is unable to acquire an accurate perception of *external* objects, resulting in problems such as reversals of letters and words.

Organization of self and of self to the environment develops from achievement of these perceptual concepts, as well as gradual mastery of gross and fine motor skills through repetition. Breakdowns in this process can interfere with development of perceptual-motor skills that prepare for functional tasks such as reading and writing. Compensations for an inadequate foundation for learning may be effective in the early school years; but when academic materials become more complex, these children find themselves working increasingly harder to learn a collection of splinter skills. They have developed adaptations to environmental demands without the necessary prerequisites. For example, both eyes may function together adequately; but when testing each alone reveals poor ocular control, the apparent binocularity was achieved by "tying" the two eyes together rather than by integrating two separate control systems, which follows a normal developmental sequence.

Figure 5.2, Feedback Mechanisms in Perception, presents Kephart's simple diagram describing the perceptual process, with input generated inside the organism by its own neural impulses, activated by external stimuli. Integration involves the processing and organization of multiple, simultaneous sensory inputs (visual, auditory, kinesthetic, proprioceptive) in preparation for a single, efficient motor response. The effects of past experiences, which alter and modify the input pattern, are also incorporated into this process. In addition, the output pattern modifies the system by feeding back sensory data, allowing constant monitoring

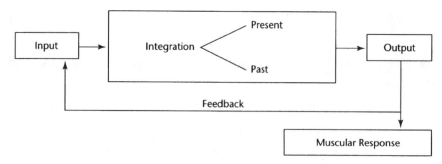

Figure 5.2 Feedback mechanisms in perception (Source: Kephart, 1960).

and alteration of output until feedback matches input exactly. Thus input and output are one perceptual process and cannot be considered separately. A breakdown of the perceptual-motor match occurs when incoming information conflicts with rather than reinforces other input. For example, if the child's eyes work together sometimes but not always, fusion may be achievable at arm's length but not any closer. Double images interfere with near-point tasks such as reading or writing. The distance at which this breakdown occurred may not always be consistent. It may depend on the child's physical or emotional state, changing from day to day or hour to hour. Ironically, if the child's eyes were uncoordinated all the time, vision would be consistently suppressed in one eye and would actually become quite efficient. Thus, unpredictable visual images could be one cause of inconsistent school performance. Children have difficulty coping with these types of transient deficits (Kephart, 1960).

Motor Control Theory

Motor control, learning, and development are considered three new approaches to understanding motor behavior. New approaches do not replace older theories but supplement them, as new research always adds to and builds on previous knowledge. For *motor control*, the question is "How is the control organized?" For *motor learning*, the question is "How are skills acquired through experience and practice?" For *motor development*, the question is "How does motor behavior change during age-related growth?" (VanSant, 1991).

As stated previously, these same issues were discussed by early pioneers such as Kephart (1960) and Barsch (1968), using similar language as current motor control theorists, who state that the coordination of motor activity and perception (perceptual-motor integration) for motor planning depends on the processing of sensory and motor feedback (Laszlo & Broderick, 1991). This processing includes kinesthetic information processing (the sensory component) and programming processing (the motor component).

Kinesthetic information processing involves intricate, ongoing sensory input from every part of the body about the prevailing posture and the movements superimposed on that posture, including extent of movement, direction of movement, timing of movement, and force produced by muscles.

Programming processing involves the activation of appropriate motor units because skilled movements must be goal-directed and flexible. Decisions are made concerning spatial boundaries (extent and direction of movement), temporal aspects (speed of movement), and the amount of force needed to overcome gravity or external resistance (Rosenbaum, 1991).

In some ways, these programming processes operate independently from each other. For example, a child may be able to move at an appropriate speed for a handwriting activity, but the movements may be in the wrong direction, so mistakes are made in the formation of letters. Or, handwriting may be accurate, but tension in pencil grasp and excessive force during hand movements may cause tearing of the paper or dark lines that are difficult to erase.

Motor planning relates to goal attainment. It is the process of choosing the starting point, the direction, the speed, the exact time to change direction, and the place to terminate the movement. For example, many children do not have a clear starting point, are confused about direction, draw too fast or too slowly, and are not able to inhibit movement in order to stop when they should (perseveration). Effectiveness of the motor plan depends not only on efficient processing but also on storage and retrieval of memory about previous movements. Different writing tasks require different degrees of motor planning skill. Drawing shapes from memory obviously requires more skill than copying. Motor planning demands for tracing are minimal, and the use of templates provides even more tangible guides. Therapists can use this sequence to plan successful steps toward task accomplishment for children with motor planning problems.

Principles of motor learning support a treatment approach that emphasizes practice of movement patterns and components of patterns in relation to functional tasks. Skill acquisition depends on both the type of task and the subject's stage of learning. Feedback (internal as well as external), facilitation, and practice are important instructional variables. Children with neurologic dysfunction are usually not motivated to practice motor patterns because the cycle of inadequate or distorted feedback causes abnormal motor output resulting in unsuccessful tasks.

Stages of motor learning have been described as cognitive, associative, and automatic. If children have difficulty moving through the cognitive and associative stages, few skills will become smooth and automatic. Research has shown that random and variable practice produce better learning and generalization for tasks such as feeding, which may take place under different conditions. Part practice is more efficient for complex tasks such as dressing. Whole practice is important for integrated timing, for tasks such as handwriting. Facilitation includes verbal instruction, demonstration, and manual guidance, always within the context of the whole task (Light, 1991; Poole, 1991).

Although these new motor control theories use a contemporary systems approach that emphasizes the heterarchy of motor behavior more than the traditional hierarchy of central nervous system function, they are not incompatible with perceptual-motor and developmental approaches because of their holistic and task-oriented nature.

Hierarchy is defined as a traditional developmental sequence, with each step following a predetermined previous one. *Heterarchy* means that task-oriented behavior is a result of the interaction of many body systems and between the person and the environment. Therefore, normal development will vary according to personal characteristics and environmental factors. Another important premise is that new movement patterns are best learned in functional contexts, where motivation and purpose produce goal-directed behaviors, within the occupational roles of childhood: play, self-care, and student (Mathiowetz & Haugen, 1994). These current practice models are actually returning to the origins of occupational therapy, when the founders of the profession developed philosophical tenets about the importance of goal-directed, purposeful treatment and the interaction of person and environment (Dunton, 1919; McNary, 1947, both as cited in Cohen & Reed, 1995).

Neurodevelopmental Treatment Concepts

Neurodevelopmental treatment (NDT) theory, originated by Berta and Karel Bobath, has been undergoing dramatic changes, as this popular model is expanded to incorporate modern motor control theory (Bly, 1992; Bobath, 1985; Bobath & Bobath, 1956; Light, 1991). NDT therapists have always considered practice to be one of the most important factors in motor learning. They have tried to ensure that it is variable, that is, done in many different ways through positioning, materials, environments, and methods. Table 5.1 illustrates an NDT interpretation of the three stages in motor learning and correlated treatment methods.

Clinical therapists, therefore, must determine what skills the patient considers important to learn because motor synergies are organized around meaningful functional tasks. Then the first responsibility of the therapist is to create an environment that allows the child to initiate and actively organize purposeful movement. Only then can the therapist fulfill the NDT goal of using therapeutic handling to provide correct alignment for muscles to work in normal synergies.

Model of Human Occupation

Kielhofner's model of human occupation is helpful in understanding functional performance deficits in children with learning disabilities. The model describes how people choose and perform everyday behaviors, operating in an open system because they are constantly interacting with

Table 5.1 Stages of Learning

Stage	Description of child's process	Therapist's treatment method
1. Cognitive	Understanding new task Exploring different strategies Performing inconsistently Retaining effective strategies, discarding others Improving significantly	Motivate by selecting meaningful task in pleasant setting Model task (verbal instruction, demo, and/or manual assistance) Give feedback for several trials Taper off feedback Ask for child's feedback
2. Associative	Determining most effective methods Making subtle adjustments Using errors to correct performance during practice Improving gradually with more consistency	Allow experimentation (no modeling, handling, demo, discussion) Provide varied feedback only during significant errors
3. Automatic	Performing task easily after many trials Ignoring distractions Accomplishing secondary task simultaneously (such as talking at same time) Attending to entire environment instead of details only	Present a variety of conditions, secondary tasks, and distractions Encourage generalization to different functional skills

Sources: Light, 1991; Poole 1991.

their environment, which is almost always changing (Kielhofner, 1985). The open system consists of four phases: intake, feedback, throughput, and output.

- *Intake*, or input, as described by Kephart in his diagram of feedback mechanisms, is the delivery of new information. A child who cannot sustain visual attention will not be able to finish reading instructions for a task.
- *Feedback*, also part of Kephart's model, gives another form of information—responses from previous output behaviors. A child whose system provides faulty feedback may be unable to critique his own performance accurately.
- *Throughput* consists of three subsystems: performance, habituation, and volition.

Performance skills (communication, perceptual-motor, and process) affect social relationships, academic tasks, and problem solving needed for planning, organizing, and executing tasks. A child with performance deficits will view new activities as frustrating rather than challenging.

Habituation is the subsystem that guides the person through routine activities, resulting in productive habits. A child with problems in self-regulation does not learn routines easily and requires supervision in many self-help tasks.

Volition is defined as the ability to invest energy in exploring and mastering one's environment to develop interests, values, and a sense of accomplishment. A child with a short attention span and disorganized behavior is unable to make thoughtful, appropriate choices in order to complete tasks successfully.

- *Output*, the motor action, is the expression of occupational behavior, according to the Model of Human Occupation. Both Kephart (1960) and Kielhofner (1992) emphasized that output always provided additional feedback to the input phase in order to integrate ongoing throughput. A child whose central nervous system is not well integrated will fail frequently and view most school, play, and self-help skills as problematic. As previously stated, many of these children develop avoidance behaviors because of low self-esteem (Knickerbocker, 1980).

If maladaptive or avoidance behaviors are caused or increased by environmental factors, intervention for these children should provide structure and reinforcement to facilitate skilled performance of life tasks, most of which require eye–hand coordination (Woodrum, 1992).

Normal and Atypical Eye–Hand Coordination and Skill Development

The Hand

The hand is able to function in different modes. It can use the power of its fingers and thumb to maintain grasp of an object in its palm, resisting gravity. It can also combine complicated blends of precise movements for all kinds of delicate tasks with or without tools (Boehme, 1988).

As a component of eye–hand coordination, the hand is an instrument for perception as well as movement. Tactile and proprioceptive sensations are used to identify size, shape, texture, temperature, and weight of objects. The high density of skin receptors in the hand provides tactile-kinesthetic spatial feedback, which is essential for ongoing direction of skilled movements (Corbetta & Mounoud, 1990). In other words, as the hand moves, the receptors tell the brain where the hand and parts of the hand are in space. Many children with sensorimotor problems are not receiving and processing that sensory information, so arm and hand motor skills do not develop normally.

Like all anatomical structures, the upper extremity has evolved in logical ways through the evolutionary process. Phylogenetically, many lower animals originally used both upper and lower extremities for functional stability as they walked on four legs. During the progression toward the human upright position, upper extremity function changed: stability was exchanged for mobility. Evolution of the shoulder illustrates how form follows function. Anatomical changes at the proximal as well as the distal ends of the arm became necessary. The forelimbs were no longer needed for weight-bearing and brachiation (swinging from tree to tree), so they were freed for prehension. Dissociation became possible, instead of the hand always acting as a unit. For example, fingers were first curved together in flexion to provide faster and better grasp of tree limbs during brachiation. The glenohumeral joint, formerly just as important for stability as the hip joint, is now the most mobile of all joints in the body. It has many axes of movement (flexion and extension, abduction and adduction, circumduction, and internal and external rotation). However, because the socket has become so shallow through its evolution, this mobility has been achieved at the sacrifice of stability. Today, the shoulder's stability is provided not by bone structure, but only by soft tissues such as muscles, tendons, and ligaments. Those soft tissues do provide adequate internal stability for most functional requirements of the upper extremity in today's human, that is, approach, grasp, manipulation, transportation, and release of objects (Kent, 1971, as cited in Erhardt, 1992). Children with low muscle tone, however, compensate for poor proximal stability at the neck, shoulder, and trunk by using many abnormal postures and movements during their attempts to reach and grasp.

Exner's model of in-hand manipulation illustrates the importance of this stability and mobility mechanism and how parts of the hand become dissociated during normal development. For example, the child who carries a block while crawling is weight-bearing on the ulnar side and grasping the block with radial digits. Exner also described how objects are moved within the hand, and how parts of objects are stabilized. For example, the ulnar fingers hold part of a pen as radial fingers push off the top (Exner, 1990, 1992). Some children with atypical or delayed development are unable to achieve these high-level manipulative skills because they cannot dissociate one part of the hand from another, or they use inappropriate points of stability. For example, the most mature pencil grasp, the dynamic tripod, requires distal mobility of the fingers and thumb, dissociated from the rest of the hand and forearm, resting on the surface.

The Eye

Although vision is usually perceived in terms of its *sensory* function, the majority of hand skills require visual monitoring, an important *motor* component of eye-hand coordination. The anatomy and physiology of vision is more complex than that of prehension. Normal physiological function of the hand can be understood in terms of general knowledge of the body's bone structure, neuromuscular function, and tactile and proprioceptive mechanisms. The study of vision, however, requires an additional understanding of the optical system as well as the neural systems and the connections between them (Erhardt, 1992).

In addition to a foundational knowledge of ocular anatomy and physiology, the therapist who works with school-age children needs to understand (a) the medical approach to visual pathology, (b) the educational view of visual perception in terms of learning, and (c) the usefulness of normal developmental sequences for planning intervention.

The medical approach to visual handicaps is based on a model of pathology. The assumption is that skilled visual function depends on intact anatomical structures and normal physiological processes of the eyes, the visual pathways, and the cerebral cortices. The medical model manages dysfunction by identifying the etiology of the injury or the disease and then attempting to remediate that pathology.

The educational view of visual perception looks at learning, adaptation, and how environmental factors affect function. *Perception* is considered an acquired skill, defined as the ability to recognize, organize, and act on information received through the senses: seeing, hearing, smelling, tasting, touching, moving, and body position in relation to space. *Visual perception* is defined as the capacity to interpret visual sensory input and assign meaning to what is seen. To process, visual information must be integrated with information derived from other sensory receptors and motor receptors (Gibson, 1970). Occupational therapists are trained to adapt the environment therapeutically to facilitate this integration process.

Developmental sequences can be useful in correlating both visual and prehensile data into an integrated model of assessment and intervention. In both fine motor and visual-motor areas of development, early reflexes and primitive movement patterns are the foundation for more voluntary refined movements. In both areas, developmental stages blend together imperceptibly during growth, and reversions to previously outgrown levels occur occasionally. During plateau periods, new skills become smoothly integrated with previous ones. These are characteristics of the developmental process (Knobloch, Stevens, & Malone, 1980).

All these models are useful for understanding the child's developing visual system. Medical evaluations describe the status of the child's optical and neural physiological systems. Educational tests and program plans state levels of function and specific objectives. Developmental assessments provide sequential structures for intervention (Erhardt, 1992).

Eye–Hand Mechanisms

Both visual and tactile sensory systems contribute similar but not identical information about objects in the environment. This information is matched and cross-matched until it is integrated. When the eye decides where the hand is to move, the direction of the eye muscle movements must agree with that of the arm muscle movements. In comparison with the eyes, the hands are limited in the quantity and quality of information they can receive. Only the areas of the skin that are in actual contact with the environment can send tactile information to the brain. The eyes, on the other hand, can respond to stimulation from much larger and more distant parts of the environment. As the young child grows, the amount of information gathered about the world gradually relies more and more on visual and less on tactile input (Hatwell, 1990; Peiper, 1963). In other words, with maturity individuals know what something feels like from past experience, without having to touch it.

The complete act of prehension contains an equally important visual component in the phases of motor operations: (a) looking, (b) reaching, and (c) grasping. Research conducted on infants revealed the importance of hand-watching as a prerequisite for eye–hand coordination during exploratory manipulation and skill development (Castner, 1932). Thus, a developmental approach can be applied to children who reach inaccurately, have immature grasps, and glance at their hands only briefly during manipulation of objects. They can be helped to move through the appropriate developmental steps toward mature approach, grasp, manipulation, and release (Erhardt, 1994). A more physiologically based approach views postural stabilization as a crucial factor, for eye–head orientation to determine correct arm and hand placement, stabilization of the trunk to ensure efficient arm transport, and controlled stability and mobility of all various arm and hand joints to achieve precise digital grasp (Paillard, 1990, as cited in Erhardt, 1992).

The prehension and vision systems have important differences in their relative positions and biomechanics affecting coordination of hand and eye movements. For example, the eyes are centrally located near the axes of the head and trunk, while the hands are peripheral to the proximal axis. The limbs, which have considerable mass and joint freedom, move through space significantly affected by gravitational pull. The eyes, on the other hand, have much less mass, and their movements are limited to rotation around a single point affected much less by gravitational forces (Duckman, 1987; Fisk, 1990, as cited in Erhardt, 1992).

According to motor learning and control theories, the visual system uses dual processing to guide arm movements: *ambient* (peripheral) and *focal* (central). Information from the peripheral field is used to analyze the direction of the moving arm in comparison to the direction of eye gaze toward a visual target. Then, acute central vision analyzes the relative positions of hand and target. The movement trajectory is constantly updated and corrected by both ambient and focal processes (Paillard, 1979, as cited in Erhardt, 1992). To get accurate and coordinated eye-hand function, the actions of the eyes and hands must be timed with consideration of their different biomechanical features. Eye movements guide hand movements at the same time that coordinated hand movements influence eye movements. This constant exchange of information is needed for adaptation to rapidly changing environmental conditions. The speed of eye movements tracking ongoing hand movements is at least doubled when the subject moves the target compared to someone else moving it, because of the prediction factor: anticipating the position of the moving stimulus (Rosenbaum, 1991). This means that eye–hand coupling facilitates efficiency of eye movements. Therefore, the development of oculomotor control in children with imperfect eye–hand coordination may be compromised.

Normally, hand movements are preceded by eye movements providing visual input such as distance, size, shape, weight, and texture. This visual information joins together with visual and tactile memory to help the hand move more accurately toward the target, where it prepares for precise shaping, rather than waiting for kinesthetic and proprioceptive data upon contact (Fisk, 1990). Piaget (1952) described this accommodation of the hand to an object as anticipatory shaping. Many children do not shape their hands during visual anticipation, only after contact. Other children cannot shape their hands to an object well enough to hold it securely without dropping, especially during arm movement.

Functional Skills

Skills have been defined as practiced abilities demonstrating dexterity and confidence in functional tasks. Skills are sequences of organized, goal-directed actions, which apply strategies proceeding to a future goal. The execution of skills depends on the individual person, the task, and the environment. This transaction between the performer and the environment is always changing. Therefore, fundamental features of skills are flexibility and problem solving, which allow generalization (Connolly & Dalgleish, 1989, as cited in Erhardt, 1992).

In their classic writings, Piaget (1952) and Bower (1966) emphatically stated that basic eye–hand patterns can be refined and expanded for functional skills only through certain prerequisite visuomotor experiences repeated many times in a variety of situations. Functional skills such as feeding, dressing, and writing require very complex and selective patterns of muscular coordination. The performance of these skills depends on an intact and mature central nervous system, as well as a foundation of basic motor patterns acquired during the first few years of life (Bobath & Bobath, 1972, as cited in Erhardt, 1992).

Theoretical Frameworks for Evaluation and Treatment of Eye–Hand Dysfunction

Physiology of Eye–Hand Relationships

Precise visual guidance of goal-directed arm and hand movements has evolved within the brain structure through specialization and organization of the parietal association cortex. As mentioned previously, the physiological approach delineates certain sequential functional movements operated by separate neural networks in different areas of the brain (Paillard, 1990, as cited in Erhardt, 1992):

- Eye–head orientation, which leads to localization and identification of an object in space, is organized at the midbrain level around the superior colliculus.
- Arm mobilization, which localizes the object following a triggered ballistic movement, is dependent on brainstem structures. A *ballistic movement* is one that prescribes in advance the direction and distance of travel; it cannot be changed in the middle of the movement.
- Grasp, which adjusts the terminal guided approach, is primarily under cortical control. When the hand gets close, the forearm, wrist, and fingers consciously prepare for grasp by orienting to the object.

Each of those motor patterns receives and uses sensory information, especially the visual feedback loops. For example, when a child reaches for a pencil, visual feedback calibrates gaze orientation. Eyes either move separately from the head, or together, whichever is more efficient in the particular situation. If the child needs to reach quite far to the side, it is more efficient to move eyes and head together rather than eyes alone. If, however, the object is fairly close, the child can look more rapidly and accurately by moving eyes only. The visual feedback also guides arm trajectory and orientation of hand grip. The shoulder and elbow joints extend just enough to reach the pencil, no further. The forearm then orients to midposition in preparation for grasp. The visual feedback also processes size and shape cues. The child remembers from past experiences how to shape finger joints for a stable grasp. After contact, tactile cues refine grasp and assist in manipulation, that is transporting the pencil to the paper, moving it across the page to write, and returning it to the surface.

When this process is disrupted in someone whose eyes may not localize accurately, visual feedback is distorted. The arm trajectory is not appropriate, resulting in overshooting or undershooting. Compensatory patterns may interfere with orientation for grasp. After contact, insufficient tactile feedback prevents the hand from adjusting grasp, so transportation and manipulation may be disrupted, with the pencil either slipping from the hand or held with excessive pressure during writing.

Developmental Sequences of Eye–Hand Components

The visual mechanism has a major role in the early development of eye–hand coordination. Stages beginning at birth and continuing to 40 weeks and beyond have been described as (a) static visual exploration, (b) active and repeated visual exploration of objects, (c) visual regulation of grasping and manipulation, and (d) refined control of eye–hand behaviors. As tactile and proprioceptive sensory input stimulates reflexive grasping, the eyes begin to explore the environment, including the hands. Vision helps to bring eye–hand coordination to higher skill levels (Williams, 1983, as cited in Erhardt, 1992). In order to develop highly refined fine motor behaviors, hand movements must be simultaneously seen and felt during interaction and exploration of the environment. Development of visual control over the hand is acquired during the first half-year of life. Visually guided reaching becomes very accurate by about 5 or 6 months of age, and it peaks at 7 or 8 months. During the last half of the first year, the need to visually monitor the hand through the entire reaching process gradually decreases. In fact, after the age of 1 year, once the hand has begun moving efficiently toward its destination, visual attention is usually transferred to another place of interest, especially after contact is made (Erhardt, 1992). For example, a baby eating small cereal bits first looks, then contacts and grasps, and usually looks away before or during grasp and transport to mouth. Table 5.2, The Development of Eye–Hand Coordination, correlates the stages of eye function and hand function and their interrelationships from 1 to 6 months of age.

Functional Relevance of Eye–Hand Skills

Performance areas in the occupations of childhood include activities of daily living, play, and productive activities such as schoolwork.

Activities of daily living include self-help skills such as feeding, dressing, and grooming. Eye–hand components of feeding begin when the eyes locate the bottle, which leads to the hands bringing it to the mouth about the middle of the first year. Finger feeding is followed by manipulation of utensils (cup, spoon, fork), requiring the eyes to direct the hands for more precise movements during the second year. As the child gets older, the ability to use a variety of tools for meal preparation tasks leads to increasing independence.

Undressing precedes dressing, and both skills are easier to manage in the lower body than the upper body because of both visual and manual access. Fasteners such as buttons, zippers, snaps, buckles, and shoelaces require sustained visual monitoring and a high level of manual dexterity. Most children have learned these skills by the time they enter school.

Grooming skills gradually improving during childhood include (a) washing hands and face (mirror awareness), (b) bathing (visually scanning body as well as monitoring hands), (c) toothbrushing, (d) hair care (mirror and use of brush or comb in hand), (e) toileting (cleansing self), and finally (f) nail care (Coley, 1978, as cited in Erhardt, 1992). During adolescence, of course, interest in appearance increases significantly, as cosmetics, hair styles, and clothes preoccupy both boys and girls. These

Table 5.2 The Development of Eye–Hand Coordination

Age	Eyes	Hands	Interrelationship
Natal	Random eye movements & passive regard of surroundings	Random & reflexive hand movements	No visual attention to hands
2 mos.	Attracted by movement in periphery (surroundings); monocular or bi-ocular fixation	Arms activate in response to stimulus; fingers open & close reflexively	Regards hand in ATNR position only with one active eye; Releases gaze to surroundings
3 mos.	Localizes noisy, illuminated, or moving targets	Swipes & contacts objects at side, not midline	Briefly regards own moving hand spontaneously; watches own hand reach and contact object
	Tracks targets with difficulty through 180°; converges & diverges on targets moving towards & away	Sustains grasp on objects placed in hand	Visually searches for object at point of disappearance but cannot combine reach & grasp
	Begins vertical tracking downward, losing target	Releases object involuntarily with awareness after sustained grasp	No retrieval of dropped or lost object
	Shifts gaze between two targets in same focal length		Alternates glances from hand to object
4 mos.	Binocular fixation	Reaches with both hands, contacts, & pulls object back against body or into mouth	Brings object to mouth without visual monitoring, then relocates after removing
	Prolonged, selective fixation on target in midline	Midline fingering	Maintains fixation on own hand or object in hand
	Visually pursues lost target outside visual field	Does not reach for lost object	Retrieval not possible when hand & object are not in same visual field
5 mos.	Fixates on tiny target (pellet)	No attempt to grasp pellet	Visually attends to pellet but doesn't approach
	Visually pursues lost target outside visual field;	Hands pursue lost object	Tries to retrieve lost object outside visual field
	Jerky vertical & diagonal tracking	Reaches with both hands to corral, grasp, & maintain grasp while shaking object, shoulder motion only	No visual attention to hand shaking (manipulating)
	Shifts gaze between targets in near and middle space		Shifts gaze (releases fixation) while grasping, manipulating, & mouthing target
6 mos.	Localizes large & small targets	Reaches & grasps with one hand & shakes object (manipulates it)	Alternately looks at, mouths, shakes object, retaining grasp
	Fixates on pellet & fixates intensely	Contacts & rakes pellet	Fixates on pellet while reaching, contacting, & raking
	Visually pursues lost target outside visual field unless distracted by another within visual field	Adjusts body position to reach objects outside visual field	Searches for lost object with eyes, hand, & body movements
	Shifts gaze in same focal length & within different focal lengths	Alternately grasps, mouths, looks, drops, grasps, transfers & shakes object, shoulder & elbow motion	Shifts gaze during adaptive interaction of eyes, mouth, & hands

Sources: Flavell (1963), McGraw (1969), and Erhardt (1992, 1994).

grooming skills require an exceptional degree of visual inspection and eye–hand coordination.

Play, another primary occupation of childhood, requires a variety of eye-hand coordination skills. It is characterized by fun, spontaneity, exploration, experimentation, imitation, and repetition of experience (Florey, 1981, as cited in Erhardt, 1992). A child shows intentionality, curiosity, and motivation when exploring the characteristics of new objects. Actions are repeated and practiced with experimentations and modifications that help the child become more efficient and competent. As skills are repeated and practiced with increasing environmental demands, mastery is achieved. Both intrinsic and extrinsic motivation are involved, as the child becomes aware of his or her own skill level, with self-evaluation and self-correction, relying less on others for help. The child continues to explore and experiment, interacting with the environment in different ways to see what happens, thus generalizing new skills (Reilly, 1974).

Schoolwork provides another occupational role: student or learner. Eye–hand coordination is essential for academic activities. Handwriting performance depends on many perceptual-motor skills, including visual perception, visuomotor integration, fine motor dexterity, and motor planning. These performance components are acquired during developmental processes in early childhood. Scribbling, coloring, and drawing give children visuomotor experiences that are prerequisites for complex writing tasks. In fact, scribbling has been described as a type of "motor" babbling, influenced by anatomical as well as perceptual factors. Although the straight line appears visually simplest, it requires complex muscular control by the multiple-jointed arm. The first scribbles are actually angular zigzag lines, which are related to the lever constructions of the arm joints. They are gradually smoothed to become circular strokes and eventually circles, which appear often in children's scribblings as well as in early cave drawings. Circles have always represented a primitive visual symbol: the eyes of animals and people (Arnheim, 1974; Cratty, 1986, as cited in Erhardt, 1992). The ability to produce letters and words depends on foundational drawing experiences with lines and shapes, evolving from normal perceptual-motor development.

An important underlying factor for these visual-perceptual-motor functions is postural control. Developmental, perceptual-motor, and motor control theoretical approaches are all based on the principle of postural stabilization and controlled stability and mobility of all various arm and hand joints to achieve precise grasp and manipulation. Children with inadequate postural control frequently perch on the edge of the seat and twist their body and legs into asymmetrical positions. Inclined desk surfaces or easels placed on flat desks facilitate optimal visual monitoring of reading and writing materials because the eyes and face are parallel with the surface (Penso, 1993).

Table 5.3, Correlation of the Stability and Mobility Mechanism and the Developmental Progression of Pencil Grasp, illustrates how young children learn to draw. First, trunk and shoulder provide internal stability for arm mobility, as the palmar-supinate grasp provides power rather than precision. Next, the elbow rests on the writing surface, which provides external stabilization for forearm mobility, as the digital-pronate grasp allows more freedom of movement. Next, the wrist stabilizes on the surface as the hand moves, with a more functional static tripod grasp. Finally, with a mature dynamic tripod grasp, the hand itself stabilizes, allowing precise finger movement dissociated from the metacarpophalangeal (MCP) joints (Erhardt, 1994).

Vision serves an important purpose in eye–hand coordination. As the child tries to sustain visual monitoring of the hands, movements slow down, and attention on the task is improved. Older children use visual feedback even more efficiently. For example, Schneck and Henderson (1990) reported that older children slowed down when coloring near the edge of a circle, while younger children tried to achieve accuracy by changing to a less mature but more stable grip.

Other school activities needing even higher levels of eye–hand coordination include computers, sports, and use of tools. Computer keyboards and monitors make some very specific demands on the visuomotor system, but computers offer many useful alternatives for children with specific learning styles or learning disabilities. Sports and games involving skills such as throwing, catching, and hitting balls challenge children to adapt to different sizes, weights, textures, speeds, direction, and so forth.

Table 5.3 Correlation of the Stability and Mobility Mechanism and the Development of Pencil Grasp

Dynamic Tripod Posture 4½–6 Years MCP joints stabilized during PIP movements	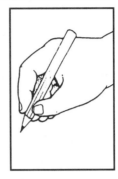
Static Tripod Posture 3½–4 Years Wrist joint stabilized while hand moves as a unit	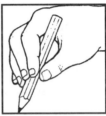
Digital-Pronate Grasp 2–3 Years Elbow stabilized while forearm moves as a unit	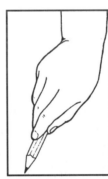
Palmar-Supinate Grasp 1–1½ Years Shoulder stabilized while arm moves as a unit	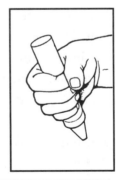

Source: Erhardt, 1994.

Both hand tools and power tools require a great deal of practice in order for the child to reach a safe level of competency in adult tasks.

An Observational Approach to Assessment and Intervention for Visual-Perceptual-Motor Function

The therapist who spends a significant amount of time observing and analyzing the performance of both typical and atypical children will experience an increase of clinical reasoning abilities and automatic improvement in therapeutic skills. The essence of the observational approach is an ongoing problem-solving process, which individualizes, adapts, and modifies activities to challenge the child's current skill level while still ensuring successful task achievement.

The Assessment and Intervention Process

Assessment begins with simple observations of the child performing selected gross motor, fine motor, and oculomotor skills. The first level of presentation is brief verbal instruction. If the child is unable to perform adequately, the next level, additional verbal instructions, is presented. The third level, if necessary, is examiner demonstration, and the fourth level is examiner assistance. The amount of assistance required is not only documented for evaluation purposes, but also serves as a guide for the intervention entry level. Some children will need a great deal of structure at first to function successfully, but the skillful therapist can gradually withdraw that structure and help the child assume as much responsibility as possible for his or her own actions and movements, as well as decisions about movements. The developing partnership relationship between therapist and child will foster that kind of responsibility and independence. The therapist guides the child in that direction by

• increasing the opportunities for complex processing of information from all sensory channels: visual (sight), auditory (sound), tactile (touch), proprioceptive (deep pressure), vestibular (movement), gustatory (taste), and olfactory (smell)

• offering experiences for exploration of body relationships in many different positions in space and time, discovery of own unique performance processes, and generalizations of tasks through variations of speed, direction, weight, size, shape, texture, temperature, and context

• integrating visual function with the gross motor and fine motor activities to achieve the highest possible levels of central nervous system integration and organization

• blending cognitively directed motor planning with automatic postural reactions to achieve accurate spatial orientation and efficient movement for complex tasks

• judging movement patterns in terms of efficient or inefficient, rather than right or wrong.

This type of occupational therapy program is designed to remediate performance component deficits and enable the child to generalize skills that can be applied to many different functional skills in performance areas of self-help, school work, and play. Increased self-esteem will lead to increased motivation to take risks by attempting new activities.

Guidelines for Intervention

Guidelines for intervention include the selection of functional tasks, preparation of therapeutic environments, and use of appropriate handling techniques, while providing opportunities for practice and generalization of new skills.

• Functional tasks must be meaningful and important to the child, so that true motor learning can take place.

• Therapeutic environments can be created that encourage the child to initiate and organize purposeful movements, first through exploration of materials, and then during structured tasks to ensure success.

• Handling techniques can include verbal as well as manual assistance and adapted equipment, if necessary, to provide positional stability and correct alignment, which allows muscles to work in normal synergies. The child's best sensory modes of learning can be matched with analysis of the task itself, so that the teaching process can be structured for easy success. Through practice new movements become subcortical, more automatic, and relatively effortless. Finally, in order for the child to generalize the new skill, it must be executed in many different ways through variable positioning, materials, environments, and methods.

Strategies to Facilitate Effective Coping Skills

The therapist who is alert to a child's particular style of coping can use several strategies to facilitate adaptations to stressful situations. These include enhancing developmental skills, changing task demands, and adapting the environment. For example, if a child has handwriting problems

• The treatment program can be geared to enhance developmental skills. Foundational activities such as chalkboard prewriting exercises use large muscle groups to avoid the learning of splinter skills. Lines and shapes can be taught in developmental sequences, using a process of decreasing structure beginning with templates, tracing, imitating, copying, and finally memory only. Templates provide both visual and tangible guides. Tracing requires the eyes to direct the hand to follow an existing visual representation. Imitating means that the eyes watch and remember another person's movements in order to repeat the same actions and production. Copying involves the eyes alternating glances between the visual representation and their own drawing in process. Production by memory only is the most difficult but can be achieved through the preceding steps.

• Task demands by therapists, teachers, and parents can be changed to match the child's current capabilities so fewer coping efforts are required. Lower goals can be temporarily set, as preparation activities are followed by handwriting practice of fewer, simpler productions.

• The environment can be adapted to achieve better postural alignment and fine motor control, if analysis has determined the need for a different chair and desk system, adapted writing utensils, and size or texture of paper.

To summarize, therapeutic goals for an observational approach to assessment and intervention are to

- teach the child to be an active effective problem solver by encouraging experimentation and analysis
- increase the child's independence by gradually reducing verbal and manual assistance
- expect the child to self-evaluate performance by tapering off external feedback and reinforcement
- help the child achieve functional competence by requiring practice in a variety of environments.

An Assessment and Intervention Model of Skill Development Based on Clinical Observations

The process of skill development follows a predictable sequence of exploration, repetition, competence, and generalization, based on the theoretical frameworks presented earlier. The motivation to *explore* is powerful in all animals, including humans. Visual and tactile senses are the primary avenues, but other senses are also used to explore. For example, young children often try to smell and taste any new object, and children at playgrounds can be observed experimenting with all sorts of kinesthetic and proprioceptive experiences. It is not usually necessary for parents to guide children's play from one developmental stage to the next; children pursue their own interests in ways that enhance skills in all areas. Children who have experienced repeated failures, however, will be hesitant to freely explore new materials and activities (Penso, 1993). *Repetition* and practice are important components of learning. An inner drive to repeat pleasurable actions can be observed in babies learning new skills, such as grasp and release into containers. Children who are not intrinsically motivated to initiate and practice new movements, however, do not move spontaneously through the stages of skill development to gain real *competence* in purposeful activities. They are not able to *generalize* skills, that is, adapt them for a variety of activities in a variety of situations.

Figure 5.3, The Process of Skill Development in Typical Children, presents several typical children, ages 2 to 7 years, using modeling clay, a rich opportunity for observations. For example, the 2-year-old, third from the left, is primarily interested in visual and tactile *exploration*, while enjoying the oral-motor input from her pacifier. The 5-year-old,

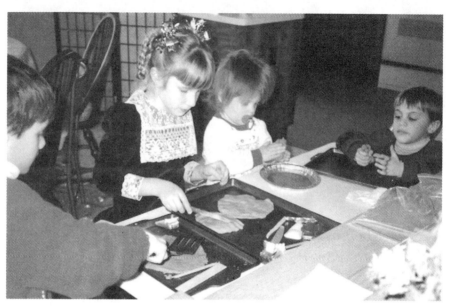

Figure 5.3 The process of skill development in typical children.

on the right, still benefits from *repetition* of this sensorimotor *exploration*. The other children, both 7 years old, are developing *competency* through *repetitive* handling of eating, cooking, and baking tools, and *generalizing* their skills to manipulate bread dough and pie crusts. Figure 5.4, Generalization of a New Skill, illustrates another way to generalize, by creating a symbolic representation (Who person from Dr. Seuss' book, *How the Grinch Stole Christmas*).

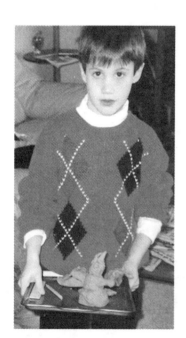

Figure 5.4 Generalization of a new skill

Clinical observations can be used to guide the process of skill development in children. As an ongoing assessment tool, observational techniques provide the information needed for adapting and modifying therapeutic activities as the child's needs change. In a way, this method incorporates the NDT approach of responding to the child's response in an ongoing sort of interactive dance (Boehme, 1988).

Figure 5.5, Clinical Observations of Skill Development, is a chart that can be used to record ongoing assessment and achievement as the child moves through the process of exploration, repetition, competence, and generalization. It documents how preparatory activities are being

Skills: sequences of organized actions, which apply strategies proceeding to future goals;
expertness in practiced activities showing dexterity and confidence in functional performances
Fundamental features : flexibility and problem-solving, transactions between persons, tasks, and environments
Key motivation for learning : self-initiated and self-directed activities

Child: _____   Skill: _____

MATERIALS/ACTIVITIES	OBSERVATIONS	DATE

Exploration: visual, tactile, auditory, proprioceptive, olfactory, gustatory

Repetition (practice): blocked, constant, distributed, massed, part, whole, random, variable (definitions below)

Competence: smooth, efficient, automatic, sub-cortical, not requiring constant visual attention

Generalization: accomplished in different environments and positions, using alternative methods, and for a variety of tasks

Blocked practice: movements always done in the same order (early learning)
Constant practice: activity practiced under same conditions each time (early learning)
Distributed practice: amount of rest time greater than amount of practice time
Massed practice: amount of rest time less than amount of practice time
Part practice: each subset of complex movement components practiced separately
Whole practice: entire task practiced to integrate timing
Random practice: movements done in different order each time (achieves generalization)
Variable practice: activity practiced under different conditions (achieves generalization)

Figure 5.5 Clinical observations of skill development.

used, the process of developing a particular skill, how components of stability and mobility interact, degree of motor control during hand use, other sensory systems recruited to supplement hand and vision, and the time lines for this progress. The model is informal, dynamic, and applicable to individuals of different ages and degrees of disability. It provides a guide for selection of strategies for adaptation, individualization, and modification of specific activities leading to new and improved skills or both.

Learning Disabilities: Definition, Etiology, and Incidence

The formal definition of learning disability, according to the U.S. Office of Education, is the standard currently applied to determine eligibility for services under the law:

> The term *specific learning disability* means a disorder in one or more of the basic psychological processes involved in understanding or in using language, spoken or written, which may manifest itself in an imperfect ability to listen, speak, read, write, spell, or to do mathematical calculations. The term includes such conditions as perceptual handicaps, brain injury, minimal brain dysfunction, dyslexia, and developmental aphasia. The term does not include children who have learning disabilities that are primarily the result of visual, hearing, or motor handicaps, or mental retardation, or emotional disturbance, or of environmental, cultural, or economic disadvantage. (National Advisory Committee on Handicapped Children, 1968; U.S. Office of Education, 1977, p. 65083)

The exact cause of learning disabilities is often unknown. Etiology is generally considered to be an interaction of environmental influences and genetic inheritance. Sometimes the family history reveals that one or both parents did poorly in school. Also contributing to the increased risk of learning disabilities is a history of minimal brain damage because of prematurity, prolonged labor, or inability to breathe spontaneously after delivery. Many children with learning disabilities exhibit low muscle tone from birth, which interferes with normal neuromuscular development. As they grow older, moving up against gravity and meeting the demands of increasing gross and fine motor tasks, tone may increase in certain parts of the body, such as the shoulders and arms, to gain stability. Hypo- or hyper-responsive sensory systems are also common in children with learning disabilities and sensory-integrative dysfunction because they lack the ability for self-regulation. These arousal states may vary from day to day or within each day, or persist at one extreme or the other, causing difficulties with behavior issues such as attention and self-control in the classroom (Oetter, Richter, & Frick, 1993). Programs have been developed to help children understand how their "engines" may run high or low at different times during the day or on different days, and what strategies can be used to modulate their systems (Williams & Shellenberger, 1992).

Traditionally, learning disability was diagnosed only in children of school age, usually second grade, because its definition implied a lag in learning skills of more than 2 years, but early identification is now the current goal (Batshaw & Perret, 1986). Infants and young children who have sensory, motor, emotional, and attentional problems are at risk for learning disabilities. They are now being served in early education programs that recognize the basis of these regulatory disorders (DeGangi, Berk, & Greenspan, 1988). In 1987, the U.S. Department of Education reported that 1.9 million, or 4.73% of all school-age children received special education services for learning disabilities defined by P.L. 94-142 (U.S. Department of Education, 1987).

However, learning disabilities are a heterogeneous group of disorders. Research into subtypes of learning disability has identified clusters of deficiencies including visual perceptual skills. Groffman and Solan (1994) reviewed seven such studies and concluded that visual perceptual deficits were present in more than 40% of the learning disabled subjects.

Case Study of a Child with Potential Learning Disabilities

The following 1-year case study of a child with potential learning disabilities demonstrates the observational approach to assessment and intervention for visual-perceptual-motor dysfunction affecting eye–hand coordination and skill development.

Kurt was referred for an occupational therapy evaluation at the age of 6½ years. His mother, a pediatric speech clinician, realized that problems he was having in kindergarten at his private school could be indicators of potential learning disabilities. She felt that early identification and intervention could prevent the need for formal educational testing, labeling, and special education services.

Teacher observations included

- inability to finish timed assignments with the rest of the class
- difficulty copying from far/near/far
- letter and word reversals
- confusion with left and right
- writing uphill or downhill
- frequent erasures
- irregular spacing of letters (see Figure 5.6, Kurt's Preschool and Kindergarten Handwriting Samples).

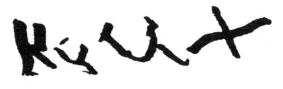

Preschool

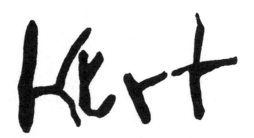

Kindergarten

Figure 5.6 Kurt's preschool and kindergarten handwriting samples.

Kurt's frequent complaints were

- blurred and double vision
- burning or itching eyes
- headaches and visual fatigue during close work.

Kurt's parents reported

- difficulty catching balls
- assistance needed for manipulating fasteners, such as buttons, snaps, and seat belts
- short attention span and distractibility
- occasional disruptive behavior and emotional outbursts
- difficulty getting to sleep and sleeping through the night.

Kurt's strengths included his social skills, memory, success through practice, and creative strategies for task accomplishment, such as inventing his own way to tie shoelaces.

Medical and Family History

Medical history included a normal pregnancy, labor, and delivery at 39 weeks gestation. Kurt weighed 6 pounds 7 ounces. Although he began talking early, he was a late walker at 16 months, with generally low muscle tone from birth. He appeared to be right-handed.

The family history included childhood optometric treatment (patching and orthoptic exercises) of Kurt's mother for amblyopia, caused by an esotropic strabismus and a significant discrepancy of acuity between her right and left eyes. Kurt's father, who had a history of reading difficulties, may have had an undiagnosed learning disability.

Occupational Therapy Evaluation of Visual-Perceptual-Motor Function

The purpose of Kurt's occupational therapy evaluation was to determine if his learning problems and delayed skill development were related to general visual-perceptual-motor dysfunction and to develop a home intervention program for remediation of missing foundational skills. Gross motor, fine motor, and oculomotor activities adapted from the Purdue Perceptual-Motor Survey were used for observational assessment. The Purdue is a standardized qualitative scale designed to detect specific errors in perceptual-motor development and to designate areas and individualized activities for remediation (Roach & Kephart, 1966).

Gross Motor Activities

Kurt's performances walking on a 2 × 4 board, through an obstacle course, and during various unilateral and bilateral jumping tasks indicated general problems with balance, postural flexibility, weight shifting, and sustaining rhythmic movements. Because he showed excellent ability to judge his body movements in relation to objects in space, the clumsiness observed can be attributed to motor control deficits rather than spatial errors. He compensated with strategies such as visually monitoring his movements and rushing through tasks. With verbal and manual assistance, his performance slowed down, showing potential for improvement with structured practice.

Strength, measured by tests of sustained prone extension against gravity, was below average, probably related to Kurt's basically low muscle tone.

Body image awareness, laterality and directionality concepts, and neuromuscular differentiation were observed during tasks such as identification of body parts, imitation of specific upper extremity movements, and directed "angels in the snow" arm and leg patterns. Kurt showed hesitancy and some confusion about single and paired parts. He exhibited abortive efforts (verifying identification with kinesthetic clues), a great deal of overflow (other parts moving), and sequential rather than simultaneous movements. Impulsivity was demonstrated by his difficulty waiting for the examiner's signal to begin each movement. An important strength, however, was his ability to recognize errors and correct them in one repetition.

Fine Motor Activities

Kurt had significant difficulties in most chalkboard drawings of lines and shapes (memory tasks), which revealed problems of directionality, laterality, and perceptual-motor matching. Arm movements were not always synchronized, and he exhibited left and right confusion and difficulty crossing midline. Again, with structure added to each repetition, his performance improved.

Paper-and-pencil drawings of shapes (copying tasks) were extremely difficult for Kurt. All forms were copied inaccurately and without discernible organization on the page (no concepts of left and right, top and bottom). These copying tasks relate significantly to reading readiness and academic achievement.

Oculomotor Activities

Kurt showed limited ability to establish and maintain visual contact with various targets (penlights, toys), essential for acquisition of reading skills. Horizontal tracking was accomplished fairly well; but as tasks became more challenging (vertical, diagonal, and convergence), his eye movements became more jerky and uneven, with eyes jumping and rolling. He lost the target frequently and had trouble regaining. However, performance improved after several repetitions. After only a few minutes of testing, signs of visual fatigue such as blinking, yawning, and muscle tensing in face and eyes indicated that a great deal of effort was being expended to perform well. Such effort required to function visually leaves little energy for cognitive processing and emotional self-regulation.

Summary of Results

- *Balance and posture:* Kurt showed consistent problems with balance and the delicate adjustments of muscle tone and small movements required to maintain balance.
- *Body image:* Kurt showed confusion about some body part placements and distinction between single and paired parts.

- *Laterality:* Kurt appeared to be right-handed, but he did not have a clear awareness of left and right within his own body.
- *Directionality:* Kurt's drawings showed the results of incomplete directionality development.

The developmental delays in Kurt's gross and fine motor skills were related to decreased physical strength and motor coordination. Because vision is part of the total body action system, his eye muscles performed similarly to the muscles throughout his body: inefficiently, inaccurately, and with limited endurance.

Consultation for Home and School Programming

Recommendations included a home program to be implemented by both parents, consultation with teachers at school, and referral to an ophthalmologist or optometrist who would consider corrective lenses to assist his visual function, especially in sustaining focus at near point. Intervention provided at the beginning of Kurt's academic learning process (kindergarten), was designed to help him develop needed skills, find useful strategies for certain deficiencies, and avoid inappropriate maladaptive compensations.

Home Program

Monthly consultations from February through May with the parents followed the January evaluation. During each session, specific treatment activities and methodology were demonstrated and videotaped for the parents, who received consultation notes, activity charts for sequencing and recording progress, and copies of the videos. They were asked to spend 30 to 60 minutes per day with Kurt exploring, structuring, and expanding at least one each of the designated gross motor, fine motor, and oculomotor activities, following the sequence designated on each chart, and applying stickers to the chart with each task completed before the next task was attempted.

Suggestions for encouraging exploration were to

- provide opportunities for information processing from all sensory channels: visual (sight), auditory (sound), tactile (touch), proprioceptive (deep pressure), vestibular (movement), gustatory (taste), and olfactory (smell)
- offer choices for experiencing body relationships in many different positions in space and time.

Suggestions for structuring activities included

- using visual, verbal, and manual assistance or a combination when needed, and withdrawing that assistance gradually as self-regulation improves, to ensure correct motor learning
- blending cognitively directed motor planning with automatic postural reactions to achieve accurate spatial orientation, efficient movement, and complex tasks
- emphasizing precise beginnings and endings of movement, including the ability to inhibit disorganized movement
- judging movement patterns in terms of efficient or inefficient, rather than right or wrong
- modifying and individualizing activities continually to ensure success for every task, but offering challenges to each next level of achievement.

Suggestions for expanding activities included

- using a variety of postures, such as prone, side lying, sitting, and standing
- adapting equipment and materials to Kurt's style of motor learning
- generalizing tasks through variations of speed, direction, weight, size, shape, texture, and context.

All activity charts given to the parents for Kurt's program were sequenced to ensure success through small increments in skill levels, with documentation of dates achieved. Gross motor activities included use of the balance beam, rocker board, scooter, and various balls. Figure 5.7, Ball Skills, shows an example of an activity chart that begins with hitting a ball suspended on a string (Marsden, 1953) and proceeds to bouncing, throwing, and catching balls with a variety of sizes, weights, and textures.

Name _____ Age _____ Date _____

The ball is suspended with string in a doorway at mid-chest level. Paper towel tube and yardstick can be marked with pieces of colored tape. Hands should hold the tube/stick at each end.

SUSPENDED ACTIVITIES   (dates completed)

1. Hit ball with towel tube (moving forward and backward) 10 times continuously.

2. Hit ball with yardstick 3 times in the middle of the stick.

3. Hit ball with yardstick 3 times on the left side of the stick.

4. Hit ball with yardstick 3 times on the right side of the stick.

5. Hit the ball 10 times, naming a different area each time.

CATCHING ACTIVITIES   (dates completed)

	beach ball	basketball	tennis ball
1. Bounce ball with two hands and catch 10 times. Count aloud.			
2. Bounce ball above head and catch 10 times.			
3. Throw ball up, let it bounce, and catch 10 times.			
4. Throw ball against wall, let it bounce, and catch 10 times.			
5. Throw ball against wall, catch, 10 times.			

Figure 5.7 Ball skills.

Fine motor activities included sensory discrimination (tactile, auditory, olfactory, visual), chalkboard drawings, clay, sorting, and block designs. Figure 5.8, Chalkboard Drawings, shows an example of an activity chart that teaches directional lines and shapes.

Oculomotor activities included flashlight tag, cops and robbers, and racetrack motility. Figure 5.9, Flashlight Games, shows an example of an activity chart that uses penlights and flashlights to improve visual tracking.

Name _____ Age _____ Date _____

MATERIALS: Chalk, chalkboard, eraser, templates

METHOD: Begin with the degree of manual and/or verbal assistance required to achieve perfect performance. Score when task can be done independently.

ACTIVITIES:

Shapes and lines	(dates completed)			
	template	trace	copy	memory
1. Circle				
2. Square				
3. Triangle				
4. Diamond				
5. Racetrack				
6. Railroad Track				
7. Ladder				
8. Hills: Down and Right				
9. Hills: Up and Left				
10. Hills: Down and Left				
11. Hills: Up and Right				

Figure 5.8 Chalkboard drawings.

This intervention program had been designed to involve the parents in (a) understanding Kurt's visual-perceptual-motor problems, (b) observing the results of intervention and effects on function, and (c) contributing new ideas to facilitate generalization of Kurt's new learning in the home environment. The formal home program was discontinued in June, when Kurt began receiving direct occupational therapy two times per week during the 3 summer months at a private agency for child development and family services. Reevaluation by the author was planned for the following December, midyear in first grade.

Name _____ Age _____ Date _____

MATERIALS: 2 penlights and 2 flashlights

METHOD: Teacher/therapist/parent moves penlight slowly in each direction starting at midline.

ACTIVITIES

Position	Direction	Dates Completed
1. Sit facing wall and follow penlight beam moving on wall with fingertip	horizontal right and left	
2. Sit facing wall and follow penlight beam moving on wall with fingertip	vertical up and down	
3. Sit facing wall and follow penlight beam moving on wall with fingertip	diagonal up right and down left up left and down right	
4. Sit facing wall and follow penlight beam moving on wall with penlight	horizontal right and left	
6. Sit facing wall and follow penlight beam moving on wall with penlight	vertical up and down	
7. Sit facing wall and follow penlight beam moving on wall with penlight	diagonal up right and down left up left and down right	
8. Sit and follow flashlight beam moving on opposite wall with flashlight	horizontal right and left	
9. Sit and follow flashlight beam moving on opposite wall with flashlight	vertical up and down	
10. Sit and follow flashlight beam moving on opposite wall with flashlight	diagonal up right and down left up left and down right	

Figure 5.9 Flashlight games.

Meanwhile, consultation at Kurt's school in April included observations of Kurt in his kindergarten class and of the first grade classroom that he enters the following year to learn its environmental features (furniture, routines, etc.) and the types of activities presented, and to share effective therapy strategies with his classroom teachers. With this information, recommendations for his summer occupational therapy program would then focus on improving the gross motor, fine motor, and oculomotor skills he needs for successful school experiences.

School Management

In the kindergarten class a mixture of the Sight Word and Phonics Approach was used to teach the alphabet. Instruction was given at an even, slow pace, with repetition that appeared to be motivating to Kurt and the other children because of its variability. Introduction of a new letter (upper case X) began with a cognitive, descriptive discussion of its components, visualization linked to known objects (sticks), references to its position in space, and comparisons with previously learned letters. The teacher slowly demonstrated how to draw the new letter, with linkage to the letter's sound, and verbally describing directionality concepts and the importance of using guide lines. All the children then went to their spots on the chalkboard, which was at the right height for their size. They each used an old sock for erasing with the nondominant arm, which not only gave them an opportunity to improve eye–hand coordination but also provided important tactile input needed for improving processing of all sensory information. Once at the board, Kurt took the time to watch the child next to him to verify the correct method of drawing the new letter (imitation). His production was then done slowly, carefully, and accurately. He repeated the letter across the board and down three rows with minimal errors in starting and stopping above or below the guide lines. However, intense cognitive effort was needed throughout the task, during which he made three errors, or rather, one error three times: starting in the wrong direction. Each time, he recognized the error immediately and corrected it. He did not spontaneously stabilize himself with his left hand on the chalkboard but responded immediately when reminded by his teacher. She expressed surprise that he was able to draw the X because in the past diagonal lines had given him trouble.

In the first grade classroom, environmental considerations included furniture, materials, and placement. Several varieties of desks were available in this classroom, with different heights, offering a selection for Kurt who would benefit from an appropriate ratio of seat to desk surface, allowing feet flat on the floor for stability, with hips, knees, and ankles at 90°. Some of the children were observed having difficulty opening their desk tops to get other materials without current materials sliding off. A variety of strategies were used, for example, grasping papers or books with the same hand that held the desk top, placing items on the floor temporarily, or using their laps. Kurt may need help exploring these problems through task analysis. If distractibility is a problem, Kurt may benefit from sitting in the front of the class to help him focus more easily.

During math, the children were required to be quiet and attend before instructions were given. Kurt would certainly benefit from a quiet classroom, because he was sometimes easily distracted and overloaded by sensory stimulation, especially sound. A hands-on activity (drawing and cutting shapes with scissors) was presented before the problem-solving workbook task.

Occupational therapy program reinforcement of the teacher's methods included

- attention to correct positioning
- cognitive description of tasks
- visualization
- references to spatial concepts
- comparisons to other tasks
- demonstration
- linking sound and hands-on concrete experiences (tactile input) to abstract concepts
- variable repetition (Kurt's special need)
- encouragement for problem solving and correction of own errors.

Optometric Examination

A standard optometric evaluation revealed clinical findings of

- visual acuity of 20/25 in the right eye, and 20/20 in the left eye, at both distance (6 meters) and near (40 centimeters)
- no refractive error
- reduced stereopsis and fusion or both at near.

Functional analysis of near-point fusion was indicative of a syndrome termed *convergence excess*. Kurt showed significant *esophoria* (a tendency for the eyes to turn inward) and suppression on positive fusional reserve testing, with very low negative fusion compensating reserves.

A complete visual perceptual evaluation was also done to evaluate Kurt's visual perceptual development. Test results indicated that he scored at or above age level in reversal frequency and visual closure.

However, Kurt scored *significantly* below age level in

- binocular function (BF), with a significant tendency for his eyes to cross
  - eye movements and fixation (OM, or ocular motility)
  - visual attention (VA)
  - visual sequential memory (VSM)
  - visual motor integration (VMI)
  - fine motor skills (FMS)
  - auditory-visual integration (AVI)

Kurt's deficiencies could account for some or all of his reported difficulties

- headaches associated with near work (BF)
- inability to do close work for extended periods of time (BF)
- inability to keep his place while reading (OM)
- inability to copy from the chalkboard (VSM)
- poor concentration (VSM)
- poor performance in handwriting, drawing, or cutting (VMI)
- inability to manipulate small objects (FMS)
- inability to sound out words (AVI).

Kurt's treatment plan was implemented in the following steps:

1. Bifocal lenses were prescribed for full-time wear in school and for all near work tasks, to address the convergence excess problem (overconverging for near).
2. Visual therapy was initiated in three main phases: (a) visual efficiency training (improving visual skills such as motility, vergence,

and accommodative facility); (b) visual processing training (techniques that will ultimately improve visual sequential memory); and (c) multisensory written language techniques (incorporated to allow transfer of improved visual skills into proficiency in written language).

Application of the Model of Skill Development

Kurt's progress during the 4-month home program was documented not only on specific *activity charts*, but also concurrently recorded on *skill development charts*, which guided him through the stages of exploration, repetition, competency, and generalization in a variety of skills requiring eye-hand coordination. Examples include Figure 5.10, Clinical Observations of Skill Development: Gross Motor Emphasis (ball skills); Figure 5.11, Clinical Observations of Skill Development: Fine Motor Emphasis (chalkboard drawings); and Figure 5.12, Clinical Observations of Skill Development: Oculomotor Emphasis (flashlight games).

Reevaluation of Visual-Perceptual-Motor Function and Effects on Eye–Hand Coordination and Functional Skills

Kurt was reevaluated in December, at the age of 7½ years, during first grade.

Gross Motor Activities

Kurt demonstrated significant improvement in balance and posture during walking board, obstacle course, and jumping tasks. He moved much more slowly, with greater control, used his arms and total body in more appropriate subtle balance reactions, and needed no manual assistance. He still had some problems shifting weight smoothly and sustaining complex rhythmic movements. Strength and muscular fitness were slightly improved but still reflected his basically low muscle tone.

Observation of body image awareness, laterality and directionality

---

Skills: sequences of organized actions, which apply strategies proceeding to future goals;
expertness in practiced activities showing dexterity and confidence in functional performances
Fundamental features : flexibility and problem-solving, transactions between persons, tasks, and environments
Key motivation for learning : self-initiated and self-directed activities

---

Child: Kurt _____   **Skill: Ball skills** _____

MATERIALS/ACTIVITIES	OBSERVATIONS	DATE
Exploration: visual, tactile, auditory, proprioceptive, olfactory, gustatory		
Balls of different sizes, textures, weights:	*Rolls, bounces, throws all the different balls, rapid*	*March*
tennis ball, basketball, beach ball, therapy ball.	*erratic movements, unaware of spatial boundaries.*	
Ball suspended from doorway, paper towel tube.	*Hits suspended ball with tube wildly, without control.*	
Repetition (practice): blocked, constant, distributed, massed, part, whole, random, variable (definitions below)		
Ball suspended from doorway, tube	*With repetition, begins to decrease force and*	*April*
with tape to mark left, right, center.	*aim tube at tape with better control and*	
	consistent visual monitoring.	
Competence: smooth, efficient, automatic, sub-cortical, not requiring constant visual attention		
Ball suspended from doorway, longer tube	*Using peripheral vision to watch ball,*	*May*
with tape to mark left, right, center.	*able to hit gently, controlling direction,*	
	10 repetitions.	
Generalization: accomplished in different environments and positions, using alternative methods, and for a variety of tasks		
Ball suspended from doorway, tube.	*Uses tube as a bat, swings at ball and hits well,*	*June*
	reports success playing softball at school.	

Figure 5.10 Clinical observations of skill development: Gross motor emphasis.

Skills: sequences of organized actions, which apply strategies proceeding to future goals; expertness in practiced activities showing dexterity and confidence in functional performances
Fundamental features: flexibility and problem-solving, transactions between persons, tasks, and environments
Key motivation for learning: self-initiated and self-directed activities

Child: Kurt   Skill: Chalkboard drawings

MATERIALS/ACTIVITIES	OBSERVATIONS	DATE
Exploration: visual, tactile, auditory, proprioceptive, olfactory, gustatory		
Standing at large chalkboard, using regular thin chalk, drawing vertical lines and using the template shapes series, at eye level.	*Chalk squeaks and breaks from heavy pressure, overshoots, copied drawings inaccurate, needs reminders to stabilize with other hand.*	*February*
Prone on hands and knees or sitting outside, using thick sidewalk chalk.	*Less breakage, larger spontaneous drawings,*	*March*
Repetition (practice): blocked, constant, distributed, massed, part, whole, random, variable (definitions below)		
Chalkboard, thin chalk, horizontal and vertical lines.	*No breakage, still squeaking, more precise starts and stops.*	*April*
Sidewalk, thick chalk, varied positions.	*Repeats movements, larger shapes, longer lines with for imaginary roads, makes circles for stop signs, squares for houses and garages.*	*May*
Competence: smooth, efficient, automatic, sub-cortical, not requiring constant visual attention		
Chalk, sidewalk, driveway.	*Shapes more accurate, stops lines neatly at intersections, more control.*	*June*
Generalization: accomplished in different environments and positions, using alternative methods, and for a variety of tasks		
Chalk, sidewalk, toy cars and trucks.	*Draws garages big enough and roads wide enough for vehicles to fit (size and shape awareness).*	*July*
Patio timbers, chalk, paint brush, water.	*Draws on wood, adapts to different texture (pressure), uses brush and water, adapts grip to different tool.*	*August*

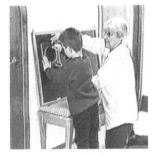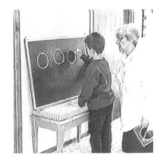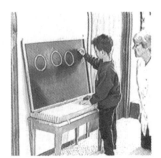

Figure 5.11 Clinical observations of skill development: Fine motor emphasis.

Skills: sequences of organized actions, which apply strategies proceeding to future goals; expertness in practiced activities showing dexterity and confidence in functional performances
Fundamental features: flexibility and problem-solving, transactions between persons, tasks, and environments
Key motivation for learning: self-initiated and self-directed activities

Child: Kurt — Skill: Flashlight games

MATERIALS/ACTIVITIES	OBSERVATIONS	DATE
Exploration: visual, tactile, auditory, proprioceptive, olfactory, gustatory		
Supine in bed at night, dark room, flashlights on ceiling, playing cops and robbers with parent.	*Moves flashlight quickly in wide sweeps, has trouble matching light to parent's light, needs verbal cues to focus on task.*	*February*
Sitting close to wall, following parent's penlight beam horizontally with fingertip.	*Avoids crossing midline by tilting trunk, more control when following light than when leading.*	*March*
Repetition (practice): blocked, constant, distributed, massed, part, whole, random, variable (definitions below)		
Sitting at wall, following parent's penlight beam with fingertip in developmental progression: horizontal, vertical, diagonal, also role reversal.	*With parent supporting trunk, less erratic movements, more accuracy, but excessive pressure moving upwards, (need to use smooth wood door rather than textured wall).*	*April*
Using penlight to follow parent's flashlight beam	*Needs slight touch at shoulders to prevent tilting.*	*May*
Competence: smooth, efficient, automatic, sub-cortical, not requiring constant visual attention		
Using penlight to follow parent's flashlight beam.	*Excellent ability to adjust speed and direction to parent's lead.*	*June*
Generalization: accomplished in different environments and positions, using alternative methods, and for a variety of tasks		
Sitting in bathtub, following parent's beam with finger, drawing shapes in shaving cream.	*Tactile feedback from shaving cream helps control speed and accuracy.*	*July*
Supine, drawing letters on ceiling with flashlight.		
Walking on campground trails, with flashlight at night to maneuver through unfamiliar areas.	*Good eye-hand coordination contributes to successful orientation and mobility.*	*August*

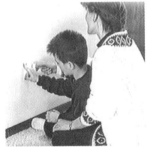 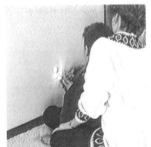 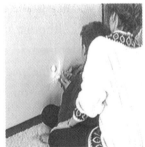

Figure 5.12 Clinical observations of skill development: Oculomotor emphasis.

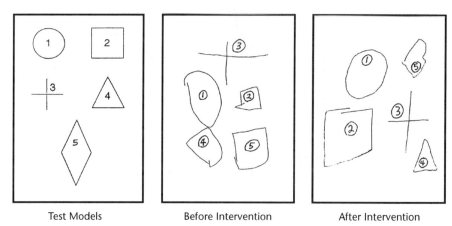

Test Models   Before Intervention   After Intervention

Figure 5.13 Test models and Kurt's drawings before and after intervention.

concepts, and neuromuscular differentiation were observed during tasks such as identification of body parts, imitation of upper extremity movements, and directed angels in the snow arm and leg patterns. Kurt demonstrated excellent effort and concentration but still showed slight confusion in single and paired parts, imprecise imitation of arm movements, and difficulty waiting for instructions. Certain complex tasks were still characterized by overflow (other parts moving), and sequential rather than simultaneous movements. Again, an important strength was his ability to recognize errors and correct them in one repetition.

Fine Motor Activities

Kurt showed impressive improvement in chalkboard drawings of lines and shapes, with much more ease, automatic movement, and accuracy. Paper-and-pencil drawings of shapes showed significant improvement. Although most of the forms were smaller than the correct size, they were copied accurately. The forms were organized in a circular arrangement on the page, which was acceptable, although less desirable than left to right, top to bottom (Figure 5.13, Test Models and Kurt's Drawings Before and After Intervention).

Oculomotor Activities

Kurt improved in all tracking eye movements. As tasks became more challenging, blinking increased and his eyes widened with effort. Convergence movements, however, showed no signs of stress or visual fatigue.

Summary of Results

- *Balance and posture:* Kurt showed significant improvements in balance and the delicate adjustments of muscle tone and small movements required to maintain balance. Intervention is still needed in learning to weight-shift smoothly and sustain rhythmical movements.
- *Body image:* Kurt judged his body movements well in relation to space but was still hesitant about some body part placements and the distinction between single and paired parts. His ability to differentiate one part from another showed improvement but required intense concentration (not yet effortless).
- *Laterality:* Kurt's hand preference (right) was well-established and his awareness of left and right within his own body showed improvement.
- *Directionality:* Kurt's drawings showed the results of more complete directionality development.

Kurt's increased gross and fine motor skills reflected improved integration of vision in his total body action system.

Functional Skills

Kurt's parents reported that he still needed to work very hard in the first-grade environment because of increased task requirements and whole days versus half-days, which sometimes contributed to increased visual fatigue, especially in the afternoons. However, he was able to maintain average grades in most subjects, below average in math, and above average in Spanish. His parents felt that improved attention span, emotional self-regulation, and sleeping habits have helped Kurt's function in school and at home.

They observed improvements in the following functional skills:

- successful experiences in the summer Little League baseball program
- complete independence in manipulating fasteners such as seat belts, buttons, and snaps

- new willingness to participate in fine motor activities such as Legos building blocks and coloring books
- improved handwriting.

Comparisons of handwriting are shown in Figure 5.14, Kurt's Productions of Letters and His Name *Before* Intervention (Kindergarten), and Figure 5.15, Kurt's Productions of Letters, Words, and His Name *After* Intervention (First Grade). The effects of reducing motor requirements for certain academic tasks are illustrated by Figure 5.16, Kurt's Solutions of Math Problems: Both Cognitive and Motor Skills Required, and Figure 5.17, Kurt's Solutions of Math Problems: Cognitive Skills Required Only.

Kurt's 4-month home occupational therapy program, followed by direct occupational therapy for 3 summer months, appears to have contributed to improvements in his visual-perceptual-motor function and increased skill development to prepare him for successful first-grade experiences. The application of prescriptive lenses addresses subtle functional optical deficits that not only cause visual fatigue but also interfere with integration of vision into total body function. Visual processing therapy remediates specific functional deficits that are interfering with visually related learning performance.

Summary

This chapter has discussed visual-perceptual-motor problems as they affect eye–hand coordination and skill development, which are viewed within the contexts of occupational performance in children, that is, self-help, play, and the role of student or learner. Clinical observations and subsequent careful analysis first determine how sensorimotor system disorganization impacts gross motor, fine motor, and oculomotor function within those roles and intervention guidelines. A model is then presented using those clinical observations to chart the process of skill development in children. The process of evaluation, consultation to home and school, referral to an eye–care specialist, and reevaluation is illustrated by a case study of a 6-year-old boy with potential learning disabilities.

Collaborative consultative relationships with eye–care specialists such

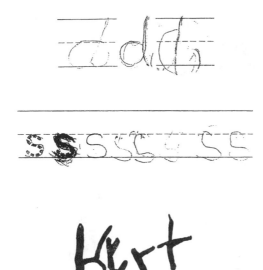

Figure 5.14 Kurt's productions of letters and his name before intervention (kindergarten).

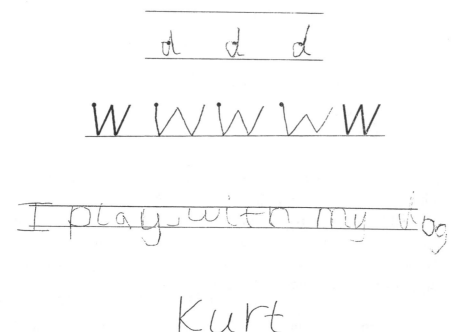

Figure 5.15 Kurt's productions of letters, words, and his name after intervention (first grade).

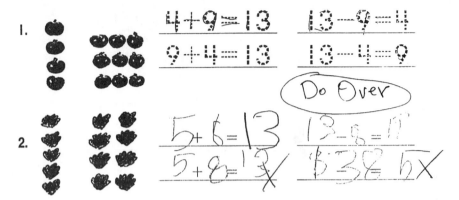

Figure 5.16 Kurt's solutions of math problems: Both cognitive and motor skills required.

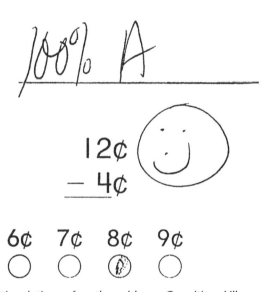

Figure 5.17 Kurt's solutions of math problems: Cognitive skills required only.

as optometrists are important in order to meet all the needs of individuals with visual-perceptual-motor problems that interfere with function in home, school, and community environments. To address these problems in effective ways, appropriate treatment depends on shared assessment data, as well as awareness of specific intervention strategies based on mutually agreed theoretical philosophies.

Activities are the occupational therapist's best therapeutic tools, used for assessment that leads directly to treatment. In other words, clinical observations of individuals during functional activities can be a primary method of determining which visual-perceptual-motor components need intervention, and just how to individualize that intervention to maximize potential for learning new skills. Informal models can be used to identify needs, plan treatment strategies, and document progress. Our role as professionals is to be facilitators of self-help, play, and learning—the occupations of childhood that lead to productive lives.

REFERENCES

Arnheim, R. (1974). *Art and visual perception.* Berkeley, CA: University of California Press.

Ayres, A. J. (1972). *Sensory integration and learning disorders.* Los Angeles: Western Psychological Services.

Barsch, R. H. (1968). *Achieving perceptual-motor efficiency* (Vol. 1). Seattle, WA: Special Child Publications.

Batshaw, M. L., & Perret, Y. M. (1986). *Children with handicaps* (2nd ed.). Baltimore: Paul H. Brookes.

Bly, L. (1992, May). What's happening with NDT theory. In *The Fifth Annual NDTA Conference.* Denver, CO.

Bobath, B. (1985, May). Changing trends in NDT. In *Symposium in Neuro-Developmental Treatment*, conducted at the meeting of the Neurodevelopmental Treatment Association (NDTA), Baltimore.

Bobath, B., & Bobath K. (1956). The diagnosis of cerebral palsy in infancy. *Archives of Diseases of Childhood, 31,* 408–414.

Bobath K., & Bobath, B. (1972). Cerebral palsy. In P. H. Pearson & C. E. Williams (Eds.), *Physical therapy services in the developmental disabilities* (pp. 31–185). Springfield, IL: Charles C. Thomas.

Boehme, R. (1988). *Improving upper body control.* San Antonio, TX: Therapy Skill Builders.

Bower, T. G. F. (1966). The visual world of infants. *Scientific American, 215,* 80–92.

Castner, B. M. (1932). The development of fine prehension in infancy, *Genetic Psychology Monographs, 12*(2), 105–191.

Cohen, H., & Reed, K. (1995). The historical development of neuroscience in physical rehabilitation. *American Journal of Occupational Therapy, 50,* 561–568.

Connolly, K., & Dalgleish, M. (1989). The emergence of tool-using skill in infancy. *Developmental Psychology, 25,* 894–912.

Corbetta, D., & Mounoud, P. (1990). Early development of grasping and manipulation. In C. Bard, M. Fleury, and L. Hay (Eds.), *Development of eye–hand coordination across the life span* (pp. 188–216), Columbia, SC: University of South Carolina Press.

Cratty, B. J. (1986). *Perceptual and motor development in infants and children.* Englewood Cliffs, NJ: Prentice-Hall.

DeGangi, G. A., Berk, R. A., & Greenspan, S. I. (1988). The clinical measurement of sensory functioning in infants: A preliminary study. *Physical and Occupational Therapy in Pediatrics, 8,* 10–23.

Duckman, R. H. (1987). Vision therapy for the child with cerebral palsy. *Journal of the American Optometric Association, 58,* 28–35.

Dunton, W. R. (1919). *Reconstruction therapy.* Philadelphia: Saunders.

Erhardt, R. P. (1971). The occupational therapist as a school consultant for perceptual-motor programming. *American Journal of Occupational Therapy, 25,* 411–414.

Erhardt, R. P. (1987). Sequential levels in the visual-motor development of a child with cerebral palsy. *American Journal of Occupational Therapy, 41,* 43–49.

Erhardt, R. P. (1990). *Developmental visual dysfunction: Models for assessment and management.* San Antonio, TX: Therapy Skill Builders.

Erhardt, R. P. (1992). Eye–hand coordination. In J. Case-Smith & C. Pehoski (Eds.), *Development of hand skills in the child* (pp. 13–33). Bethesda, MD: The American Occupational Therapy Association.

Erhardt, R. P. (1994). *Developmental hand dysfunction: Theory, assessment, and treatment* (2nd ed.). San Antonio, TX: Therapy Skill Builders.

Exner, C. E. (1990). The zone of proximal development in in-hand manipulation skills of nondysfunctional 3- and 4-year-old children. *American Journal of Occupational Therapy, 44,* 884–892.

Exner, C. E. (1992). In-hand manipulation skills. In J. Case-Smith & C. Pehoski (Eds.), *Development of hand skills in the child* (pp. 13–33). Bethesda, MD: The American Occupational Therapy Association.

Farrell, W., & Schultz-Krohn, W. (1990). A computer program for enhancing visual-motor skills. *American Journal of Occupational Therapy, 44,* 557–559.

Fisk, J. D. (1990). Sensory and motor integration in the control of reaching. In C. Bard, M. Fleury, and L. Hay (Eds.), *Development of eye–hand coordination across the life span* (pp. 75–98). Columbia, SC: University of South Carolina Press.

Flavell, J. (1963). *The developmental psychology of Jean Piaget.* Princeton, NJ: Van Nostrand.

Florey, L. L. (1981). Studies of play: Implications for growth, development, and for clinical practice. *American Journal of Occupational Therapy, 35,* 519–528.

Gesell, A., Ilg, F. L., & Bullis, G. E. (1949). *Vision its development in infant and child.* New York: Paul B. Hoeber.

Getman, G. N. (1962). *How to develop your child's intelligence.* Luverne, MN: Research Press.

Gibson, E. J. (1970). The development of perception as an adaptive process. *American Scientist, 58,* 98–107.

Groffman, S., & Solan, H. (1994). *Developmental and perceptual assessment of learning-disabled children: Theoretical concepts and diagnostic testing.* Santa Ana, CA: Optometric Extension Program Foundation.

Hatwell, Y. (1990). Spatial perception by eyes and hand: Comparison and intermodal integration. In C. Bard, M. Fleury, & L. Hay (Eds.), *Development of eye–hand coordination across the life span* (pp. 99–132), Columbia, SC: University of South Carolina Press.

Hung, S., Fisher, A. G., & Cermak, S. A. (1987). The performance of learning-disabled and normal young men on the test of visual-perceptual skills. *American Journal of Occupational Therapy, 41,* 790–797.

Kephart, N. C. (1960). *The slow learner in the classroom.* Columbus, OH: Charles E. Merrill.

Kielhofner, G. (1985). *A model of human occupation: Theory and application.* Baltimore: Williams and Wilkins.

Kielhofner, G. (1992). *Conceptual foundations of occupational therapy.* Philadelphia: F. A. Davis.

Knickerbocker, B. M. (1980). *A holistic approach to the treatment of learning disorders.* Thorofare, NJ: Slack.

Knobloch, H., Stevens, F., & Malone, A. (1980). *A manual of developmental diagnosis: The administration and interpretation of the revised Gesell & Amatruda's developmental and neurological examination.* New York: Harper & Row.

Laszlo, J. I., & Broderick, P. (1991). Drawing and handwriting difficulties: Reasons for and remediation of dysfunction. In J. Wann, A.M. Wing, & N. Sovik (Eds.), *Development of graphic skills* (pp. 259–285). London: Academic Press.

Light, K. (1991, May). Applied concepts of motor control and learning. In The Fourth Annual NDTA Conference, Atlanta, GA.

Marsden, C. D. (1953). The Marsden ball. In *Visual training at work, Optometric Extension Program Papers, XXV,* 8. Santa Ana, CA: Optometric Extension Program.

McGraw, M. B. (1969). *The neuromuscular maturation of the human infant.* New York: Hafner Publishing.

McNary, H. (1947). The scope of occupational therapy. In H. S. Willard & C. S. Spackman (Eds.), *Principles of occupational therapy* (pp. 10–22). Philadelphia: Lippincott.

National Advisory Committee on Handicapped Children. (1968). *First annual report, special education for handicapped children.* Washington, DC: U.S. Department of Health, Education and Welfare.

O'Brien, V., Cermak, S. A., & Murray, E. (1988). The relationship between visual-perceptual motor abilities and clumsiness in children with and without learning disabilities. *American Journal of Occupational Therapy, 42,* 359–363.

Oetter, P., Richter, E. W., & Frick, S. M. (1993). *M.O.R.E. integrating the mouth with sensory and postural functions.* Hugo, MN: PDP Press.

Paillard, J. (1990). Basic neurophysiological structures of eye–hand coordination. In C. Bard, M. Fleury, & L. Hay (Eds.), *Development of eye–hand coordination across the life span* (pp. 26–74). Columbia, SC: University of South Carolina Press.

Peiper, A. (1963). *Cerebral function in infancy and childhood.* New York: Consultants Bureau.

Penso, D. E. (1993). *Perceptuo-motor difficulties.* London: Chapman & Hall.

Piaget, J. (1952). *The origins of intelligence in children.* New York: International University Press.

Poole, J. L. (1991). Application of motor learning principles in occupational therapy. *American Journal of Occupational Therapy, 45,* 531–537.

Reilly, M. (1974). *Play as exploratory learning.* Beverly Hills, CA: Sage.

Roach, E. G., & Kephart, N. C. (1966). *The Purdue Perceptual-Motor Survey.* Columbus, OH: Charles E. Merrill.

Rosenbaum, D. A. (1991). *Human motor control.* New York: Academic Press.

Schneck, C. M., & Henderson, A. (1990). Descriptive analysis of the developmental progression of grip position for pencil and crayon control in nondysfunctional children. *American Journal of Occupational Therapy, 44*(10), 893–900.

Schrock, R. E. (1978). Research relating vision and learning. In R. M. Wold, (Ed.), *Vision: Its impact on learning* (pp. 29–50). Seattle, WA: Special Child Publications.

Suchoff, I. B., & Petito, G. T. (1986). The efficacy of visual therapy: Accommodative disorders and non-strabismic anomalies of binocular vision. *Journal of the American Optometric Association, 57*(2), 119–124.

U.S. Department of Education. (1987). *Ninth annual report to Congress of the implementation of the Education of the Handicapped Act.* Washington, DC: U.S. Government Printing Office.

VanSant, A. (1991). Motor control, motor learning, and motor development. In P. C. Montgomery & B. H. Connolly (Eds.), *Motor control and physical therapy: Theoretical framework and practical applications* (pp. 13–28). Hixson, TX: Chattanooga Group.

Williams, H. G. (1983). *Perceptual and motor development.* Englewood Cliffs, NJ: Prentice-Hall.

Williams, M. S., & Shellenberger, S. (1992). *An introduction to "How does your engine run?": The alert program for self-regulation.* Albuquerque, NM: Therapy Works.

Williamson, G. G. (1987). *Children with spina bifida.* Baltimore: Paul H. Brookes.

Wold, R. M. (1978). *Vision: Its impact on learning.* Seattle, WA: Special Child Publications.

Woodrum, S. C. (1992, December). Understanding attention deficit hyperactivity disorder using the model of human occupation. *Developmental Disabilities Special Interest Section Newsletter, 15*(4), 1–2.

SUGGESTED READINGS

Bly, L. (1994). *Motor skills acquisition in the first year.* San Antonio, TX: Therapy Skill Builders.

Bobath, B. (1971). Motor development, its effect on general development, and application to the treatment of cerebral palsy. *Physiotherapy, 57,* 526–532.

Coley, I. L. (1978). *Pediatric assessment of self-care activities.* St. Louis, MO: C. V. Mosby.

Erhardt, R. P., Beatty, P. A., & Hertsgaard, D. M. (1988). A developmental vision assessment for children with multiple handicaps. *Topics in Early Childhood Special Education, 7*(4), 84–101.

Goble, J. L. (1984). *Visual disorders in the handicapped child.* New York: Marcel Dekker.

Mathiowetz, V., & Haugen, J. B. (1994). Motor behavior research: Implications for therapeutic approaches to central nervous system dysfunction. *American Journal of Occupational Therapy, 48,* 733–745.

Paillard, J. (1979). Distinctive contribution of peripheral and central vision to visually guided reaching. In D. Ingle, M. A. Goodale, & R. J. W. Mansfield (Eds.), *Analysis of visual behavior* (pp. 367–385). Cambridge, MA: MIT Press.

Warren, M. (1990). Identification of visual scanning deficits in adults after cerebrovascular accident. *American Journal of Occupational Therapy, 44,* 391–399.

6 Visual Perception

Development, Assessment,

and Intervention

Carol Coté Loikith, MA, OTR

Introduction

The purpose of this chapter is to provide a framework for understanding visual perception, its development, and the nature of deficits—particularly as children are concerned. First, however, the term *visual perception* needs to be defined. In reviewing the literature, two general categories of definitions emerge. The most commonly found definitions consider perception to be "stimulus-driven" (see Table 6.1). The perceptual process begins with the visual stimulus and then proceeds through to higher level cognitive processes (Warren, 1993). Ayres (1974) used this approach in her definition: "Perception refers to the use made of sensations rather than the raw sensations in themselves ... perception is a function of afferent neural interaction for the purposes of interpretation and organizing sensory stimuli for insight and use" (p. 14); Bouska, Kauffman, and Marcus (1990) said perception involves " ... the dynamic process of receiving the environment through sensory impulses and translating those impulses into meaning based on a previously developed understanding of that environment" (p. 706).

The other general way of defining visual perception is as a "goal-driven" activity. This view is most likely found in the psychology literature and includes, for example, Piaget, who described visual perception as an activity—one must mentally act on a visual scene (Ginsburg & Opper, 1969). According to Piaget, perceiving information is dependent on the ability to know what to look at (Grobecker, 1992). Yantis (1992) found evidence supporting a goal-driven visual attention theory in which attention is directed to objects with attributes that are relevant to a current perceptual goal. In goal-driven theories, it is the perceiver's cognitive abilities and intentions that initiate and regulate perception. Here, vision is a tool, directed by cognition, for seeking and providing some needed information.

Cognitive psychologists would use the terms "bottom-up" and "top-down" (Yantis, 1992) to describe these different perspectives. It is possible that the two approaches are describing different phenomena with some perceptual activities being more strongly one type of processing or the other. For example, a stimulus-driven or bottom-up experience could be a sudden flash in the room that commands visual attention. The image would be processed and a memory match or recognition occurs—a fire. Other tasks may involve a greater degree of goal-driven or top-down processing. Such a task could be searching through the refrigerator for a jar of mayonnaise. The memory match is already in mind, the possibilities of location have been considered and a plan of action—including a motor plan for eye movements—has been made. The role of vision is now only to fill in the last bit of information, the exact location of the jar.

Table 6.1 Visual perception: Two conceptual approaches

Stimulus-driven Bottom-Up processing	*Goal-Driven* Top-Down processing
↑ Higher level cognitive functions Perceptual processing Selective attention Image processing Image transfer—receptor centers **Object in the visual field**	**Goals or task demands** Knowledge or expectations Strategies and procedures Attention allocation Commands to ocular motor control ↓ centers

Many visual perception tasks are done without actual vision, for example, using the "mind's eye" to plan the arrangement of furniture, or a child determining which crayons will be needed to make a certain picture. Visualization, or imagery, may seem to be a purely top-down process, involving only higher cognitive functions. However, there are arguments regarding the nature of this skill. Stimulus-driven accounts portray imagery as recreated visual scenes that are in essence the same as actual visual scenes, and processing proceeds from there (for discussion, see Kosslyn, 1990). In a top-down approach, imagery is seen as the application of what an individual knows about an object or scene rather than an actual "viewing" (for discussion, see Pylyshyn, 1986).

Visual perception is likely to involve both bottom-up and top-down processing. Aleksandr Luria (1966) emphasized the interplay between a visual stimulus and higher cognitive processes. He wrote: "The main obstacle in the way of a correct understanding of optic perception has been the receptor theory of sensation and perception" (p. 149). He defines the "receptor theory" as the excitation of the retina directed to the receptor centers of the cortex, where it acquires the character of sensations combined into perceptions, which in turn are analyzed and converted into the more complex units of perceptual activity (see Table 6.1 "Bottom-Up Processing"). Instead, Luria describes the *visual analyzer*, a dynamic interaction between the sensory receptors and the higher cognitive processes. On a neuronal level, every act of visual perception incorporates both afferent and efferent mechanisms. Afferent pathways originate at the eyes and send messages to the higher cortical centers. Efferent pathways originate in the higher cortical visual centers and communicate directly with the ocular motor control centers (Bronson, 1994; Luria, 1966). As the visual stimulus activates the higher cognitive processes, these cognitive areas in turn influence the direction of the eyes. If we consider the example of the sudden flash that initiated perceptual activity (afferent or stimulus-driven), immediate decisions are made about how to use the eyes in order to satisfy the need for more information—how big? how close? (efferent or goal-driven).

For this chapter, a definition of visual perception is used taking both aspects into account: *visual perception is the point at which an individual's knowledge meets environmental opportunities.* "Knowledge" comes first because, with the exception of occasional attention-grabbing events such as a flash, vision is directed to a scene with some intention. The term visual *opportunities* is used rather than *stimuli* because specific images become stimuli only after certain cognitive activities have occurred.

This definition forms the framework for the rest of the chapter, with particular emphasis on the nature and development of the knowledge, skills, and procedures that constitute the top-down aspect of visual perception. Evidence from research will be presented on the nature of that knowledge, how it is acquired, and how good (or mature) perceivers differ from poor (or immature) perceivers in terms of the knowledge the individual brings to a visual task. Other chapters in this book address the more purely visual aspects of perception. The ultimate aim of this chapter is to consider the practical implications for visual perception deficits or developmental delays in children.

The Dynamic Cognitive Activity of Visual Perception

Three very general and overlapping cognitive components of visual perception are described in this section: memory, attention, and encoding. Current theory and research in each general area are reviewed to provide an overall picture, then specific findings on visual perception and, where possible, evidence of how these areas change through childhood and differ from normal to perceptually impaired children.

Memory

Current theorists (Baddeley, 1986; Cowan, 1988) define memory as the total of an individual's knowledge base, with short-term memory the very small portion of the base that is currently active. This knowledge base can be thought of as consisting of two general types. Domain-specific knowledge is the store of specific memories of images, events, or facts, whether acquired recently or long ago. Procedural knowledge is a memory store for "how to" knowledge and includes strategies for accomplishing a task and knowing when to apply which strategies (Glover, Ronning, & Bruning, 1990). These strategies are highly individualized methods for organizing, understanding, and remembering information in order to accomplish a task.

Long-term memory has an unlimited capacity (Cowan, 1988). But how can a structure of limited size have an unlimited capacity? Current theoretical models depict knowledge as connections among simple processing units rather than as exact copies of the image or sensation. To learn new material is to make new connections or associations among previously learned elements. *Recall* is reconstructing the image from these elements. With the increase in number and strength of connections comes a greater opportunity for more connections—*the more you know, the more you can know.* Since there are no limits to the connections, there is no limit to memory capacity (see Figure 6.1).

Short-term memory (STM) is no longer considered a separate storage area. Rather, it is the part of the knowledge base that is currently active and being addressed. Cowan (1988) refers to STM as elements from the long-term store brought into a heightened state of awareness. Using the definition of perception as the point at which knowledge meets environmental opportunities, STM may be that point. In this model, STM is *not* a temporary store of images *from* the visual scene; it contains the active memories aroused *in response to* the visual scene. To illustrate this difference, consider how difficult it would be to remember a briefly presented image that is meaningless or unfamiliar compared to remembering one that is familiar. If STM is a storage area of environmental stimuli, then the familiar and unfamiliar would be similarly stored and equally available for use. Obviously that is not true. The familiar image

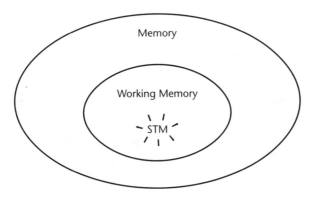

Figure 6.1

is immediately apprehended with little cognitive effort. The unfamiliar requires some time and effort to make "sense" of it, which means finding relevant traces from memory to be able to connect with the image. If sufficient memory is not found, the image is "nonsense." Attempting to hold a nonsensical image (or sound or other stimulus) in STM is a very difficult and frustrating task.

An accident scene provides a classic illustration of how STM is made up of associated stored knowledge. If three people witness the accident, three very different accounts of what happened would likely emerge; three different knowledge bases with three different sets of expectations, assumptions, and emotional reactions derived from three different life-time experiences would be activated in response to the current scene. In short, what we see has much to do with what we know, and who we are.

Letter reversals in the work of young children is another illustration of the role of memory in active perception. Kindergartners often show an increase in letter reversals as they learn to write. When they first draw letters, they are copying lines and curves. Once the letters become more familiar, they are produced from memory even though a model to copy may be present. At this young age, the direction of the letters may not be a relevant part of that memory, therefore, more errors are made. This is not regression—it is actually progress.

Perhaps the most fundamental and stable property of memory is the very limited capacity of STM (Chase & Ericsson, 1981). In a classic article, Miller (1956) put the limit of STM capacity at seven bits of information, plus or minus two. Although there is some debate as to what constitutes a "bit" of information, this theory largely holds today (Baddeley, 1994). There is no evidence that through any sort of training or practice this capacity can be enlarged (Shiffrin & Dumais, 1981), nor does it appear to change with age (Baddeley, 1986). How then can we account for obvious differences in STM ability between younger and older children? The likely answer to that question lies in the concept of *working memory*. Working memory consists of elements that have been brought into aware-ness but are not the current focus of STM. The material held in working memory is available for direct attention. To illustrate the concept of working memory, consider the example of someone making a telephone call. STM would first be totally consumed with remembering the telephone number (seven bits!). Once dialed, the caller can easily retrieve the knowledge about who and why the party is being called. If the call is to make plans for an event, the possibilities and constraints are available in working memory and activated in response to the newly learned information. Levine (1987) refers to this as "holding data in mind" (p. 104).

In his work on the limitations of STM, Miller (1956) also introduced the concept of *chunking*, whereby information can be categorized or held together by some meaningful association and stored in memory, with the category being one bit of information in STM, and the specific details held in working memory to be retrieved when needed. As a child develops, his or her knowledge base increases and consequently there are greater possibilities for categorizing, or chunking, related bits, thus allowing for more information to be available in working memory.

What exactly is a "bit" or "chunk" of visual information? Most research in this area investigates verbal knowledge. In some classic studies, a bit might be a single number, with seven numbers being about the limit for STM to retain. Numbers can be grouped in some meaningful or familiar pattern, for example an area code, and that group (or chunk) could now constitute one bit to be held in STM. However, it is also important to realize that the single digit could also be considered a chunk that can be broken down into smaller bits: the sounds within the word, the image of the figure, associated quantities, and personal meanings such as a house number or child's age. When a spoken number is heard, it is easily retained in STM because it carries the strength of all those associations and is further strengthened through repetition. A number spoken in an unfamiliar language would not be so easily retained because it does not elicit meaningful associations. Any effort to remember this foreign number would likely depend on phonetic associations, and STM would be able to hold about seven of these phonemes at once.

Unfortunately, relatively little has been done on the concept of chunking visual information (Baddeley, 1994). However, we can consider how the concepts from the verbal domain might apply to visual knowledge and visual memory. The image of a stop sign carries very strong long-term-memory traces for the shape, color, size of letters, scenes where

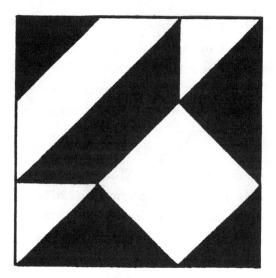

Figure 6.2

found, and motor reactions associated with it. A stop sign is easily recognized and held as a bit in STM. An unfamiliar figure, such as the one in Figure 6.2, would not likely be held as a single bit because as a whole it has no meaning (like the foreign number). Meaningless images may be held in STM through observable bits that may have some meaning to an individual: the line thickness, angles, colors, pattern regularity, and association with more familiar objects. A viewer who may have a good knowledge base for finding such meanings would have an easier time holding this image in STM than a viewer who does not. So, although the stop sign and the strange figure may be similar in size and complexity, the ability to recognize and hold each image would be quite different and would vary with individual knowledge bases.

This model of memory portrays a critical role of previously acquired knowledge in all aspects of memory, including immediate STM, and suggests that we see (perceive) with our memory as much as, or perhaps even more than, with our eyes. In the following discussions on attention and encoding, the importance of the knowledge that an individual brings to a task will be referred to repeatedly.

Visual Attention

The topic of attention is vast, with many theories and descriptions of levels and types. Here, attention will be addressed specifically as it is involved in the acquisition and use of visual information. Those aspects include limitations on attention, the development of automatic processes, types of attentional task demands (simultaneous or sequential), attention to the scene (scanning), attention to meaning (attentional shifts), and maintenance of attention (attention deficits).

Limitations on Attention Capacity

A discussion on attention is very much a continuation of the discussion on STM. The terms are often used interchangeably. Both depict the point at which the cognitive action is happening. Attention might be viewed as the outside of this point, facing the environment, and STM as the inside, coming from the knowledge base. However, they should not be considered as separate entities because, as James Gibson noted, it has not been possible to find out when perceiving stops and remembering begins (Riesner, Garing, & Young, 1994).

As with STM, attention is very limited. It is probably not possible to pay attention to more than one cognitive task at a time, or at least not very skillfully. More likely when a situation demands, one will shift attention rapidly between tasks. If attention is so limited, how are we able to do the many skilled, complex cognitive tasks we do? With learning and practice we develop *procedures* (Anderson, 1981, 1987). Procedures are long-term-memory productions created through practice and repetition that can be automatically executed without active attention. Procedures can be motor in nature—walking, postural control, and handwriting are familiar examples of highly practiced routines that can be executed without active attention, once learned. Ocular motor skills such as binocular vision or scanning patterns could be described as motor procedures. Cognitive associations can also become automatic—one can recognize familiar objects and make judgments about size or distance while active attention is given to an entirely different activity.

The strength of these procedures becomes apparent when we execute them by mistake. Changing from a standard transmission car to an automatic transmission car requires a period of relearning while the left foot automatically goes for the nonexistent clutch petal. Magicians make use of their audience's automatic visual processing to direct attention to the expected while performing the unexpected.

Proceduralization is essential to functioning with a limited attention capacity. Once a procedure develops, however, it is very difficult to change. People, particularly children, are problem solvers. They will find a way to achieve a goal using the skills available to them; this may not necessarily be the best or standard way (see Bly, 1991, and Mathiowetz & Haugen, 1994, for review of this concept in motor learning). Procedures may develop that are inefficient, ineffective, or even counterproductive to the task. A child with weak ocular motor skills may find early in life that a successful way to focus on close objects is to shut off visual information coming from one eye and view only with the other. Soon, whenever close objects are viewed, this procedure is automatically executed.

Procedures are involved in many aspects of a perceptual task. For example, a left-to-right processing procedure is used for certain scanning or matching tasks by adults and children old enough to be reading. This procedure, though likely developed in reading, is applied to other tasks (Elkind, 1975; Schwantes, 1979). On these same tasks, people in Israel show a right-to-left processing procedure, reflecting their reading practice (Elkind, 1975). Procedures may have developed for how much attention to allocate to a task. Even emotional reactions can become associated with certain stimuli and be automatically retrieved.

Each time a procedure is used its connections are strengthened, particularly if it results in a satisfactory outcome. The therapist who wishes to change a learned "habit" will need to bring the task back to a conscious attentional focus in order for the child to learn a new procedure. This new procedure must result in an equally satisfactory outcome or the child will never use it. This is not an easy undertaking!

Simultaneous and Sequential Information

Many theorists studying learning have divided the perceptible world into two general categories described by various names: simultaneous and successive (Das, Kirby, & Jarman, 1979), visual and verbal (Paivio, 1990), parallel and serial (from computer model cognitive theorists), and right-hemisphere and left-hemisphere (Ayres, 1974; Rourke, 1989) are examples. Levine's terminology—simultaneous and sequential—will be used in this chapter because of its descriptive quality (Levine, 1987). Sequential information has a time-ordered nature where the order in which pieces of information are processed is critical to understanding. This is usually language based. Simultaneous information, generally visual, is available all at once, and its appreciation requires analysis and understanding in a way that maintains the whole picture (relative positions, size, and organization). The Gestalt concept of the whole being more than the sum of its parts is testament to the difference between simultaneous and sequential processing. For example, it is not likely that a familiar face would be recognized if the information is presented in sequential bits—first an eyebrow, then the bridge of the nose, and so forth. In order to make adequate use of the information, the whole picture must be available at once.

While these are two distinct forms of information, each has aspects of both simultaneous and sequential processing. Perception requires a connection or integration of both. Language, in order to be understood, must be reconstructed in working memory to create an image where the later words can be related to earlier words. Visual, or simultaneous, information also has a sequential nature. Although a visual image is available all at once, the fovea of the eye is capable of focusing only on a very small area of any scene. We scan with our eyes over the image with a series of rapid fixations, with each fixation encoding a small bit of information. The visual scene does not provide the viewer with a scanning sequence or organization; the viewer must impose this structure.

Locher and Worms (1977, 1981) investigated children's scanning of visual stimuli and compared the performance of children with learning disabilities (LD) with nondisabled (ND) children. Observing the strategies used by these children provides some information about how they search, what critical features they attend to, and their method of sequentially encoding this information. In viewing items on the Bender-Gestalt test, ND children used scanning patterns that were characterized by efficiency in selection and organization (Figure 6.3). They systematically selected

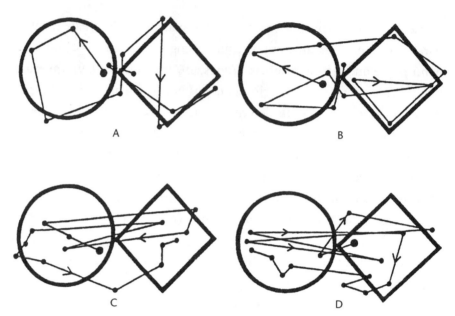

Figure 6.3 Eye movement scanning pattern of two ND children (A and B) and two LD children (C and D) viewing Bender design A.

parts of a design to be encoded and focused on parts that were high in information content. LD children used more fixations, encoded fewer salient features per design, and exhibited scanning strategies that were less well organized in terms of the structural organization of the stimulus. They frequently fixated on noninformative areas of the stimulus and areas previously examined. Average scanning time and duration of fixations are significantly longer for LD children.

So, there is evidence that the sequential organization of this simultaneously available information was less efficient in children with known learning disabilities. Are these poor scanning strategies a characteristic of the learning disability, which causes inefficient intake of information (top-down argument)? Or, do the ineffective scanning patterns provide faulty information which leads to or contributes to learning difficulties (bottom-up argument)? In keeping with our definition of perception, each visual task is likely to involve both aspects, creating a cycle that reinforces inefficient procedures and ineffective learning. Ultimately, however, scanning is a goal-driven activity. Bronson (1994) made an interesting observation of the scanning patterns of infants. He found that 6-week-old infants display stimulus-driven scanning patterns as evidenced by prolonged fixations on very salient features. A change in pattern is noted in infants of only 12 *weeks* of age. At that age fixations are briefer, scanning is more extensive, and patterns indicate some searching and expectation. Bronson argues for a very early change to goal-directed or top-down scanning. Noton and Stark (1971) discovered that there are different characteristics to scanning a familiar object than an unfamiliar object, indicating that knowledge and goals regarding the object are directing the scanning patterns. So, if scanning patterns are goal-driven processes, then the disorganized scanning strategies of the LD children would likely be a symptom of a more general cognitive disorganization.

Attention to the Meaning

In Figure 6.4, the arrow draws your attention to a dot. You will recognize this as familiar, having a certain size and color. As a skilled perceiver you immediately and automatically scanned the other three dots and now your attention to the target dot has shifted. You now see it as the top dot, a dot belonging to the group because it shares common size, shape, and color. You can also attend to the regularity of spacing, which may evoke memory traces of possible meanings—the tips of a diamond or perhaps compass points. Which of these possibilities reaches STM or attention would depend on the task demands, which at this point are not apparent. If you were asked, "What does this mean?" you would not know. However, if asked, "What time is it when both hands point to here?" the meaning of the dots changes and your attention shifts to those aspects that will satisfy this task demand. It is now obvious that the top dot is the "12" on a clock face. Your perception of these dots shifts in response to changing task demands.

Another type of attentional shift is part-to-whole perception. A central

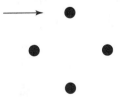

Figure 6.4

tenet of several theories of perceptual development is that young children's perception is holistic or unitary, while older children's and adults' perception is featural and analytic (Shepp & Barrett, 1991). However, according to Piaget, what a young child attends to is determined by the organizational characteristics, or *field effects*. These field effects capture and dominate a young child's perception. His or her attention is "centered." For example, a young child viewing a picture may be centered on the properties that define the whole scene if those characteristics catch his or her attention. Although young children are biased toward holistic properties, they can attend to the features of the stimuli if directed to either by instruction or by varying which aspect of the stimulus is most salient (Ruskin & Kaye, 1990). Toward the end of the preoperational period, when the child is about 7 years old, he or she develops perceptual regulations and can begin to act mentally on the visual material by attending to various aspects of a stimulus and integrating them into an "operative whole."

Elkind (1975), in a classic study of these Piagetian concepts, illustrated this change in ability to make attentional shifts. Children ages 3–12 were shown stimulus items that consisted of a familiar image made up of other familiar objects (see Figure 6.5). The younger children tended to see the parts (fruit), with some seeing the whole (man), but they were not able to see both aspects. In order for a child to see "a man made of fruit," he or she had to shift attention between two different meanings. This part-to-whole integration was found to be present in 75% of children by the age of 9 in this study. Younger children could be shown, or discovered the parts and wholes, but did not process both rapidly enough to see "a man made of fruit." The mature observer could be expected to gain almost equal access to both holistic and featural properties. A major developmental achievement might be the child's learning to attend to the property that optimizes performance (Shepp & Barrett, 1991).

Shifts of attention are involved in other visual perception tasks. Figure-ground tests require the subject to keep an image of a target figure in working memory, then to scan a scene containing the target, plus distracters. The successful performance of this task is sometimes described as maintaining focus of attention on the target figure. However, scanning and therefore attention does shift from target to distracters. So, success

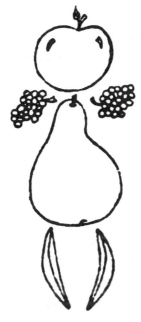

Figure 6.5

would depend on making attention decisions that best satisfy the goal of matching the target in working memory rather than in purity of attention. If the subject cannot make these shifts and becomes centered on a distracting feature, he or she will lose attention to the target and likely be unsuccessful.

Selective Attention

Using the concept of visual attention as having a front side of vision and a backside of knowledge, the importance of meaning in a visual task is apparent. Visual opportunity must be met by memory traces in order for attention to occur. This is critical to understanding children who may be having difficulties with visual perception. It is no easy task to sense what a child is seeing. As mature perceivers, adults automatically make associations, find relevant meanings, consider various possibilities, and attend to those aspects that satisfy a task demand. This is done without conscious effort and responses to a visual task seem obvious. A child given the same visual opportunity and task demands may not possess similar knowledge and skill. Although his or her gaze is directed appropriately, the backside of attention may not find relevant connections. Levine (1987) describes children with secondary attention deficits who have intact attentional focus, arousal, and selectivity in general, but are likely to become inattentive because their selective attention does not elicit useful information. If a stimulus is not meaningful or interesting, it becomes habituated; that is, it will no longer hold active attention (Cowan, 1988).

A normal, intelligent adult who is forced into a situation where he is expected to pay attention to a scene that is not meaningful—a football game or ballet, perhaps—will exhibit characteristics of secondary attention deficits. The person may become fidgety or distracted, may pay attention to the light fixtures rather than the action, or may simply fall asleep. The enthusiasts in the audience cannot understand this person's lack of interest. Similarly, a child who is confronted with a task or learning situation in which he or she does not possess adequate knowledge (both domain specific and procedural) likely will not be able to pay attention. The child may also develop an automatic procedure for tuning out in such situations. In this case it would be wrong to assume that the child's problem is inattentiveness. More likely the problem is inadequate knowledge. (There are many children with general attention deficits that do interfere with learning; however, this is not specifically addressed in this chapter.)

Piaget recognized the importance of sufficient knowledge in even a very young child's attention to the visual world. He observed curiosity of the physical world in infants, but their curiosity was selective. They showed preferences for moderately novel events or objects; not too new because this does not correspond to anything in their present knowledge base, and not too familiar because that is not affording any new information (Ginsburg & Opper, 1969). In infancy all the way through adulthood, attention to information requires enough knowledge to be able to relate to the new information in a meaningful way, as well as enough novelty to hold interest.

Encoding

In the preceding sections, the vital role of knowledge in perception has been emphasized. *Encoding* is the process of placing knowledge into memory (Glover, Ronning, & Bruning, 1990). This may well be thought of as the process of learning. Encoding is not only the acquisition of long-term-memory structures to be retrieved at a later time; it also includes more immediate memory, which can be used in the present situation. As new information is encoded, it becomes available to provide a meaningful reference for further attention and encoding processes.

Dual Coding: Visual-Verbal

Paivio (1990) proposed a dual-coding theory that describes two separate systems for verbal and nonverbal information that are independent and additive. When both are used, memory improves. Simultaneous and sequential aspects of tasks as described above can be purposefully connected to create stronger memory traces. Paivio cited numerous studies that demonstrated improved performance when subjects used dual coding. For example, in remembering a list of words, subjects who make a visual image of each word in their minds consistently remember significantly more words than subjects who do not make use of the visual code.

The effect of dual coding in remembering visual information has not been investigated as thoroughly as with verbal information. The following study, summarized here, provides some evidence and illustrates the concept of dual coding in children's processing of visual information.

Developmental changes in children's encoding strategies were investigated by Hitch, Woodin, and Baker (1989). Five- and 11-year-old children were presented with sets of pictures that had to be remembered in serial order. The 5-year-olds made the greatest number of errors on the set of pictures that were visually similar, whereas 11-year-olds had greater difficulty remembering the sequential order of the pictures that were phonemically similar (i.e., rat, bat, hat). This provides evidence of a difference in method of encoding between the younger and older children. The younger children retained the items in some form of visual store and apparently made no use of phonological storage. They made more mistakes on visually similar pictures because the similarity of the images would lead to confusion on the correct sequence. The older children, it appears, used a dual-coding memory strategy: image with name. The phonological storage dominated, leading to errors of confusion with phonemically similar pictures. As would be expected, the older children made fewer mistakes in total. A third subject group was used in this study, comprising of 11-year-olds who were under an articulatory suppression condition (i.e., repeating "the, the, . . ." throughout the trials). They were thus prevented from making use of phonological coding, and in remembering, performed very much like the 5-year-olds. They made more errors in the *visually* similar picture sets and the absolute number of errors was similar to that of the 5-year-olds. So, without the use of the second code, their memory performance looked very much like that of a younger child. This lends support to the idea that STM capacity does not change with development; rather, children gain access to more sophisticated processing strategies (Baddeley, 1986).

Dual Coding: Visual-Kinesthetic

The literature on the topic of dual coding generally focuses on the visual-verbal connection (more likely, the verbal-visual connection). However, there are other methods of making a cross-reference to encode new information. Visual-kinesthetic connections may also be quite powerful and are perhaps more important than verbal codes in learning and internalizing the properties and relationships of the observable world.

Early learning, in Piaget's terms, is sensorimotor. Knowledge is acquired by making connections between movement or touch and vision. Only later do children elaborate on this information with language. The young child, according to Piaget, looks at things, handles them, and acts like them, thereby incorporating a great deal of information about them (Ginsburg & Opper, 1969). Perceptual development of the young child involves acquiring domain-specific knowledge of objects, their topology, actions, proximity, order, separation, and continuity. This is accomplished through actions—to act on an object is to understand it (Grobecker, 1992). The visual-kinesthetic connection is arguably the method of first learning from which other learning arises. Piaget further proposed that development of imagery results from action. First, the child overtly imitates the actions of things or people. Later this imitation becomes internalized. It is through this internal activity that images arise, and these images are not separate from the activity the child experienced (Ginsburg & Opper, 1969). Piaget saw a greater role of action than vision in the development of imagery and considered it an intellectual ability rather than a product of perceptual familiarity. In a visual perception task, imagery is involved in anticipating, transforming, and comprehending movement or changes as continuity of the same scene. As we are directly viewing a scene, imagery is actively involved in perception as we act upon the scene in response to a particular goal. Imagery also allows us to think, plan, and problem solve about visual information in the absence of the actual stimulus.

An experiment by Rieser, Garing, and Young (1994) illustrates the visual-kinesthetic connection in an imagery task. They found that in even quite young children, dynamic (transformational) imagery (to create a remembered image and mentally move, or transform, the scene) was possible if accompanied by related movements, but not possible if children remained static. Each child was asked to picture his or her classroom (or other familiar, but not present room) and describe what he or she could see from his or her seat. All children were able to do this quite easily. Next they were asked to describe what they could see from the teacher's desk. Five-year-olds were correct on only 2% of trials, 9-year-olds on 27%, and adults were 100% correct. However, when the same subjects actually moved—that is, stood up and walked to the place that would correspond to the new viewing point—accuracy was virtually 100% for all ages, and for adults responses were more rapid. The authors concluded that children's action, imagination, and perception are tightly linked.

Visual-kinesthetic coding can also be a powerful tool for learning procedures on visual tasks as illustrated in the following study. Locher (1985) found a relationship between visual scanning patterns and haptic scanning (sequence of movements used to explore an object using hands and no vision) in children. These children were identified as having attention deficits, and their impulsivity was reflected not only in their behavior, but also in their visual and haptic scanning strategies. Locher devised a 15-week training program targeting haptic scanning strategies. With vision occluded, the children were taught, using hand-over-hand techniques, verbal cuing, and demonstrations, to use more systematic "fixations" and to attend to the most salient features of the form in their hands. Their goal was to visually locate the match to the shape in their hands. Following the training program there was measurable and significant improvement in scanning with hands *and* similar improvement in visual scanning patterns even though visual scanning was never directly addressed. Here, the children appear to have learned new procedures, or strategies, for encoding information and were able to apply these strategies to another sensory domain. Locher attributed success to the sequential nature of haptic scanning, which provides an opportunity to teach sequential strategies, and to the fact that this less practiced modality is easier to modify. The subjects also made fewer errors in posttest trial task items indicating that there was an improvement in information-gathering skill as well.

Context Specificity

All knowledge is acquired in a context (Glover, Ronning, & Bruning, 1990). Context can include external variables: physical surroundings, instructions or cues, incidental irrelevant stimuli, distractions, and so forth. Anything that is perceived at the time of encoding will become part of the memory trace. Context also includes internal variables: strategies or procedures used, evoked memories or associations, emotional state, and attention processes. All of the issues discussed in memory and attention are involved now in creating a context for learning.

At the time a particular memory trace is to be retrieved, recreating the context in which it was originally encoded can be facilitative. For example, a child trying to remember which letter comes next in the alphabet may sing the "ABC" jingle to find the letter in that context. Most people can relate to the problem of trying to retrieve the name of a person seen "out of context," or needing to pantomime the pushing of buttons on a telephone in order to say a familiar telephone number. Many behaviors and skills can be tied to context. The more skilled the learner is in a particular domain, the less dependent he or she is on context. Knowledge can then be attained, retrieved, and applied in a variety of contexts. Less skilled or younger learners may be more dependent on context. This has far-reaching implications for teaching new skills. If a skill is learned in a quiet therapy room, with one-on-one instruction, certain cues, and special materials, it would not be very surprising if that skill is not applied when working independently in a busy classroom.

Cognitive Activity Summary

This section provides a definition and framework for understanding visual perception based on current learning theories and research. A definition of visual perception is proposed: the point at which an individual's knowledge meets environmental opportunities. The knowledge one brings to a perceptual task includes not only specific related information but also strategies and automatic procedures. The point of perception is a very limited, active cognitive effort that includes, at once, attention to the visual array and evoked memories related to the stimulus. Perceiving visual information involves many cognitive activities: systemic scanning procedures, associations of stimuli with memories, decisions about which aspects satisfy a task demand, and encoding of new information into memory within the context it was perceived. The connection between visual information and the movement or action is very important, particularly in early learning of visual perception.

As a child develops, he or she has access to more sophisticated strategies for learning and understanding visual information. The child has a greater knowledge base from which to find meaning in a visual experience. He or she also becomes increasingly able to consider more than one aspect of a scene—the process of decentering. With decentering, the child can see relationships such as part to whole.

Developmental Assessment of Visual Perception

Overview

Efficient and effective perception of visual information is an important aspect of school performance for students at any age. Younger children who are learning to recognize and differentiate letter and number forms rely heavily on their visual processing skills. Math and science concepts involve the ability to perceive relationships between objects. Art instruction and in-class construction projects are particularly demanding of these abilities (Levine, 1994). In addition, as students grow older, visual imagery is important to reading comprehension (Bell, 1991) and in planning, problem-solving, and organizational skills (Levine, 1994). Occupational therapists, school psychologists, and learning consultants are often asked to assess the visual perception ability of children who are having difficulty learning or managing school requirements.

The preceding section of this chapter views visual perception as a dynamic cognitive effort that at once involves memory, strategic knowledge, short-term memory, and attention to satisfy a visual task demand or goal. The goal of assessment is to discover what knowledge a child brings to a visual task. This leads to the treatment goal of adding to or changing this knowledge base. There are two general types of knowledge: domain-specific and procedural.

Domain-specific knowledge includes the store of specific facts related to a task, such as knowledge of specific features that allow recognition of relative size, positions, familiar shapes, patterns, colors, or any bits of information that are related to the current visual scene. Knowledge of task demands, goals, consequences, and what constitutes success are also part of the domain-specific knowledge base.

Procedural knowledge is "how-to" knowledge that can be cognitively directed procedures or automatic procedures not consciously executed, including "bad habits." Strategic knowledge is part of procedural knowledge, including organization of visual intake, methods of information gathering, methods of encoding new information and monitoring progress. Knowledge of how to direct attention for successful completion of a task, regulation of competing demands, and maintenance of vigilance can also be considered part of this knowledge base. (In other literature some of these processes are called "executive functions.")

The factors that may be underlying or contributing to the child's current performance status also need to be considered, although these will not be reviewed in detail here. These may include

- *visual dysfunction:* visual or oculomotor skills that do not serve as efficient tools for learning
- *general attention deficits:* impulsivity or poor regulation of attention that may not be conducive to learning
- *neurological deficits:* decreased intellectual abilities in general
- *sensory integration deficits:* decreased ability to encode information through interaction with environment
- *conflicting or competing demands:* emotional problems, fear of failure, lack of security or support, deprivation, and so forth.

Caution must be used, however, in ascribing a cause-effect relationship between an "underlying" problem and a skill deficit. It may be that the relationship is actually reversed. For example, we might assume that attention deficits have a causal relationship with visual perception skill acquisition when it may be that a lack of skill or knowledge results in a situation that is not affording enough meaningful information to hold attention. Sensory integration problems seem to be related to, but are not necessarily the cause of, visual perception problems (Murray, 1991). Also, both the underlying factors and skill deficits may be the result of a more general processing deficit. In planning intervention, it is very important to keep this in mind and to be certain that the visual perception skills are being directly addressed.

Testing is a highly structured situation from which a score is derived. Assessment is a multifaceted approach to gaining an understanding of a child's skills and of how those skills might be improved. Testing can be part of assessment, but scores alone can never offer understanding of problems or implications for treatment. It is fairly easy to determine that there is a discrepancy between a child's achievement on visual perception tasks and what is expected for that child's age. Standardized tests provide measurable tasks from which to make these comparisons. The more difficult part of assessment is determining why this discrepancy exists and what it means to a child's daily functioning. Standardized tests usually do not provide this information in their theoretical constructs or in the categorization of subtest scores. To understand the nature of a child's difficulty, the specific test requirements must be understood in terms of the general development of cognitive skill, which is the basis of perception. Piaget's theory of development provides such a theoretical framework and is consistent with the definition and supporting research put forth earlier in the section on cognitive activity.

This section begins with a brief description of the characteristics of developmental stages and is followed by a discussion of the various types of standardized tests of visual perception. It also contains ideas for obtaining even more information through "testing the limits" and using everyday activities for observation of skills. A case study on Joey will begin with a summary of his assessment.

Development of Cognitive and Perceptual Processes Based on Piaget's Theory

The following developmental stages are based on Piaget's theory of cognitive development. Included here are brief summaries of the cognitive abilities that are available at each stage, the visual perception abilities that can be expected, and appropriate testing activities. The reader can obtain more detailed discussion of these stages from any of the numerous books on Piaget's theory that are widely available. The ages listed are general and vary from child to child. Even with an individual child, developmental stages may vary from task to task. However, Piaget believed very strongly that the sequence is universal.

Ages 0–2 years (sensorimotor). First, the very young child develops a knowledge base of the properties of objects and their uses by making connections among touch, movement, and vision. Perception is tied to the child's immediate scope of vision. Perceptual characteristics include curiosity, exploration, and imitation. Assessment at this stage would best be accomplished by careful observation of the child's interaction with objects, perhaps guided by standardized developmental checklists (not covered in this chapter).

Ages 2–4 years (preoperational). Piaget proposed that as a result of both neuromaturation and the numerous and varied experiences, imitation of objects becomes internalized and now the child can use one object (including words) to represent another. Now the capacity for symbolic thought develops, making it possible for the child to operate on new levels. He or she is no longer restricted to the immediate environment because symbolic functions allow him or her to evoke the past. The child can imitate internally both actions and visual images. Perceptually, the child is centered on only one aspect of any task or scene.

Standardized tests of visual perception for this age group generally use manipulatives for recreating exact copies of simple structures or imitations of the examiner's actions. These tests can be unreliable, however, since it is difficult to know if the child truly understands the task demands. Being centered limits a child's ability to switch procedures in response to changing task demands. Here, too, observations of interactions with objects, level of curiosity, and evidence of symbolism (e.g., using a block for a car), are important adjuncts to standardized testing.

Ages 5–7 years (preoperational, continued). After considerable practice with symbolism and internal imitation, as well as continued neuromaturation, the child becomes more efficient in these processes and is now able to hold more information at once. The ability to see relationships between objects or events develops as long as these are closely related in terms of time or proximity. Reversal errors decrease toward the end of this stage because letter forms can be perceived in relation to each other. A child can see more than one aspect of a situation, but is still limited in ability to coordinate these separate perceptions or relate them to more distant objects or events. He or she is less centered, but not fully able to integrate parts and wholes. Static imagery, an internal reproduction of an object or scene that is unchanged from the original, develops. To the child, things are exactly as they appear.

Assessment tasks generally tap the child's ability to decenter from singular aspects by requiring reproductions of increasingly complex figures, which must be analyzed according to the relationship of the parts. However, this ability is limited to the relationship of one part to another and not to a larger, overall structure. The ability to hold an image in memory and use that image is also commonly assessed. It would not be expected that the child could visualize outcomes or changes.

Ages 7–11 (concrete operational). Gradually, the child develops the ability to think simultaneously in terms of the whole and its parts. He or she becomes decentered. Toward the end of this stage, imagery can now be anticipatory (picture outcomes, plan ahead) and transformational (image changes rather than static states). With these abilities the child is able to reverse processes, that is, reconstruct transformations to get back to the original point. Spatial problem solving (e.g., what size box is needed for some objects) and planning are possible due to anticipatory imagery. Imagery is still concrete, however, involving objects and situations actually seen or experienced.

Assessment tasks include even more complex designs to be reproduced, matched, or remembered. Figures that must be analyzed, deconstructed into parts, and reconstructed, maintaining overall configuration, are now possible. However, although this stage is characterized by the development of dynamic processing abilities, most standardized tests provide only static tasks (e.g., requiring exact copies of a stimulus).

Standardized Testing

Standardized tests (see Table 6.2) are highly structured assessments in which the variables that could influence performance are constrained as much as possible. Physical settings, materials, and instructions are held constant so that a child's performance can be compared with those of other children. In general, these tests are either "motor" or "nonmotor," depending on the nature of the responses required. The tests covered here are described by their authors as visual or visual-perceptual assessments. Many general tests of intelligence or achievement used by psychologists or learning consultants also have a visual perception component, often described as nonverbal intelligence. In keeping with the research presented in the section on cognitive activity as well as Piagetian principles, it is not possible to separate perception from intelligence. Therapists may find the test results from psychological testing helpful in understanding visual perception skills and should be aware that psychologists or learning specialists may use some of the same tests that are available to therapists. It is important to coordinate efforts so a practice effect will not result.

Table 6.2 Standardized tests of visual perception

Test	Age	Subtests	Type of Output
Developmental Test of Visual-Motor Integrations (VMI or "Beery")	4–17	N/A	Motor, direct copy
Test of Visual Motor Skills (TVMS)	2–13	N/A	Motor, direct copy
Pediatric Extended Examination at Three (PEET)	3–4	Copy Figures Stick Construction Block Construction Figure Matching Draw a Person Object Recall	Motor, direct copy Motor, construction Motor, construction Nonmotor, direct match Motor, from imagery Nonmotor, memory
Pediatric Examination of Educational Readiness (PEER)	4–6	Visual Matching Manipulate Sticks Copy Figures Draw from Memory Block Construction	Nonmotor, direct match Motor, construction Motor, direct copy Motor, memory Motor, construction
Pediatric Early Elementary Examination (PEEX2)	6–9	Pencil Control Draw from Memory Pattern Learning Visual Vigilance Vis Whole:Part Form Copying	Motor Motor, memory Nonmotor, memory Nonmotor, match Nonmotor, match Motor, direct copy
Pediatric Examination of Educational Readiness at Middle Childhood (PEERAMID2)	9–15	Visual Vigilance Visual Recognition Visual Retrieval Form Copying Graph Paper Copying	Nonmotor, match Nonmotor, memory Motor, memory Motor, direct copy Motor, direct copy
Rey-Osterreith Complex Figure Test	8+	Copy production Memory Production	Motor, direct copy Motor, memory
Miller Assessment for Preschoolers (MAP)	2.9–5.8	Figure Ground Puzzle Eye–Hand Coordination Block Design Object Memory Draw a Person	Nonmotor, match Nonmotor, construction Motor Motor, construction Nonmotor, memory Motor, from imagery
Sensory Integration & Praxis Tests (SIPT)	4–8.11	Space Visualization Figure-Ground Percept Design Copying Construction Praxis	Nonmotor, match Nonmotor, match Motor, direct copy Motor, construction
Test of Visual-Perceptual Skills (TVPS)	4–12	Visual Discrimination Visual Memory Spatial Relationships Form Constancy Sequential Memory Figure-Ground Visual Closure	Nonmotor, match Nonmotor, memory Nonmotor, match Nonmotor, match Nonmotor, memory Nonmotor, match Nonmotor, match
Developmental Test of Visual Perception (DTVP-2)	4–10	Eye–Hand Coordination Position in Space Copying Figure-Ground Spatial Relations Visual Closure Visual Motor Speed Form Constancy	Motor Nonmotor, match Motor, direct copy Nonmotor, match Motor, grid copy Nonmotor, match Motor, speed Nonmotor, match
Detroit Tests of Learning Aptitude (DTLA)	6–17	Design Reproduction Design Sequences Picture Fragments	Motor, memory Nonmotor, memory Nonmotor, identification

Visual-Motor Tests

Paper-and-Pencil Tasks

Certain visual perception tests include a motor output response to a visual stimulus. Most often the task is to copy a form exactly with a pencil.

These tests may provide useful information, particularly since copying figures on paper is closely related to many types of school demands. Pencil drawing is by nature a sequential effort, so the examiner has an opportunity to observe how the child organizes the visual information for reconstruction. All but the simplest items on these tests include perception of the parts as related to the whole, which can be reflected in the child's production. Do the parts touch where they should or are they separate entities? Are the relative size and alignment maintained? These may be indications of ability to shift attention between meanings and to hold and compare relevant information in working memory in order to maintain the integrity of the figure. Placement of the drawing on the paper can also show part-to-whole processing. Can the child attend to both the boundaries of the paper and the figure? Or, is the drawing all in one corner, or do the lines go all the way to the edges of the paper? The Copying Test (DTVP-2) includes as part of scoring an assessment of the child's ability to grasp the "Gestalt," or the basic idea of the design, in addition to accuracy.

Some tests require construction of a figure exactly on coordinates, such as a dot grid or on graph paper. For some children the coordinates add to the challenge as they must attend to both the figure—its components, direction, overall shape—and to the coordinates on which it is placed. Other children find this structure helpful. It is important to observe how the child accomplishes the task. Does he or she proceed line by line, counting or figuring out the coordinates for each segment in isolation? Or, does the child see the whole configuration and draw lines as tangents sharing coordinates? The Design Copy Test (SIPT) provides the examiner with specific observation guidelines to assess method of production.

Limitations. Motor output problems may interfere with accurate assessment of the visual perception skills involved. Even with close observation it is difficult to know if poor performance is due to perception of the stimulus or to planning and executing the motor act. If a child has motor impairment, these tests may not be valid or informative. Also, scores are usually based on final product only and, as such, cannot account for method or organization. On some tests, scoring criteria are quite demanding of precision. So, an impulsive child, or one who does not appreciate the importance of precision, may score poorly even though his or her perception was adequate.

Construction Tasks

Some visual-motor tests involve construction tasks such as block designs or stick designs rather than pencil-and-paper output. These tasks are particularly appropriate for preschool or young school-age children (or those operating on this level) because perception of actual objects is more familiar to them than two-dimensional representations. Also, manipulation incorporates actions with visual perception, which is characteristic of this stage of development. Construction tasks allow for observation of method and organization. For younger children, trial and error may be an appropriate level of organization.

Limitations. Again, tests requiring motor responses involve many sensory, motor, and cognitive abilities; it may be difficult to make judgments regarding specific visual perception skills. The test scores alone do not provide any information on how the child proceeded. It is possible for a child who used haphazard, disorganized methods but managed to make the final product to get a higher score than the child who used good strategies and was organized but missed the exact final copy.

Complex Tasks

The Rey-Osterreith Complex Figure Test (see Figure 6.6) is a design copying task, originally designed for use with adults, but it also presents a challenge to an older child's ability to organize and reconstruct a large amount of information. The Constructional Praxis, Part 2 subtest of the

SIPT provides a very complex structure that is to be recreated. Such tasks would require the ability to perceive part-to-whole, not only of pieces close in proximity, but also to the whole structure. It is not a reasonable expectation that a child in the preoperational stage of cognitive development would be very successful on these tasks.

Tests of Visual Retrieval—Motor Response

These tests include drawing a figure, or part of a figure, from memory. Test items may provide some context (part of the figure) and require the child to fill in what is missing. Other test items require total recall or delayed recall.

Drawing from a remembered image can give some insight into how the child encoded the stimulus figure. Which aspects did he or she find meaningful? Did he or she see part-to-whole relationships or only isolated segments? Could the child find meaningful "chunks" that could be retrieved as one thought? If only some parts were remembered, which were they—the most familiar, recognizable shapes? Did the child make errors that transformed the stimulus figure into something more meaningful to him or her?

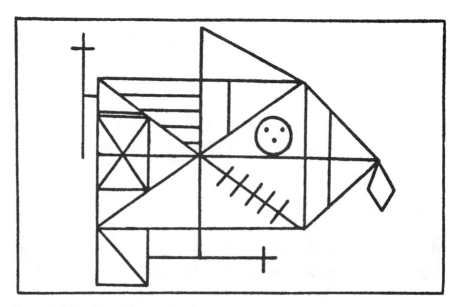

Figure 6.6 Rey-Osterrith complex figure.

Strategies for encoding simultaneous (i.e., figures) or sequential (i.e., row of letters or numbers or shapes) stimuli can be observed. For example, verbal strategies such as vocalizing nameable items or relating images to something familiar, or kinesthetic strategies such as tracing the figure with a finger, may be spontaneously used by a child to help him or her to remember. These should not be considered "cheating." They are positive signs of metacognition—an awareness of one's own limitations and need for a strategy.

The memory aspect of these productions cannot be separated from the original perception, discrimination, and encoding of the stimulus figure. A lack of organizing methods may become obvious during memory production. A relationship has been found between organization of original perception and memory productions. For example, on the Rey-Osterreith Complex Figure Test, those children who can see and draw the basic structure (rectangle, bisecting lines) to organize the production on the direct copy part of the test are more successful on the memory production part than those children who see and draw isolated fragments (Loikith, 1994).

Occasionally one may find a child who performs better on memory tests than on direct copy. Here, a more thorough visual assessment may be indicated.

Limitations. Poor scores are not necessarily a deficit of STM. The issue actually may be deficits of attention or encoding strategies, discrimination ability, or knowledge of task demands. Also, motor output is a consideration as with all visual-motor tests.

Visual-Motor Independent Drawing

Draw-a-Person or House-Tree-Person tests are commonly used psychological tests. Here, the child has no stimulus to copy, only the image in his or her own mind that he or she can work from. Guidelines for scoring can be found in the MAP. Interpretation of these drawings should be done in conjunction with psychological test results.

Visual-Motor (Eye–Hand) Tasks

Many test batteries include visual-motor control tasks that are generally considered indicators of motor, not perceptual, ability. However, they can provide an opportunity to observe gaze control and visual attention in monitoring work. Test items that involve keeping a pencil line within certain boundaries demand visual and attentional shifts between the pencil point and boundary lines, as well as between the pencil point and where it is going. Success on these tests requires *vigilance,* or maintaining attention, for the constant monitoring of progress. Figure 6.7 is an example of a child's performance on a pencil control task. This child was unsuccessful because his attention was captured by the center dot and he was not able to shift his attention back to where he was. (This conclusion was based on this and other observations).

The Visual-Motor Speed test (DTVP-2) is greatly dependent on perception and vigilance, perhaps even more than motor skill. This is a complex task and is discussed below under "visual vigilance."

Nonmotor Visual Perception Tests

Nonmotor tests are designed to directly measure visual perception without involving planning and executing a motor response except for pointing to or circling an answer.

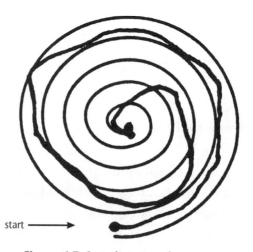

Figure 6.7 Sample test performance.

Direct Matching Tests

On several nonmotor tests, the child must indicate the correct item out of several choices with the correct response usually being a direct match of the target. Different visual perception skills are thought to be assessed as the matching tasks are varied from identical match, to match with distracters, match from memory, or match with deformations of the target. As difficulty and, consequently, age-expected performance increases, there is an increase in complexity of the figures, in subtlety of differences, and in the presence of greater distracters.

Nonmotor tests are particularly beneficial for use with children who have known or suspected motor impairments. They provide an opportunity to assess certain visual processes. As with motor tests, observation of strategy use can be made. Examiners can closely watch how the child surveys the choices. Is he or she systematic? Does he or she have a consistent strategy, such as proceeding left to right? Is he or she impulsive or disorganized, choosing randomly, or not scanning all possibilities? One strategy found to be consistently used by normal children over age 5 is to encode the target figure into working memory as an image, then scan the options (Das, Kirby, & Jarman, 1979; Locher & Worms, 1981). Does the child appear to use such a memory strategy or does he or she frequently look back at the target? Does the child enlist verbal or kinesthetic strategies, such as naming, or tracing with a finger the figures to be compared or remembered?

Limitations. Scores on these tests should be interpreted with caution. While they often have very general names such as "visual discrimination" or "visual memory," the tasks are only an instance of this type of skill, in black and white, two-dimensional, and in a constrained context, and as such are not necessarily representative of that domain in general. Also, the subtests do not assess skills in isolation. Visual memory requires adequate visual discrimination. "Figure-ground" involves visual discrimination and part-to-whole perception. All require knowledge and understanding of task demands. It is more difficult to observe the thought processes and problem-solving skills in a nonmotor test than in one which has a motor output. Also, on multiple choice tests a child can be right by guessing. If the child is incorrect, it is difficult to know how close he or she was to being right.

Other Nonmotor Tests

Visual Vigilance (PEEX2 and PEERAMID2) is different than other direct matching tests because the child must find repeated matches through several lines of possibilities. Observations can be made, not only of discrimination, but also of procedures, attention maintenance, and self-monitoring. A young child may be able to make good comparisons to find matches among choices near the target; but with the choices becoming further from the target in both time and proximity, he or she may not be able to keep both target and choices in mind at once.

The Visual-Motor Speed test (DTVP-2) is quite demanding of visual vigilance as the child must find target shapes from among eight rows of densely printed shapes and distracters. In addition, the child must make appropriate markings in each of two different target shapes, within time constraints, and the task must be done neatly (no score for lines extending outside the shape). Such complex integration of perceptual, attentional, and motor skills provides an appropriate challenge for older children but is too difficult for a preoperational child. Even though the standardization of this test includes 4-year-olds, the expected performance of the younger children is so poor that it is questionable whether this is an appropriate experience for them.

The Puzzle Test (MAP) involves a very practical, age-appropriate application of part-whole construction. A simple puzzle (two or three pieces) requires some ability to decenter from the isolated pieces to see a whole structure, but allows for piece-to-piece comparison. This is an expected ability for children around the age of 4, according to Piagetian stages.

Visual closure tests vary in task demands. The Picture Fragments subtest of the Detroit Tests of Learning Aptitude (DTLA) uses line drawings of familiar objects but with some of the lines broken or missing. This is believed to measure the Gestalt function of closure in which familiar objects can be recognized with only some information provided. Research and theories abound on the topic of object recognition; however, it is not clear what it means if a child (or adult) cannot perform well on this task. It could be that the child is centered on the fragments and cannot shift attention to the whole picture. Or it is possible that the figure is not familiar enough to a child to elicit recognition with sparse details.

Another type of visual closure task is found on the TVPS and DTVP-2. Here the child is provided with pieces of an abstract design that he or she must mentally connect to arrive at a completed design and match to one of four choices. Keeping in mind the developmental stages outlined earlier, it is clear that this would be a very difficult task for young children. It requires them not only to decenter from the fragments provided in order to see a whole picture, but also the choices must be viewed and considered separately. Visualizing how the fragments would be connected probably involves transformational imagery. We would not expect such processing from a preoperational child. This is confirmed by the standard scores provided on the TVPS, which show that up to age 6 years 3 months a child can score within normal limits (within one standard deviation) by getting only two correct answers. Considering that there are only four possible choices in each item, chance may account for those two correct answers (there is a 25% chance of guessing right).

Pattern Learning on the PEEX2 does, to some degree, assess the more dynamic aspects of visual perception. Here the child is given a rather complex configuration to reproduce from memory but is given up to four trials to get it correct. The process of learning completely new visual information can be observed, including strategies for remembering, learning to discriminate new forms through repeated exposure, recognizing mistakes, and modifying strategies accordingly.

Interpreting Standardized Test Scores

If a child does well on standardized testing, we know only that he or she is able to do those particular tasks in a manner similar to other children the same age. If a child does poorly on standardized testing, what does that mean? Unfortunately, the answers to that question are not easy. There are many factors that can influence the outcome of a testing situation.

Tests are usually designed to expose a lack of the cognitive or perceptual abilities necessary to perform the task adequately. It may be frustrating to the therapist who is trying to understand the nature of these abilities because the test manuals provide only descriptions of the task behaviors. Using the theories and research presented in this chapter, we can identify some of the basic abilities, such as

• sufficient knowledge to find tasks and stimulus items meaningful, or to be able to hold specific information in memory
• ability to shift attention between meanings at an age-expected level and make good decisions about which meanings will help with task demands
• decentering at an age-expected level in order to consider part-to-whole relationships and maintain these relationships across time and space
• age appropriate use of imagery to anticipate or make transformations of complex information.

It is important to consider that other factors may also, or alternatively, be involved. These may include

• impulsivity resulting in inadequate search or insufficient consideration of possibilities
• lack of understanding the task demands—either because of the language used or no appreciation of the difference between a correct and incorrect answer
• attention is not on task because of the stress of testing, fear of failure, other conflicting emotional problems
• inability to shift from one mode of thinking to another in response to changing task demands.

Altering Testing Procedures for Further Investigation

Going beyond the standardized administration of a test can be helpful in understanding a child's abilities that may not be readily observed with strict adherence to testing procedures. It is very important that the entire test be administered according to standardized procedures if the results are to be reported. However, once administered, the examiner can always go back and "test the limits" (Beery, 1989; McLoughlin & Lewis, 1986) to find out how close the child is to success and what types of intervention might bring about success.

The following are some suggestions for ways to use tests after scores have been obtained. A skilled examiner may make note of questionable performance during testing and go back to explore further in whatever manner will provide useful, treatment-relevant information. The aim is to create an optimal situation for skill performance by eliminating obstacles or providing guidance or assistance.

1. *Permit a second try.* If a subtest changes task demands with no warning, or if the child seems distracted, or if the child seems unaware of task demands initially but catches on later, a second try may be more indicative of ability.
2. *Prompt.* The child can be prompted to start in the right place or have attention directed to relevant information, then can proceed independently from that point.
3. *Demonstrate.* The child can be shown how to do one test item or have procedures or strategies demonstrated. The examiner can observe if the child is able to learn by example and apply these strategies to other test items.
4. *Extend or remove time limits.* Allow the child to complete the task or remove the time component entirely if this causes distraction or stress.
5. *Impose time limits.* Some children may be more motivated to focus on the task if a stopwatch or egg timer is running.
6. *Change instructions.* Use language or gestures that are more comprehensible to the child. Make sure he or she understands the task requirements.
7. *Change the presentation.* Place the test on a vertical surface to eliminate the added demands of plane integration (interpreting horizontally presented information from a vertical position). Cover extraneous material or point to choices in order to direct attention. Allow a glance at choices before presenting a figure to be matched

from memory so the child has an idea of what will be expected or what details will be relevant.

Another way to enhance the testing situation is to *question* the child about his or her responses or methods. Can the child see his or her mistakes? If the child can see them, can he or she fix them? Can the child devise a method for checking accuracy? Can the child structure the test more to his or her liking? Can he or she figure out a way to "cheat?" Is there awareness of his or her own limitations? Such questions can reveal the extent to which the child is able to interact with the test information and find it meaningful, even though his or her responses may not be exactly correct.

Going even beyond the concept of testing the limits is *dynamic assessment*. Dynamic assessment was developed by Dr. Reuven Feuerstein (Feuerstein, Rand, & Rynders, 1988) and refers specifically to the assessments he has devised. However, some basic concepts might be applied to other testing situations. As defined by Lidz (1991), "Dynamic assessment follows a test-intervene-retest format [that] focuses on learner modifiability and on producing suggestions for interventions that appear successful in facilitating improved learner performance" (p. 6). This type of assessment is not used for judging skill level; rather, it is used for planning intervention. Dynamic assessment is a very long, intense process. The reader is referred to the references for additional information.

Observations

The overall goal of therapy is always to help a child improve in areas that are relevant to school or home functioning. Thus, an important part of assessment is observing a child's performance in those natural situations where visual perception is an integral part of age-appropriate activities.

When a child is referred for evaluation because of problems in areas related to visual perception, it is important to differentiate between a problem with perception and a problem with output production or another cognitive area. Here, the results from standardized tests that separate perception and output can be helpful in determining the nature of a problem. Careful observation of activities also provides some clues. Observations can be made of the procedural knowledge and strategies, the domain-specific knowledge the child possesses, attention skills, and use of mental images.

Procedural knowledge includes the child's method of intake of visual information. Scanning procedures, thoroughness of search, organization of search, and use of working memory to hold information while completing a search are some possible observations that can be made. It is helpful for the assessor to sit across from the child and try to observe how he or she scans and searches. For example, a child may be observed while making a shape or form puzzle. Efficient visual intake could be characterized by the child looking first at the target to be matched, then systematically searching (e.g., left to right, or near to far) while holding the target image in working memory, until a possible match is found and tried. Clues that intake might be inefficient or ineffective may be seen in random selection rather than an organized search; in not searching all possibilities; in not maintaining the target in working memory, resulting in frequent rechecking; or in changing target or repeatedly making the same mistake. Through such observations, it is possible to get a sense for how well the child uses his or her eyes for gathering information. An evaluation by a developmental optometrist can provide valuable information about the child's visual skills.

Verbal or kinesthetic strategy use can be observed. For example a child may cue himself or herself verbally ("I'm looking for a square;" "I tried that already"). Pointing to objects or using a finger to guide a search or to focus on details are examples of incorporating kinesthetic strategies to help organize visual intake.

Observation of the child engaged in activities can also provide some information about the *domain-specific knowledge* that the child possesses. Familiarity with objects, shapes, and features that allow for recognition and differentiation from other objects is part of this knowledge base. This can best be observed when language and motor components are eliminated. For example, a young child may not "know" his or her letters. However, it needs to be determined if this is a visual perception issue or a labeling issue. A form board with letter shapes can reveal how readily a child can match up the letters without a verbal label.

Domain-specific knowledge also includes concepts about object relations—relative size, position, and sequence, for example. A game of "memory," in which cards are turned over two at a time to try to find matches, can be very difficult for a child who has weak concepts of relative position. During the game, the child may be observed to be allocating appropriate visual regard, may recognize and remember the picture on the upturned card, but may not be able to remember its position in relation to the other cards. His or her guesses may be close, but repeatedly miss finding the match.

Knowledge of task demands and what constitutes success should not be overlooked. Does the child know what is meant by "stay on the line" while cutting? Can he or she tell the difference between a poor attempt and a better attempt?

The use of *mental images* might also be observed in natural situations. A child who is given a loosely structured activity will need to create an image of the task in order to plan his actions. Given the task of drawing a picture of his family, the child needs to picture family members in his or her mind, how they should look, what color crayons to choose, and where to start. A child may be observed looking off into space conjuring up a mental image to plan his or her next step. Children who have not yet learned to use their "mind's eye" will have great difficulty with these unstructured tasks.

Countless activities can be used for observing a child's visual perception. The assessor needs to analyze the task according to what types of knowledge, procedures, and strategies are involved. Using a variety of activities and looking for patterns of problem areas are helpful in the detective work of teasing out a child's particular problems and needs.

Assessment Summary

To gain an understanding of a child's ability and skill development in the area of visual perception, an assessment should include three settings:

CASE STUDY: JOEY: Assessment Summary

Joey is a 7-year-old boy who came to occupational therapy following recommendations of a pediatric neurologist who described him as having developmental dyspraxia. He has a history of school difficulties and has been moved into a self-contained class for most of the school day. The following is a summary of the assessment done on Joey in the area of visual perception. Other areas of concern such as motor and attention exist but are not reviewed here. In the next section, areas addressed in treatment will be described along with anecdotes of activities and progress.

Standardized Test Results: Test of Visual–Motor Integration   7%ile

Test of Visual–Perceptual Skills (nonmotor):

Visual Discrimination	25%ile	Visual Sequential Memory	1%ile
Visual Memory	50%ile	Visual Figure Ground	2%ile
Visual–Spatial Relations	9%ile	Visual Closure	16%ile
Visual Form Constancy	9%ile		

Pediatric Early Elementary Examination:

Visual Vigilance: poor performance, many errors of reversing pattern, lacked persistence

Visual Discrimination: poor, but in general did better on items where single designs rather than sequences were involved

Visual Retrieval: poor; some errors included making an N instead of only the diagonal, and T instead of the inverted form given

Pencil Control: poor, lacked persistence (see Figure 6.7 for sample)

Adaptive Skills:

Shoe tying: with great difficulty

Handwriting: knows letters and can form recognizable letters but formations are incorrect; has trouble with line placement and consistency of letter size; teacher feels writing is poor

Scissoring on line: starts well but moves too quickly to the end; does not stay on line

Discussion:

Many types of visual information seem to be not very meaningful to Joey. He has trouble identifying shapes, understanding component parts and how they go together, and understanding directionality of lines, letters, and shapes.

Joey has difficulty with tasks that require attention to two or more visual aspects (e.g., cutting on a line so that he must attend to where he is cutting as well as to where he is going). He also seems to lack persistence on certain tasks and is not able to maintain the visual attention necessary to complete the task or to be accurate. However, he does not seem inattentive or impulsive in general and will usually stay on task, even if it is difficult.

It is difficult to know if there is a specific visual memory problem because memory is dependent on attention and understanding. Joey's judgment about the correctness of his work is often faulty. On several occasions he said, "Oh, now I see," when in fact he did not. This may be the result of lack of understanding of the task demands, or it may be a cover-up for frustration or boredom, or may evidence fear of looking "bad."

natural, structured, and optimal. A natural setting includes age-appropriate and relevant task observation in the context of the child's everyday environment. Structured settings involve standardized testing and are used to look more closely at specific skills and how these skills compare to other children of the same age. Test situations can be altered following completion of administration in order to create a more optimal situation to observe the child's ability. In all of these settings, it is possible to observe the strategies a child uses to attend to, organize, and perform a visual task.

Interpretation of test scores must be done with respect to developmental abilities. Therapists need to be aware that simply because a test item has been standardized for a certain age group does not necessarily mean that the item is developmentally appropriate. Piaget's developmental stages provide a useful framework for understanding the cognitive abilities that give rise to visual perception skills. It is through this understanding that therapists can try to answer the question of why a child can or cannot perform a certain perceptual task.

The purpose of assessment is to plan intervention to improve performance on age-appropriate tasks. If assessment focuses on discovering what knowledge a child brings to a task, this will lead to ideas of what new knowledge is needed and what procedures and strategies might be learned or modified.

Intervention

In planning treatment for children who have not developed adequate visual perception, it is important to know and incorporate the normal developmental sequence of skill acquisition. However, a realistic view would be that if, through the normal progression of development within a rich environment, these skills did not emerge, then treatment will have to draw on other avenues for learning. Developmentally sequenced activities may be used in therapy, but mere exposure and practice along a developmental sequence is only pursuing abilities that did not work in the first place. Treatment must address not only the product of the child's effort, but also the procedures, strategies, knowledge, and cognitive development that will make the product possible and meaningful.

Children who may also have underlying or contributing factors, including vision and oculomotor abilities, general attention deficits, or other cognitive or emotional issues that may interfere with perception or performance in this area, will certainly benefit from having them addressed. However, even if the underlying problems can be corrected, the child remains with the same knowledge base, procedures and habits, and automatic associations that he or she had prior to the correction, which will need to be changed in order to use new skills effectively. So, intervention cannot involve only underlying problems; visual perception must be directly addressed.

Remediation, Strategies, and Adaptations

Three general types of intervention can be considered: remediation, strategy use, and environmental adaptations.

Remediation refers to efforts aimed at "fixing" the problem. The goals are to improve deficit skills so that the child can function normally and independently. This can involve intervention of underlying causes, or structured practice of specific skills so skills can develop and become more automatic.

Strategy use overlaps with remediation because certain deficits may be due to ineffective strategy use. Strategies for search, scanning, attention to details, maintaining attention, monitoring work, and encoding information might be taught and can enable the child to function more competently. Other strategies can be used to bypass deficits where remediation looks improbable. These can be "tricks" or ways to use other avenues to achieve a desired outcome, such as using verbal prompts or mnemonics, or imposing structure.

In adaptation of the environment, an adult (teacher, parent) changes the task as an accommodation to a child's limitations so success is possible. An example of an adaptation might be to substitute a pull-over smock for the one that ties in back, or precued work papers for organizing written work.

Intervention plans are likely to incorporate all three types in an effort to improve skills through remediation but also make necessary adaptations so as not to miss out on age-appropriate learning activities.

JOEY—GENERAL AREAS TO BE ADDRESSED IN THERAPY

1. Improve visual perception skills such as those that are measured on standardized tests
   a. Improve ability to attend to all relevant aspects (parts and whole) of objects or scenes.
   b. Improve understanding of the relationship of objects, such as directionality, relative size, and sequences.
   c. Improve ability to accomplish increasingly complex tasks that require planning, organizing, monitoring progress.
2. Improve awareness of accuracy of work
   a. Learn self-questioning techniques and other verbal self-cuing.
   b. Learn to check both details and overall structure of productions for accuracy.
3. Improve functional skills
   a. Improve handwriting—learn better, more consistent formations and improve attention to lines.
   b. Improve scissoring skills—improve ability to maintain visual attention throughout cutting task.
   c. Shoe tying—increase speed and consistency of tying laces.

General Principles of Intervention

Task Demands

Activities must be chosen or designed to be most successful when the child uses the strategy or procedure he or she is being taught. In keeping with the idea that visual perception is mainly a goal-driven activity, the goal must be attainable and meaningful (refer back to importance of meaning for attention and STM) to the child so that he or she can experience a successful implementation of new or modified procedures. Interest and curiosity, the hallmarks of learning, are most likely to arise from a situation that has a combination of familiarity and novelty.

JOEY—BUILDING ON TASK DEMANDS

Erector Set Jr. was introduced as an activity. The set contains large, plastic, color-coordinated pieces with a booklet of step-by-step directions. First, only the nuts, bolts, and a few structural pieces were used in order to practice the basic movements and concepts of fastening nuts and bolts to hold pieces together (Goals 1a and 1b). Shapes, "weapons," and stick figures were created and practiced until Joey became bored. Then the simplest race-car structure was presented, and Joey found the prospect of building it inviting, but too hard. Joey was shown strategies for proceeding with the project: organizing strategies such as finding all pieces needed for one step, placing the pieces in the same orientation as the picture, finding landmarks on the picture and the corresponding place on the structure, and counting holes in pieces to check correctness (Goals 2a and 2a). With these strategies, the task was possible, although challenging. This became Joey's favorite activity. Independent use of strategies, and consequently skill, improved (Goal 1a). A race car was produced in about four sessions, and Joey used it in some other activities.

Encoding Strategies

Encoding is the act of acquiring new knowledge, either domain specific or procedural. In keeping with the theoretical model described earlier, the acquisition of knowledge involves making new associations with previously acquired knowledge. It has also been demonstrated that learning, or memory, improves with "dual coding" or cross-referencing to another modality (refer back to "Dual Coding" in the section on cognitive ability). Incorporating verbal and kinesthetic codes helps to structure the sequential organization of visual tasks. In intervention we can make use of dual coding to help a child gain new knowledge. The codes could be

1. *Visual-verbal:* using a verbal label to identify, categorize, and remember a visual stimulus, or use verbal cues to guide and learn procedures.
2. *Visual-kinesthetic:* involving movement or touch in processing visual information. For example, using a finger to direct attention, cue, or facilitate planning. Learning the properties of visual material can be facilitated with kinesthetic techniques. Manipulatives such as string to go from point to point may help with learning procedures for line drawing. Simple construction activities can facilitate attention to part-whole relationships. Painting an object on all sides or covering it completely with putty can draw attention to all aspects of the object and incorporate movement with object perception.
3. *Visual-visual:* relating new visual information to well-learned visual knowledge or images, for example, "bed" image to remember direction of "b" and "d," in which the child envisions the headboard as the "b," which comes first, and the footboard as the "d."

JOEY—VISUAL-KINESTHETIC ENCODING

Joey's handwriting (Goal 3a) is a highly practiced, automatic procedure at this point and is reinforced daily in school. Change will be difficult. Writing activities that avoid overlearned habits were devised to bring active attention to the lines on the paper. Paper with raised lines was used to provide a kinesthetic connection—Joey could see and feel the line as his pencil reached it. Activities included making colorful line patterns of "short" (from dotted middle line) and "tall" lines. The feel of the bump helped direct visual attention to the lines. When letters or letter-like forms, such as an "o" were introduced, Joey easily reverted to his habitual patterns of letter formation, which did not include attention to line. Redirection of attention through verbal cues (first the therapist, then Joey self-cued) and alternating with nonhabitual formations led to improved maintenance of attention to the accuracy of his work. Generalization to everyday writing tasks will take much time and practice.

Context Specificity

All learning, all encoding of information, occurs within the context in which it was perceived. Treatment approaches that grade difficulty without changing the context may reinforce context dependency (Toglia, 1990). Just as recognizing letters or shapes in a variety of contexts is part of perceptual skill, recognizing the need to apply certain strategies in a variety of settings and conditions is a main goal of therapy.

Generalization

Toglia (1990) describes a "multicontext treatment approach" for generalization of therapeutic goals. This approach involves practicing a targeted *strategy* in multiple environments with varied tasks and expectations. Transfer of skill is accomplished through four stages: near transfer—an alternate form of the original task, with one or two characteristics changed; intermediate transfer—additional task characteristics are changed, similar to original task but similarities are less obvious; far transfer—task similar in concept, that is, in the strategy involved, but is physically different; and very far transfer—the spontaneous application of what has been learned to everyday tasks. (See Table 6.3.)

Awareness or Metacognition

Often, a part of perceptual deficits lies in the child's lack of awareness of his or her own limitations, of what is necessary to accomplish the

JOEY—AWARENESS

A string design board (made with pegs or nails placed in a grid so a string can be wrapped around them to create a design) was used with Joey to develop an understanding of line direction with a kinesthetic connection (Goal 1b). First, very simple line designs were made without following a sample in order to learn the motor procedures of the task. Then designs to be copied were introduced. Joey was taught the "two-finger check" technique, which involved using his left index finger for the design card and his right index finger for the design he created (Goal 2b). Starting at the first dot and corresponding peg, then proceeding segment by segment, accuracy was checked and line direction was further reinforced. A very positive occurrence was when Joey became confused in the middle of a design and independently chose to use the technique to see where he went wrong. Similar methods were applied to other situations where Joey had to create something and then check accuracy.

Table 6.3 Sample activity: DLM pegboard designs

Task	Strategy	Transfer	Far Transfer/Classroom
Search for pegs scattered on table	Left-right and top-down sweep Use finger to cue or pace	Start with fewer pegs, progress to many	Search for puzzle piece Search for hidden pictures
Gaze Control: Look for necessary peg in box	Maintain gaze until needed peg is in hand	Start with needed peg on top, progress to peg that is buried	Maintain gaze throughout cutting task Search for red crayons in a box
Sequential Organization: Where to start design	Therapist provides suggestions and rationale, child finds suggested starting point on card and corresponding hole	With new design card, independently points to starting	On cutting task, student points to best starting point
Planning next steps	Verbalize or trace different possible plans to proceed with design and choose one	Same strategy on different design card Same strategy on different construction task as block design	Picture tracing, plan for being sure every part is traced, decides on sequence Coloring design patterns in organized way
Attentional Shifts: Attention to parts	Count to find coordinates of correct hole to place peg, then ...	Independently checks correctness of design by checking both pieces and whole configuration	Collage with pieces placed with each in correct orientation but also balances or fills paper
Attention to whole	Judge if it looks right, (i.e., makes straight line or joins at right place)	Uses method to check correctness on other tasks (i.e., block design)	

task, of what resources he or she has, or of the ability to recognize the need for help. Successful performance and independence may depend on learning to recognize when and where a strategy (or trick) is needed. An example is the child who uses a finger to help space between words. The child knows (although may not fully understand) that spacing between words is necessary, recognizes the point at which a space is needed, and uses the finger strategy. With experience, as the child develops the ability to see words as a whole instead of as isolated letters and the knowledge that words have a relationship to each other and to the page (a decentering process), the strategy will be dropped. Not all strategies are dropped, however, and many become automatic procedures. Children with perceptual impairments may never be able to drop some strategies, but if they can be applied and lead to success, then they are certainly worth keeping.

Sample Activity

Table 6.3 provides an analysis of a sample visual perception activity that is commonly used in therapy settings—pegboard designs. However, it is not intended to be a recommendation for this particular activity; any activity that affords an opportunity to learn and practice strategies could be used. In the sample, the task is analyzed according to the strategies involved, which could be taught using verbal or kinesthetic references and suggestions for possible transfer of skill tasks. Generalization of skill requires much practice in a variety of situations. Here, only a few samples are given for the purpose of illustration.

Intervention Summary

Intervention in the development of visual perception can include *remediation*, in which deficit skills are improved, and teaching *strategies* for encoding new information, directing attention, and monitoring progress. In designing intervention activities, task demands must be created that are attainable and meaningful, and that are successful when the target strategy is applied. All learning must include generalization to a variety of contexts if the child is to achieve independence.

REFERENCES

Anderson, J. R. (1987). Skill acquisition: Compilation of weak-method problem solutions. *Psychological Review, 94,* 192–210.
Anderson, J. R. (1981). *Cognitive skills and their acquisition.* Hillsdale, NJ: Erlbaum.
Ayres, A. J. (1994). *The development of sensory integrative theory and practice.* Dubuque, IA: Kendall/Hunt.
Baddeley, A. D. (1986). *Working memory.* Oxford, England: Clarendon Press.
Baddeley, A. D. (1994). The magical number seven: Still magic after all these years? *Psychological Review, 101,* 353–356.

Beery, K. E. (1989). *Developmental test of visual-motor integration manual.* Cleveland, OH: Modern Curriculum Press.

Bell, N. (1991). *Visualization and verbalization for language comprehension and thinking.* Paso Robles, CA: Academy of Reading Publications.

Bly, L. (1991). A historical and current view of the basis of NDT. *Pediatric Physical Therapy, 3,* 131–135.

Bouska, M. J., Kauffman, N. A., & Marcus, S. E. (1990). Disorders of the visual perceptual system. In D. A. Umphred (Ed.), *Neurological rehabilitation.* St. Louis, MO: Mosby.

Bronson, G. W. (1994). Infants' transitions toward adult-like scanning. *Child Development, 65,* 1243–1261.

Chase, W. G., & Ericsson, D. A. (1981). Skilled memory. In J. R. Anderson (Ed.), *Cognitive skills and their acquisition,* Hillsdale, NJ: Erlbaum.

Cowan, N. (1988). Evolving conception of memory storage, selective attention, and their mutual constraints within the human information processing system. *Psychological Bulletin, 104,* 163–191.

Das, J. P., Kirby, J. R., & Jarman, R. F. (1979). *Simultaneous and successive cognitive processes.* New York: Academic Press.

Elkind, D. (1975). Perceptual development in children. *American Scientist, 63,* 533–541.

Feuerstein, R., Rand, Y., & Rynders, J. E. (1988). *Don't accept me as I am: Helping "retarded" people to excel.* New York: Plenum.

Ginsburg, H., & Opper, S. (1969). *Piaget's theory of intellectual development, an introduction.* Englewood Cliffs, NJ: Prentice-Hall.

Glover, J. A., Ronning, R. R., & Bruning, R. H. (1990). *Cognitive psychology for teachers.* New York: MacMillan.

Grobecker, B. A. (1992). *Spatial perception and imagery in learning disabled children.* Unpublished doctoral dissertation, Rutgers University, New Brunswick, NJ.

Hamill, D. D. (1991). *Detroit Tests of Learning Aptitudes* (3rd ed., manual). Austin, TX: Pro-ed.

Hitch, G. J., Woodin, M. E., & Baker, S. (1989). Visual and phonological components of working memory in children. *Memory and Cognition, 17,* 175–185.

Kosslyn, S. M. (1990). Mental imagery. In D. N. Osherson, S. M. Kosslyn, & J. M. Hollerbach (Eds.), *Visual cognition and action, invitation to cognitive science* (Vol. 2). Cambridge, MA: MIT Press.

Lerner, J. (1985). *Learning disabilities: Theories, diagnosis and teaching strategies* (4th ed.) Boston: Houghton Mifflin.

Levine, M. D. (1987). *Developmental variation and learning disorders.* Cambridge, MA: Educators Publishing Service.

Levine, M. D. (1994). *Educational care: A system for understanding and helping children with learning problems at home and in school.* Cambridge, MA: Educators Publishing Service.

Lezak, M. D. (1983). *Neuropsychological assessment.* New York: Oxford University Press.

Lidz, C. S. (1991). *Practitioner's guide to dynamic assessment.* New York: Guilford Press.

Locher, P. J. (1985). Use of haptic training to modify impulse and attention control deficits of learning disabled children. *Journal of Learning Disabilities, 18,* 89–93.

Locher, P. J., & Worms, P. F. (1977). Visual scanning strategies of neurologically impaired, perceptually impaired and normal children viewing the Bender-Gestalt designs. *Psychology in the Schools, 14,* 147–157.

Locher, P. J., & Worms, P. F. (1981). Visual scanning strategies of perceptually impaired and normal children viewing the Motor-Free Visual Perception Test. *Journal of Learning Disabilities, 14,* 416–419.

Loikith, C. A. (1994). Assessing children's organizing strategies on the Rey-Osterreith Complex Figure Test. Unpublished master's project. Montclair State University, Department of Communication Sciences and Disorders.

Luria, A. R. (1966). *Higher cortical functions in man* (2nd ed.). New York: Basic Books.

Mathiowetz, V., & Haugen, J. B. (1994). Motor behavior research: Implications for therapeutic approaches to central nervous system dysfunction. *American Journal of Occupational Therapy, 48,* 733–745.

McLoughlin, J. A., & Lewis, R. B. (1986). *Assessing special students* (2nd ed.). Columbus, OH: Merrill.

Miller, G. A. (1956). The magical number seven, plus or minus two: Some limits on our capacity for processing information. *Psychological Review, 63,* 81–97.

Murray, E. A. (1991). Hemispheric specialization. In A. G. Fisher, E. A. Murray, & A. C. Bundy (Eds.), *Sensory integration theory and practice.* Philadelphia: F. A. Davis.

Noton, D., & Stark, L. (1971). Scanpaths in eye movements during pattern perception. *Science, 171,* 308–311.

O'Hare, C. B. (1987). The effect of verbal labeling on tasks of visual perception and experimental investigation. *Educational Research, 29,* 213–219.

Paivio, A. (1990). *Mental representations: A dual coding approach.* New York: Oxford University Press.

Piaget, J. (1969). *Mechanisms of perception.* New York: Basic Books.

Pylyshyn, Z. W. (1986). *Computation and cognition, Toward a foundation for cognitive science.* Cambridge, MA: MIT Press.

Rieser, J. J., Garing, A. E., & Young, M. F. (1994). Imagery, action and young children's spatial orientation: It's not being there that counts, it's what one has in mind. *Child Development, 65,* 1262–1278.

Rourke, B. P. (1989). *Nonverbal learning disabilities: The syndrome and the model.* New York: Guilford.

Ruskin, E. M., & Kaye, D. B. (1990). Developmental differences in visual processing: Strategy versus structure. *Journal of Experimental Child Psychology, 50,* 1–24.

Schwantes, F. M. (1979). Cognitive scanning processes in children. *Child Development, 50,* 1136–1143.

Shepp, B. E., & Barrett, S. E. (1991). The development of perceived structure and attention: Evidence from divided and selective attention tasks. *Journal of Experimental Child Psychology, 51,* 434–458.

Shiffrin, R. M., & Dumais, S. T. (1981). The development of automatism. In J. R. Anderson (Ed.), *Cognitive skills and their acquisition.* Hillsdale, NJ: Erlbaum.

Toglia, J. P. (1990). Generalization of treatment: A multicontext approach to cognitive perceptual impairment in adults with brain injury. *American Journal of Occupational Therapy, 45,* 505–516.

Warren, M. (1993). A hierarchical model for evaluation and treatment of visual perceptual dysfunction in adult acquired brain injury (Part 1). *American Journal of Occupational Therapy, 47,* 42–54.

Yantis, S. (1992). Multielement visual tracking: Attention and perceptual organization. *Cognitive Psychology, 24,* 295–340.

SOURCES OF STANDARDIZED TESTS

Developmental Test of Visual-Motor Integration (VMI). Author: Keith E. Berry. Publisher: Modern Curriculum Press. Available from: Slosson Educational Publication, PO Box 280, E. Aurora, NY 14052-0280.

Developmental Test of Visual Perception, Second Edition. Authors: Donald D. Hammill, Nills A. Pearson, and Judith K. Voress. Publisher: Pro-Ed, 8700 Shoal Creek Blvd, Austin, TX 78757-6898.

Detroit Tests of Learning Aptitude, Third Edition. Author: Donald D. Hammill. Publisher: Pro-Ed, 8700 Shoal Creed Blvd, Austin, TX 78758-6897.

Miller Assessment for Preschoolers (MAP). Author: Lucy Jane Miller. Publisher: The Psychological Corporation, 555 Academic Court, San Antonio, TX 78204-2498.

Neurodevelopmental Examinations (PEET, PEER, PEEX2 and PEERAMID2). Author: Melvin D. Levine. Publisher: Educators Publishing Service. Available from: OT Ideas, Inc, 124 Morris Turnpike, Randolph, NJ 07869.

Rey-Osterreith Complex Figure Test. Source: Lezak, M.D. (1983). *Neuropsychological assessment.* New York: Oxford University Press.

Sensory Integration & Praxis Tests (SIPT). Author: A. Jean Ayres. Publisher: Western Pscyhological Services, 12031 Wilshire Blvd, Los Angeles, CA 90025-1251.

Test of Visual Motor Skills (TVMS). Author: Morrison F. Gardner. Publisher: Psychological & Educational Publications. Available from: Sammons, Inc., PO Box 386, Western Springs, IL 60558.

Test of Visual-Perceptual Skills, Non-Motor (TVPS). Author: Morrison F. Gardner. Publisher: Psychological & Educational Publications. Available from: Sammons, Inc., PO Box 386, Western Springs, IL 60558.

Part II. Acquired Visual Dysfunction

Evaluation and Treatment of Visual Dysfunction

An Osteopathic Approach

Viola M. Frymann, DO, FAAO, FCA, MB, MF Hom (Eng.)

Frank, age 6, shown in Figures 7.1–7.4, could maintain only a forward gaze in the horizontal plane by holding his head bent forward onto his chest. When asked to look to the right or left, Frank had to incline his head, and his eyes turned upward as they moved sideways. He was hyperactive and was having academic difficulties in school. He had been dropped as a baby, causing his head to "crack on the cement." He had been hospitalized with very severe allergic reactions, once to a rug cleaner at age 18 months and once to eggs and cheese at age 23 months. Allergic manifestations are common in children with learning and perceptual problems. Osteopathic manipulative treatment, which restores optimal structural relationships within the musculoskeletal system, will overcome the allergic state. This, in turn, contributes to overall well-being.

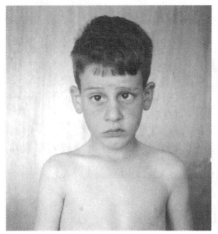 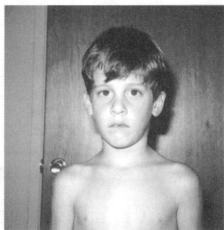

(a) April 3   (b) After 9 treatments

Figure 7.1 a) Frank, age 6 years, hyperactive, strabismus, scoliosis, severe incoordination. b) After treatment no evidence of strabimus, excellent progress in school.

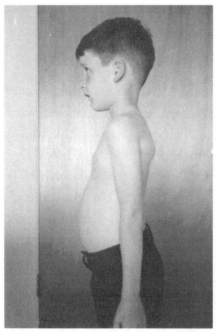 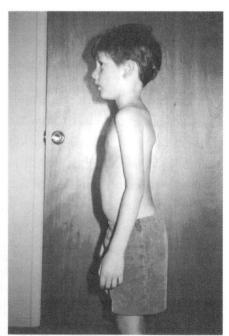

(a) April 3   (b) After 9 treatments

Figure 7.2 a) Note lumbar lordosis, thoracic kyphosis and forward position of head. b) After treatment posture improved.

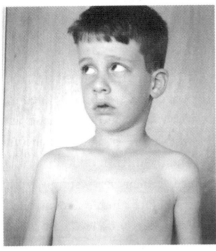
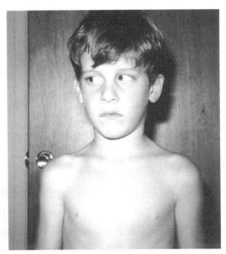

(a) April 3   (b) After 9 treatments

Figure 7.3 a) Unable to look right on horizontal plane. Eyes turn upward. b) After treatment pure motion to right horizontally.

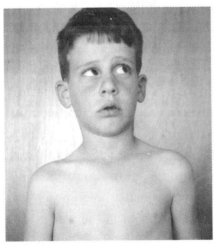
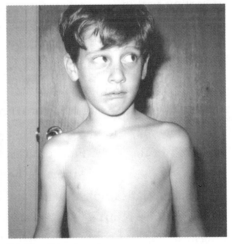

(a) April 3   (b) After 9 treatments

Figure 7.4 a) Unable to look left on horizontal plane. Eyes turn upward. b) After treatment improved motion to left.

At 6 years of age, Frank's family brought him for an osteopathic evaluation of his visual and learning problems. He was treated osteopathically for 3 months. The before-and-after photographs show the significant improvement in Frank's visual skills and posture. In order to understand Frank's problem and its resolution, a new look at the anatomy and physiology of the visual apparatus is necessary.

Anatomy of the Eye

The eyeball is the instrument through which visual images are received, providing information on form, size, shape, color, light, shade, and position in space. This information is then processed and interpreted by the brain. Six precisely positioned muscles move the eyeball in exact integration with the six muscles of the other eye. The superior rectus, inferior rectus, and medial rectus muscles and the inferior oblique muscle (which turns the eye up and outward) receive their nerve supply from the third cranial nerve (III). The superior oblique muscle is controlled by the fourth cranial nerve (IV). The lateral rectus muscle is controlled by the sixth cranial nerve (VI).

These cranial nerves pass from the brain to the eyeball in the bony orbit by an interesting anatomical journey; but in order to appreciate the significance of this anatomy, it is essential to recognize the component of motion within the cranial mechanism. Two distinct types of motion can be recognized in a living being. One type of motion may be called voluntary motion, such as walking, holding an object, and looking up or down and right or left. The other type of motion is essentially involuntary motion. An example of involuntary motion is that of the circulatory system. The heart beats in accordance with its own inherent rhythm so that blood may circulate to deliver oxygen and essential nutrients to every cell in the body. Furthermore, the blood carrying carbon dioxide returns, by the same rhythm, to the heart to be pumped into the lungs to discharge its carbon dioxide and be reoxygenated once more. This renewed blood returns to the heart for the next tour of the tissues. The lungs expand and contract in their inherent rhythm, about one-fourth the rate of the heart. As the lungs expand, they are filled with oxygen-rich air from which the oxygen is transferred to the blood. After receiving the carbon dioxide from the blood, in exchange, the lungs contract to squeeze the air out into the atmosphere and provide space for the next inhalation and oxygenation.

Rhythm of the Brain and Central Nervous System

An inherent rhythm of the brain and central nervous system (CNS) is remarkably unchangeable. This motion, induced by the inherent rhythmic motion of the brain, is transmitted through the cerebrospinal fluid and the dural membranes to the bones that make up the skull and face. This rhythmic motion of the cranial bones has been recorded in human beings and monkeys and has been palpated in dogs, ducks, a hummingbird, and even an injured cormorant. The CNS rate is slower than that of the heart or the lungs, but in any one individual in health the rate remains constant whether one is sleeping in bed or running a marathon. This physiologic function is called the *primary respiratory mechanism*: *respiratory*, because it is concerned with that exchange of gases and electrolytes at the cellular level, known as cellular respiration; *primary*, because it forms the foundation for and controls all the other physiologic mechanisms in the body; and *mechanism*, because it manifests through the intricate articular arrangement of the skull bones.

The *orbit* (see Figure 7.5), the cavity that contains the eyeball, its muscles, nerves, and blood vessels, is composed of eight bones that articulate with each other in a very delicately integrated fashion. These bones move rhythmically with the primary respiratory mechanism and thereby rhythmically change the shape and dimension of the orbit. This in turn influences the shape of the eyeball, which in turn affects its *acuity*, or the clearness of vision. Is vision equally efficient at near and far points? Is vision better at a near point, which is myopia, or is it better in the distance, which is hyperopia. A student complained to me that in the previous 6 weeks his vision had rapidly deteriorated, requiring one diopter of change in his glasses. A fellow classmate had forcefully squeezed his head a few weeks earlier. By a palpatory examination I could identify a strain in the cranial mechanism that caused the orbit to become shorter and wider, thereby making the eye farsighted. When the traumatic force was corrected by a gentle, perceptive technique that restored his anatomical structure to its optimal state, the student no longer needed the extra diopter of correction.

In the perfect eye, the image of the object seen enters the eye and focuses on the light-sensitive retina at the back of the eye. In the *myopic*, or nearsighted eye, the image focuses in front of the retina. In the *hyperopic*, or farsighted eye, the image focuses beyond the retina. The eyeball is a soft, fluid-containing sphere held by a cone of muscles but influenced by changes in the form and motion of the component parts

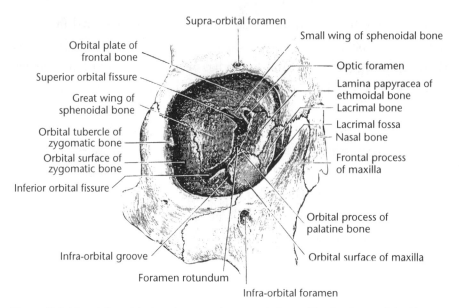

Figure 7.5 The right orbital cavity, anterior aspect. From *The Anatomy of the Human Body* (25th ed.), (p. 116, fig. 127), by H. Gray, 1948, Philadelphia: Lea and Febiger. Copyright 1948 by Lea and Febiger. Reprinted with permission.

of the bony orbit. These bony changes can affect the shape of the eyeball, causing the refractive errors of myopia and hyperopia, and can affect the blood and nerve supply, affecting visual functioning.

The orbit is a cone-shaped cavity at the apex of which most of the muscles that move the eyeball have their origin. Looking down on the contents of the orbit from above, a precise geometric relationship between the right and the left orbit is apparent (see Figure 7.6). If the axes of the orbits from their apices are projected forward, the axes diverge symmetrically from the midline; if projected backwards, they will reach the midpoint of the opposite quadrant of the posterior part of the head. Four rectus muscles move each eye: (a) the superior rectus that turns the eye upward and slightly inward, (b) the inferior rectus that turns the eye downward and slightly inward, (c) the medial rectus that turns the eye inward toward the nose; and (d) the lateral rectus that turns the eye outward on a horizontal plane.

While this arrangement seems very simple, the function of these muscles is a most delicate, complex, and integrated activity. For example, in order to look to the right, the right lateral rectus must contract and be

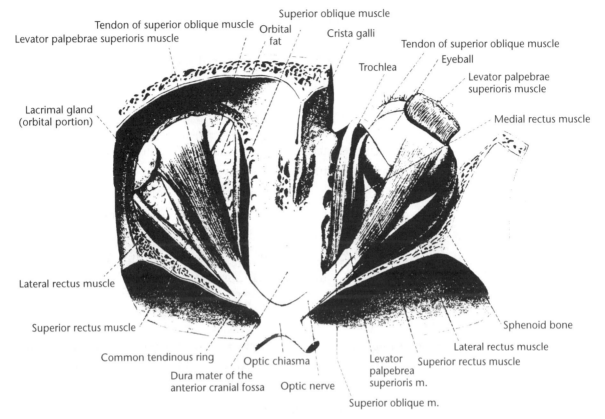

Figure 7.6 The muscles of the orbital cavity as seen from above. From *Anatomy: A Regional Atlas of the Human Body* (fig. 492), by C. D. Clement, 1975, Philadelphia: Lea and Febiger. Copyright 1975 by Lea and Febiger. Reprinted with permission.

NOTE: 1) the orbital plates of the frontal bone have been removed from within the cranium. On the left side, only the bony roof of the orbit has been opened and the muscles, orbital fat and lacrimal gland have been left intact.

2) on the right side, the levator palpebrae superioris muscle has been resected and the orbital fat removed in order to expose the ocular muscles.

balanced by an appropriate degree of relaxation of the right medial rectus. Since accurate vision, including an awareness of position and depth, requires the exact coordinated movement of the two eyes, that is, binocular vision, positive contraction of the left medial rectus and relaxation of the left lateral rectus must occur in perfect harmony with the activity in the right eye. Furthermore, the superior oblique of the right eye, which contributes to turning the right eye both outward and downward, must be precisely coordinated with the inferior oblique, which turns the eye both outward but also upward, and with the lateral rectus if the eye is to turn laterally on a horizontal plane. (Notice the problem of the patient in the photographs.)

Similarly, the superior and inferior recti of the left eye must be coordinated in this delicate harmony of muscular activity because in addition to turning the eye upward or downward respectively, these muscles also contribute to the turning of the left eye to the right, that is, toward the nose.

This precise geometrically programmed movement of the eyes is dependent on the innervation of these muscles by their respective nerves. These nerves pass from the brainstem by an anatomical pathway that takes them under, over, or through important bony or membranous structures. If these structures are injured during the birth process or in sports, in bicycle or car accidents, or in the various falls during the process of growing up, the injuries may compromise the function of one or more of these nerves.

Such injuries may distort bony relationships, the shape of the orbit, or the geometric axes of the orbits within the head. Of even greater clinical significance is the impairment of that inherent motion of the primary respiratory mechanism. Disturbance of that motion can disturb blood circulation, both arterial and venous, and the rhythmic fluctuation of the cerebrospinal fluid. One of the critical areas of this anatomical pathway of the nerves to these muscles is that of the developmental articulation of the sphenoid bone. Figure 7.7 shows a developing sphenoid bone. The sphenoid, like most of the other large bones of the head, is

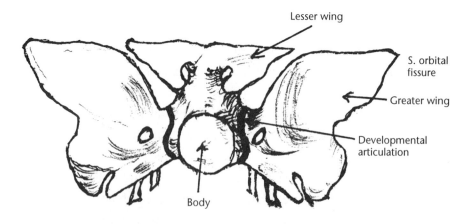

Sphenoid at Birth

Figure 7.7 Sphenoid at birth.

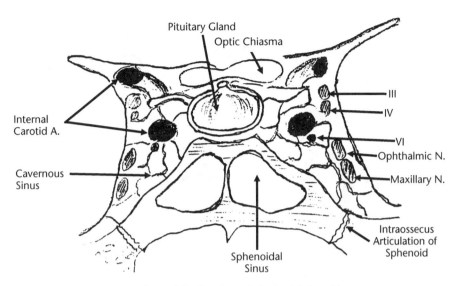

Pituitary Gland
Optic Chiasma

III
IV

VI
Ophthalmic N.

Maxillary N.

Internal
Carotid A.

Cavernous
Sinus

Intraossecus
Articulation of
Sphenoid

Sphenoidal
Sinus

Coronal Section through Body of Sphenoid

Figure 7.8 Vertical section through body of sphenoid.

still in its developmental stage at the time of birth. Note the central body that carries the lesser wings contributing to the roof of the orbit. On either side is the greater wing, forming a major part of the lateral wall of the orbit. Between these two parts on each side of the body is a developmental articulation that has micromobility in infancy and retains flexibility and resilience in later years. The nerves to the muscles of the eye, namely III, IV, and VI, accompany the ophthalmic vein, carrying blood from the eye over and in close proximity to this articulation (see Figure 7.8). These nerves with the vein pass through the fissure between the lesser and greater wings of the sphenoid. Thus it becomes apparent that trauma that distorts the relationship of these developmental parts of the sphenoid and impairs their physiologic inherent mobility may compromise the function of the extraocular muscles and their nerves.

Vision Impairment and the Birth Process

Studies of children with learning disabilities or perceptual dysfunction have revealed that at least 80% of these children have had difficulties during the birth process (Fackelmann, 1981; Frymann, 1976; Hoffman, 1971; Rossborough, 1963). These difficulties may include an unusually long labor or a period of false labor before productive labor began. The

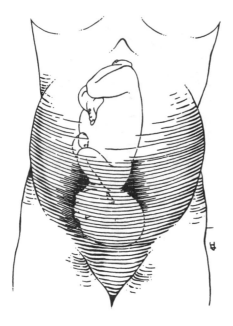

Abdominal view.

Figure 7.9 Mechanism of labor: median vertex presentation. Note: Baby's head extended on the neck. From *Human Labor and Birth*, by H. Oxorn-Foote, 1986, Norwalk, CT: Appleton-Century-Crofts. Copyright 1986 by Appleton-Century-Crofts. Reprinted with permission.

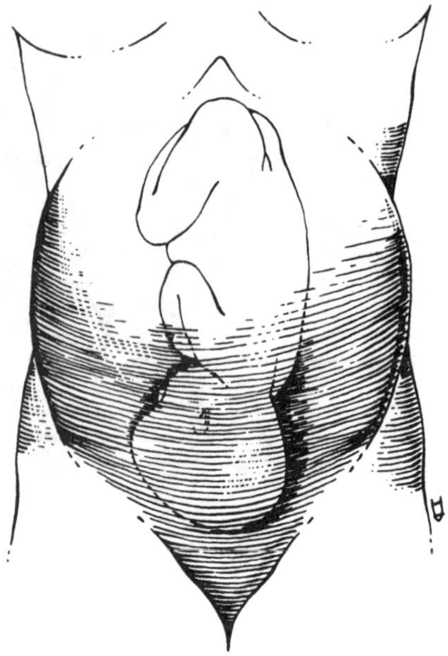

Abdominal view.

Figure 7.10 Left occiput anterior: LOA. Note: Baby's head well flexed on to the chest. From *Human Labor and Birth*, by H. Oxorn-Foote, 1986, Norwalk, CT: Appleton-Century-Crofts. Copyright 1986 by Appleton-Century-Crofts. Reprinted with permission.

Figure 7.11 Note: Baby's head passing between the sacrum and the pubis. From *Human Labor and Birth*, by H. Oxorn-Foote, 1986, Norwalk, CT: Appleton-Century-Crofts. Copyright 1986 by Appleton-Century-Crofts. Reprinted with permission.

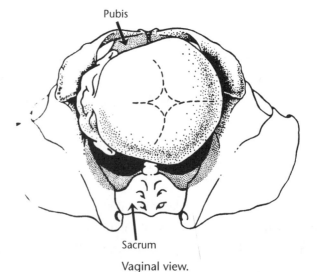

Vaginal view.

baby may have presented with the face forward instead of backward or with the head partially extended on the neck (see Figure 7.9) instead of fully flexed on the chest (see Figure 7.10) or the mother's pelvis may have been relatively small from front to back, causing the baby's head to be compressed from side to side as it passed between the promontory of the mother's sacrum (posterior) and her pubic symphysis (anterior) (see Figure 7.11).

Other dimensions may exist in which the baby's head is disproportionately large relative to the mother's pelvis, thereby making delivery more difficult. If the baby is presenting in the breech position, that is, the buttocks present first, the head may suffer undue stress as it follows through the birth canal. Some conditions demand assistance with the delivery, and forceps must be applied. This may be a valuable lifesaving measure; but even when forceps are applied expertly and with great care, some compression of the baby's head from side to side may be unavoidable. Other factors impairing the supply of oxygen to the brain, as for example the cord being coiled one or more times around the baby's neck, may compromise the neurological integrity of the CNS. Furthermore, as babies mature and mobility increases, curiosity motivates exploration; children begin climbing before they learn safe descent, creating innumerable opportunities for injuries to occur. Not all injuries are significant, and young children are resilient in their ability to overcome the effects of minor injuries. Significant injuries, however, are not necessarily accompanied by lacerations, fractures, or loss of consciousness. How then can the significant injury be identified?

The details of the birth history may be suggestive, but these questions can give conclusive answers about potential birth-related trauma.

1. Did the baby take hold of the nipple immediately and suck effectively? If delays or difficulty in nursing satisfactorily were present, even if all was well within a few days, suspect some trauma at birth.
2. Did the baby spit up frequently or vomit?
3. Did the baby cry excessively?
4. Did the baby have difficulty sleeping?
5. Did the baby arch the back or throw the head back when held over the shoulder?

6. Did the baby roll from back to side at only a few weeks of age because of extensor spasms occurring in the neck or back?

7. Did the baby insist on standing in the mother's lap instead of sitting?

If an affirmative answer is made to questions 2–7, you have evidence that the anatomical mechanism of the head, pelvis, or vertebral structures probably suffered some trauma during birth, which is manifesting in dysfunction in related areas of the CNS. These are critical questions for parents of a child who has perceptual or learning difficulties. If a fall or injury occurred after birth, were any behavioral changes, sleeping difficulties, or new problems with academic performance noted? If the answer is yes, consider that accident as a significant traumatic event. The whole body may be involved in the response to trauma.

Evaluation of Children with Academic Difficulties

In evaluating the child with academic difficulties, one must recognize the high probability of visual-perceptual dysfunction as a significant part of the problem. Visual-perceptual dysfunction may have a somatic or whole-body structural component, resulting from trauma before, during, or after birth and may also have a neurological developmental component. To elaborate, the development of efficient, integrated visual perception is delicately programmed into the comprehensive neurological development of the whole child. Neurological developmental integration refers to the process in which mobility, language, and manual dexterity develop concurrently with visual perception, auditory perception, and tactile perception. If any one of these aspects is obstructed, distorted, or hindered, the other phases of the process may reflect the inadequacy to some degree.

Figure 7.12 illustrates the integration of early mobility skills with visual perception. When the baby is placed face down on the floor, his or her head is turned to one side. The first movements forward should be a combat crawl in which the body is flat on the floor while one hand is raised beside the face and one leg and knee are flexed on the floor (see Figure 7.12, Stage 2, a–d). In a short time this becomes an efficient system of forward travel in which the head turns toward the advancing

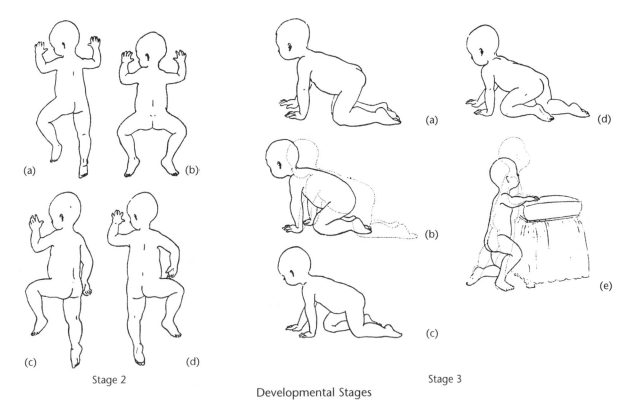

Stage 2

Developmental Stages

Stage 3

Figure 7.12 Mobility: Stage 2. Level II Crawling. (a) without pattern; (b) homologous pattern; (c) homolateral pattern; (d) cross pattern.
Mobility: Stage 3. Level III Creeping. (a) without pattern; (b) homologous pattern; (c) homolateral pattern; (d) cross-pattern; (e) rising from creeping to cruise.

hand. At this stage, the baby generally uses one eye to look at the hand. In the next developmental stage, the baby creeps on hands and knees, now coordinating the two eyes into efficient integrated binocular vision (Stage 3, a–d). Progressively, depth perception in three dimensions develops, enhanced by pulling to a standing position (Stage 3, e), cruising sideways, and eventually walking. If mobility progresses from the symmetrical motions of the newborn through crawling, creeping, cruising, and well-integrated cross-pattern walking, visual-perceptual function is enhanced. Conversely, if deficits in this gross motor development exist, they may have a negative effect on optimal visual-perceptual development.

Osteopathic Evaluation and Treatment

The body has, however, a remarkable capacity for adaptation and accommodation to overcome inadequacies and to function efficiently. Recognition of structural problems as described above and their successful treatment as soon after birth as possible will permit optimal development in all these vital functions as growth progresses. The following example illustrates the interrelationship between mobility and vision. I evaluated a group of medical students on their walking, creeping on hands and knees, and crawling flat on the floor. One man in that group was totally unable to perform crawling flat on the floor. He had no history of a learning disability as a child. After a few moments' reflection he said, "But I'm unable to copy a diagram." He had grown up in a culture where babies were not put on the floor. Thus, part of the evaluation of perceptual function must be the evaluation of the child's ability to crawl, creep, and walk with smooth, integrated head, arm, and leg movements. If those activities were competently performed in infancy, they still can be demonstrated in childhood or even adult life.

The osteopathic evaluation includes

1. thorough history of pregnancy, labor, delivery, and immediate state of the newborn
2. history of health, developmental progress, and trauma or illness during infancy and childhood
3. structural examination standing and supine for asymmetries in anatomical landmarks, such as head, facial features, dental occlusion, ears, shoulders, scapulae, spinal curves, rib cage, pelvis, knees, and feet
4. functional evaluation by gentle, manual palpation of the inherent motions within all parts of the body
5. standard medical evaluation of ears, throat, heart, lungs, and abdomen
6. standard test of developmental movement patterns (crawling, creeping, and walking) as described previously
7. screening examination for visual acuity and oculomotor function.

In my office I have a wall hanging that I will ask a child to look at while I examine his or her back in the standing position. The wall hanging has three circles, the middle one has a mother panda cuddling a baby and the other circles each have one panda. When I asked one 4-year-old boy how many pandas he saw, he stepped up to the wall and at about 4 inches away said, "There are four." He had a very severe degree of myopia! Such a simple test will be suggestive; a more detailed test of acuity will give a more precise evaluation.

Assess the tracking of the eyes laterally, vertically, and diagonally, and note whether the child has to move the head. Assess the child's ability to follow a moving object in erratic directions. This assessment provides information on the ease of motion of the eyes within the orbits, on the ability to keep the eye on a moving object, and on the attention to the task or distraction to other objects or people. Note convergence. Does one eye diverge (*exotropia*) or converge (*esotropia*) inappropriately as one object is brought from a far point toward the nose? Test for dominance by instructing a child to hold a small kaleidoscope with both hands. The child puts the kaleidoscope to his or her dominant eye, for example, the right eye. The child is then given the kaleidoscope in the opposite hand, left hand in this example. If the right eye is dominant, the child will again put the kaleidoscope to the right eye.

Testing for the presence of crossed dominance can provide further evidence of impaired neurological integration. Crossed dominance may be developmental, the result of efforts to change a left-handed child into a right-handed child, or the result of some traumatic event. Note the posture of the child at a desk when a dominant left eye endeavors to respond to a dominant right hand! As adults, such inconsistencies may be overcome or at least accommodated; but if a well-integrated total body function and structure can be established at the beginning of life, academic performance, athletic performance, and even social skills will develop more easily, more competently, and with less stress.

This screening process will reveal the structural problems that require osteopathic treatment, visual problems that may be completely resolved or significantly improved by the osteopathic treatment, and neurological developmental inadequacies that may also be completely resolved or significantly improved by osteopathic treatment. (Frymann, Carney, & Springall, 1992). At the conclusion of the treatment program, in perhaps 8 to 12 treatments, a reevaluation is made to determine whether the need exists for a program of vision development or neurological developmental stimulation.

The human body is a delicately designed and remarkably integrated unit of function from the head to the feet. The osteopathic physician uses highly trained perceptive manual palpatory skills to make the initial diagnosis and to monitor tissue changes as the gentle process of manipulation is performed. Treatment includes all regions and parts of the body. Manipulation is comfortable, and it gives a sense of well-being, manifested by the smile and confidence in the child when he or she emerges from the treatment room. The treatment is designed progressively to optimize the structural integrity, to improve fluid motion throughout the body—blood, lymph, and cerebrospinal fluid—and to enhance the inherent healing forces within.

An analogy may illustrate the importance of the osteopathic evaluation and treatment relative to other modalities for children with perceptual dysfunction. You intend to give piano lessons to a musically gifted child by a highly competent piano teacher. No matter how talented the child or how competent the teacher, the child will be unable to produce harmonious, melodic music if the piano, the instrument, is out of tune. First, tune the instrument and then teach the child how to play it. The physical body is the child's instrument: the osteopathic physician tunes and perfects that instrument. Then perceptual training and academic tutoring will rapidly lead this child to efficient performance.

REFERENCES

Fackelmann, K. A. (1981). Birthing trauma linked to diminished IQ. *Science News, 13,* 295.

Frymann, V. M. (1976). Learning difficulties of children viewed in the light of the osteopathic concept. *Journal of the American Osteopathic Association, 76,* 46/103–61/118.

Frymann, V. M., Carney, R. E., & Springall, P. (1992). Effects of osteopathic medical management on neurologic development in children. *Journal of the American Osteopathic Association, 92,* 729–744.

Hoffman, M. S. (1971). Early indications of learning problems. *Academic Therapy, 7*(1).

Rossborough, P. M. (1963). *Physical fitness and the child's reading.* Problem Exposition Press.

8 Vision Rehabilitation Following Acquired Brain Injury

Rosamond Gianutsos, PhD, FAAO, CDRS

Visual Problems Following Acquired Brain Injury

Why Is Visual Function Such an Important Concern After Brain Injury?

A supreme achievement of neurological functioning, vision is both precious and, unfortunately, vulnerable to central nervous system injury. This vulnerability stems in part from the fact that anatomically the visual system is a large target. The optic pathways extend from the eyes toward the back of the brain, partially crossing at the optic chiasm, forming a junction at the lateral geniculate bodies and then fanning out in the optic radiations before reaching the occipital cortex in the rear of the brain. A secondary visual system departs from the lateral geniculate bodies toward the superior colliculi. Many association areas and cortical circuits also are involved in visual perception and in planning and directing eye movements. In contrast, smell and hearing are controlled by pathways and centers that are proximal (near) to the sense organs themselves; the primary sensory pathways do not cross from one hemisphere to the other.

Vision tends to dominate the other senses, so that when information conflicts, visual information will be relied on over information from the other senses. For example, in driving simulators, nausea (so common that it is called simulator sickness) occurs when visual information suggests turning and weight shifting that do not actually occur.

Sensory information has primacy in the flow of information through the human nervous system. If information is lost or distorted on entry into the system, this loss or distortion becomes a problem when the individual attempts to perform a task that requires the use of that information. As computer people say: garbage in, garbage out. Clinically, I have observed people who have survived brain injury who became extremely frustrated, or languished in confusion, which abated when their visual problems were successfully treated. Sometimes, helping the visual problem is the key that unlocks the system—the reverse of the straw that breaks the camel's back.

Vision and Activities of Daily Living

Vision is, of course, integral to many daily living functions, including activities requiring distance vision and peripheral awareness, such as environmental mobility, and activities requiring near-point acuity and sustained visual attention, such as reading and paperwork.

Mobility includes walking around familiar locations, for instance in one's own home, as well as ambulation in more public or less familiar environments, such as guiding a cart around the supermarket. In this regard, fans of comedian W. C. Fields will recall the blind Mr. Muckraker, whose approach with his white cane struck terror into the greengrocer, who knew he would soon have to rebuild his mound of kumquats. The most prized of the mobility activities of daily living (ADL) is operating a motor vehicle. Here, the integrity of the visual fields is of paramount importance. Ranking a close second (among visual factors in driving) is far-point depth perception. Acuity, the only visual function routinely measured for licensure, is of somewhat lesser importance. Many sports activities also call for good far-point depth perception, for example, catching or hitting a ball and target shooting.

Near-point visual ADL include reading, working with numbers and charts, and maintaining eye contact in interpersonal situations. At near point, *acuity* (seeing detail clearly) and *accommodative skill* (ability to adjust focus) are especially important, for instance, in assembly work in a factory. Under- and over-reaching are also common visually related problems. However, unless one is a surgeon, sculptor, or welder, depth perception at near point is not likely to be a major factor in daily living.

Clinically, near-point vision becomes more significant when one is confined to a wheelchair, especially in the early stages of recovery when overall mobility is limited. It is unfortunate that the far-point acuity chart is the standard first step in testing vision and in some rehabilitation facilities is the only step. One acute medical rehabilitation setting had a policy that *near-point refractions* (optical corrections for poor near-point acuity) were only to be done in the outpatient clinic. Hence, while people were inpatients and most likely to be in a wheelchair, their most significant visual acuity needs were given the least attention! The occupational therapist's finely tuned appreciation of functional needs is frequently required to counter such policies.

Metavision

Remarkable as is the automaticity of visual system function, a negative aspect exists, namely, a lack of awareness of how one's own visual system is functioning (or, more significantly, *not* functioning). In other cognitive domains there is *metacognition*, meaning a person has knowledge about his or her own cognition. In the domain of memory, for example, it is metamemory that suggests that one might not remember something and should, therefore, write a note or apply some other mnemonic technique. In vision, by extension, we can speak of metavision. Let us take a minute to develop this concept and to show why it is important.

The human visual system is very sensitive to glare. Glare causes people to take such actions as wearing dark glasses, limiting driving, and going to the eye doctor for help. When it comes to glare, in other words, the human visual system is very well tuned. The opposite is true for several other visual functions, including oculomotor dysfunction, accommodation problems, and, especially, visual field losses. In the latter instance, the human system has a tendency to fill in the gaps to complete the image. The best example is the physiological blind spot associated with the area where the optic nerve exits the retina. This area is one of total blindness and is about the size of a fist at arms length. What is interesting is that, although we all have such blind spots, we are not aware of them. One can demonstrate that these areas exist (see Figure 8.1), but people do not experience them as missing, blank, or empty spots.

L   R

Figure 8.1 A demonstration of the physiological blind spot. Instructions:
1. Hold at arm's length.
2. Close your left eye.
3. Look at the L with your right eye.
4. Slowly bring the page towards you.
5. Keep looking at the L, but notice what happens to the R.
6. At some point you will realize that the R is no longer visible.
7. Keep moving the paper closer and the R will reappear.
8. Repeat the process with the other eye.

Notice: Although the letter disappears, the paper does not. This phenomenon is known as the *completion effect*. The brain fills in gaps in the visual field with predictable patterns or surfaces.

Clinically, substantial visual field losses can exist yet the individual will staunchly deny that any visual problem exists, all the while complaining that things get in the way or that they cannot be found. People may report symptoms, such as headaches, frustration, and difficulty concentrating, but do not connect these symptoms with underlying visual dysfunction. Vision problems can cause behavioral symptoms like anger secondary to frustration and misattribution, similar to the case of a person who is hard of hearing but complains that everyone is mumbling. Accommodation problems can be experienced as frustration when attempting certain activities like watching a moving object come toward you or maneuvering in visually stimulating environments.

The person with a visual field loss often has a dual disability: the loss of vision and a lack of awareness thereof (metavision). People who are unaware of a partial loss of vision will feel little need to compensate.

Impact of Hidden Visual System Dysfunction

Unappreciated or underappreciated visual system problems will often appear as frustration or inability to sustain a work effort. For example, difficulty with sustained near-point work such as reading and studying may be reported as an inability to concentrate, resulting in avoidance or dislike of such activities. Clinically, it is easy to miss breakdowns in visual system functioning that are brought on by extended use. Some such instances may even be diagnosed as attention deficit disorder. However, one can often infer visual problems from self-report and observations.

On a social level, relations can be disrupted by poor eye contact, especially when the two eyes are not aligned. A person who bumps into people in a crowd because of a visual field loss may be regarded as rude. Similarly, poor acuity can impede facial recognition.

How Do You Know What to Expect?

Occupational therapy is a clinical endeavor in which it is important to know what kinds of individuals are at risk for which kinds of visual system breakdown. All such diagnoses will fall under the umbrella of *acquired brain injury* (ABI). *Acquired* means that the person began neurological development normally but that something happened to bring about brain injury. *Injury* includes, but is not restricted to, *traumatic brain injury* (TBI). *Stroke* (cerebrovascular accident or CVA) is a very common form of ABI and is third in the list of life-threatening conditions (after heart disease and cancer) prevalent in the United States. Anoxia (often caused by near drowning, near electrocution, attempted suicide, and surgical mishap) and brain infections belong in the ABI category, as do chronic debilitating disorders of the central nervous system such as multiple sclerosis, Lyme disease, and AIDS-related encephalopathy. Much of the author's experience is with the nonprogressive forms of brain injury; these will be the focus of the discussion in this chapter. It is likely, however, that the same principles will apply to debilitating progressive conditions as well.

Some empirical data on the incidence of different kinds of problems are offered by Gianutsos, Perlin, and Ramsey (1988); however, a more comprehensive study with systematic sampling of different etiologies and controls for medication side effects is clearly needed. On the basis of clinical experience, people with TBI are likely to have accommodative problems, binocular dysfunction, and eye movement dysfunctions, while people after having a CVA are more likely to experience losses in the fields of vision. Patterns of incidence and underlying neuropathology notwithstanding, in the rehabilitation clinic all kinds of visual problems need to be investigated.

In the author's opinion, visual field impairment is the most disruptive to the safe and effective performance of ADL. Diller and Weinberg (1970) have documented falls and other mishaps following visual field loss or neglect. The safety factor is compounded by impaired metavision—the individuals frequently do not perceive a problem. By underestimating their visual loss and overestimating their ability to compensate, for example, people with visual field losses often do not anticipate any difficulty with driving.

People with TBI are much more likely to have problems with the dynamics of visual system function—anything that involves the muscles

in and around the eye, including maintaining fixation, pursuit and saccadic eye movements, accommodation of the lens to different focal distances, and maintaining binocular alignment. Eye movement dysfunction
and incoordination in the use of both eyes may often lead to patient
reports of headaches, difficulty keeping the eyes focused, dizziness, and
balance problems. Accommodative insufficiency or infacility is often
manifest as frustration; while binocular dysfunction will result in inability
to sustain visual work. When driving, accommodative problems make it
difficult to shift focus from the road ahead down to the dashboard and
back. Binocular dysfunction often brings on road fatigue. These problems
can be devastating and may be misunderstood or misinterpreted. Recognition of the problem is often itself therapeutic, and it is crucial that such
patients receive a visual evaluation by an optometrist who has expertise
in rehabilitation.

Current Practices and What Is Needed

Acute Medical Care

In the acute medical setting, eye care is typically ophthalmological. For
people who have survived brain injury, the emphasis is on the immediate
effects of the trauma with an evaluation of the patient's ocular health
(e.g., eye infections, detached retinas, cataracts), distance visual acuity,
and refraction. Neuro-ophthalmologists address the neurological integrity
of the visual system and will order tests to help localize injury. However,
the author's experience is that in the United States ophthalmologists are
rarely trained, experienced, or interested in visual system rehabilitation
or function. In medical settings, the commonly held presumption that
ophthalmologists offer complete eye care for rehabilitation patients needs
to be addressed. Important as ophthalmologists are, their specialty shares
little with brain injury rehabilitation.

Optometry

In the United States optometrists are eye doctors (doctors of optometry,
or ODs) who have completed a four-year postgraduate training curricu-

lum that addresses all aspects of eye health and function. An increasing number of optometrists have experience and interest in rehabilitation, which represents a natural extension of the emphasis within optometry on visual function and training (Cohen & Rein, 1992). We can offer some practical suggestions for developing a list of referrals that will take you beyond the yellow pages. In addition to local colleges of optometry, national professional associations such as the American Optometric Association and the Academy for the Advancement of Optometry are such a source for referrals. Specialty organizations exist within optometry for optometrists who have particular concerns with rehabilitation and training. Members of the College of Optometrists in Vision Development (COVD), the Neuro-Optometric Rehabilitation Association (NORA), and the Optometric Extension Program (OEP) are likely to have experience and interest in treating people who have survived brain injury. Similarly, optometrists who have expertise in low vision, vision therapy, or behavioral optometry may be helpful. Contact information for these organizations is given in the Resources at the end of this chapter.

Perhaps the ideal setting for outpatient rehabilitation optometric services is a specialized clinic like the Head Trauma Vision Rehabilitation Unit at the State University of New York State College of Optometry in New York City. Here several optometrists and a neuropsychologist (the author) work as an integrated team. Each patient is given a thorough eye exam, addressing both near- and far-point acuity, eye health, eye movements and binocular function, visual fields, and perception. This evaluation can be followed with specialty evaluations of eye movements, low vision, and functional visual fields. Interventions include not only conventional spectacle correction but also various kinds of prismatic lenses, vision training, and computerized exercises. It is hoped more such treatment centers will become available in the future, and a logical way to look for one is by contacting your nearest college of optometry.

Many head injury rehabilitation facilities have developed relationships with individual optometrists in their community. In some instances, the optometrist makes rounds within the facility, and in other cases arrangements are made for the patients to go to the optometrist's office.

Finding a suitable optometrist and developing a collaborative relationship takes time and effort (Gianutsos & Ramsey, 1988). Interest and flexibility are important; experience, though highly desirable, may be a luxury. When approached, most optometrists will be quite receptive. However, some kinds of optometric practices are not likely to prove suitable, for example, large practices in which much pretesting is done by technicians, or where a heavy emphasis is placed on contact lenses.

Finding an optometrist may involve helping an optometrist in general practice to work with people who have survived brain injury. Typically, little explicit training is offered in the general optometric curriculum for rehabilitative optometry. The occupational therapist should not be bashful about offering help and feedback to the optometrist. If the optometrist is responsive to this input, it bodes well for the collaboration between the occupational therapist and the optometrist and, ultimately, for the patient. Not all optometrists will show a special interest in or talent for working with people who have survived brain injury. Sometimes it will be necessary to find another eye care professional who will work with these people.

The single most useful question to ask is, How often have you worked with people who have survived brain injury (TBI, stroke, etc.) in the last year? If the answer is not at all, then you have to consider the alternatives, as well as try to assess the professional's receptivity to your input. A doctor who listens and communicates well can often make up for limited experience.

A few patients need to be seen at home or in the hospital. Although this may limit the tools the optometrist has at hand, many optometrists will extend themselves to meet this need. Institutional settings may have a home-care program for this purpose. If you are asking an optometrist to go into a hospital or nursing home, you will have to obtain the facility's permission. Most hospitals will offer optometrists privileges, although this practice is not yet common. Some optometrists are eager for this kind of medical recognition, and the occupational therapist may be able to lend support from within the medical setting.

Rehabilitative Optometric Consultation—Sooner or Later

Underdiagnosis and consequent lack of treatment are significant problems in brain injury rehabilitation. For example, the Gianutsos, Perlin, and Ramsey (1988) study found that half of the residents in a long-term head injury rehabilitation center had significant, yet mostly treatable, visual system dysfunction. Each of those patients had been in at least one other hospital, and most were many months post-onset. Despite this care, their visual problems were undiagnosed and most likely would have remained so if we had not done our vision screening. These visual problems would have persisted, unrecognized and undermining the intensive rehabilitative efforts in other areas. We can speculate on why this happens: Acute care is rendered in medical settings where eye care is focused on disease and eye health rather than on visual system function. Not all eye exams are alike.

Further, because some people do not experience visual disorders for what they are (the metavision problem), they do not articulate their concerns or seek help. For this reason, one should not wait for the patient to complain of a visual field problem: Aggressive evaluation is needed because of the safety implications of visual field problems combined with a total or partial lack of awareness.

A final consideration is the cost efficiency of rehabilitation optometric services. The evaluation itself may involve two or three office visits. In the majority of cases, treatment may be limited to one or two sets of lenses. Even if custom-made lenses are needed, these are a relatively small expense, especially in view of the advantage the lenses convey for other therapies. In my clinical experience, I have seen many people who went through comprehensive rehabilitation with poor acuity, balance problems caused by untreated binocular dysfunction, and inability to sustain a work effort and concentrate because of binocular system dysfunction. One can only speculate how much quicker these people would have completed their therapies had their visual dysfunction been recognized and treated earlier.

Professionals often disagree on when to initiate rehabilitation optometric services. Logically, the earlier it is begun, the better. Gianutsos, Perlin,

Mazerolle, and Trem (1989) state that rehabilitation optometric services can be offered even to persons who are in coma. Sometimes the argument is made that the visual problems may resolve spontaneously and that rehabilitation optometric services should be deferred for up to 6 months. This argument fails to take into account the fact that without treatment patients may adapt in an ultimately undesirable manner. For example, to deal with double vision, people learn to squint or adopt other ways to suppress visual input from one eye. They become functionally monocular and lose the three-dimensional awareness most efficiently achieved by binocularity. Waiting 6 months for visual problems to resolve or stabilize makes as much sense as waiting 6 months to see if patients who have had a stroke can learn to walk again before doing a physical therapy evaluation.

What Occupational Therapists Can Do

Occupational therapists situated in acute and rehabilitative care settings have a key role to play in drawing attention to the possible presence of visual problems and facilitating optometric diagnosis and treatment. Occupational therapists can also provide follow-up activities that give individuals the opportunity to use vision functionally after participating in optometric exercises. (For more detailed discussions on this topic, readers may refer to the following sources: Arnsten, 1994; Bouska & Gallaway, 1991; Bouska, Kauffman, & Marcus, 1990; Gianutsos et al., 1988; Hellerstein & Freed, 1994; Suter, 1995; Warren, 1990; Warren, 1993a; Warren, 1993b; Warren, 1994).

Occupational therapists have taken a leading role in bringing visual problems after brain injury into focus. The author remembers well the workshop Clinical Vision Assessment by the late Mary Jane Bouska that became a professional turning point for her and for many others in the field. In this course, practical methods for vision screening were offered, along with guidelines for working with optometrists. Some years later a similar presentation by Laurie Ritter, OTR/L, and Joel Warshowsky, OD, attracted several hundred therapists.

Not only do occupational therapists need to communicate with each other about vision after brain injury, but they also need to communicate with other professionals with expertise in brain injury rehabilitation. Unless an occupational therapist speaks up, the physicians who manage acute care often may not appreciate the relationship between vision and functional activities. Further, medical doctors are likely to prescribe ophthalmological services unless an occupational therapist conveys the need for a *functional* rehabilitative orientation. Neuropsychologists, especially those trained in clinical psychology, may have very little training in clinical vision assessment. They may acknowledge visual problems but not take them seriously enough even to ask for, or look for, a patient's glasses before launching into their assessment.

One way to assure that vision is addressed properly is to develop policies and procedures that mandate that visual problems be carefully addressed, including local screening, consultation with appropriate eye-care practitioners and systematic follow through on treatment recommendations.

Occupational Therapy Vision Screening

For the therapist, the beginning of the clinical process is a good time to begin vision screening with questions concerning the patient's ability to perform functional tasks requiring visual skills such as reading, shopping in stores, and locating items. Attention should be given to headaches and dizziness following certain activities. The formal assessment includes near and far acuities, binocular function, visual fields, and perception. Many of these issues can be addressed at the bedside with simple tools and good clinical skill. However, for many patients a stereoscopic vision screener, such as the Keystone VSII, Titmus, or Stereo-Optical vision testers, can provide needed answers in a few minutes. I would also recommend computerized testing of the functional visual fields, which can be done using software I have developed (PERFIELD and CENFIELD, available through Life Science Associates, Bayport, NY).

The primary purpose of this screening is to rule out visual problems, if possible. If the possibility of any such problems is present, expeditious referral to an optometrist is in order. Extensive vision screening is rarely appropriate in suburban and urban settings where an eye care professional may be available. An important purpose of the occupational therapy vision screening is to offer a timely alert to the existence of problems and to serve as a basis for an informed referral. Screening not only identifies referrals for rehabilitative optometric services, but it also helps the occupational therapist ascertain that the relevant vision issues have been addressed. For example, in a hospital cited earlier, eye care was the responsibility of the ophthalmology department, which had a policy of doing near-point refractions only on outpatients. Using their own screening data that showed problems with near-point vision, occupational therapists were able to convince the ophthalmology service to be responsive to the near-vision needs of the inpatients undergoing brain injury rehabilitation.

Occupational therapy screening for visual system dysfunction is used primarily to identify those patients who can benefit from referral for rehabilitative optometric services. An additional benefit is that visual screening can begin the process of educating patients about the current status of their visual system. This educational process is especially important because visual disorders are often not obvious to the person who has the problem—the issue of metavision discussed earlier.

Is Occupational Therapy Vision Screening Always Necessary?

I believe that every person who has survived brain injury should be evaluated optometrically. The thoroughness and type of occupational therapy vision screening will, of course, depend on the kinds of other services available. If optometrists are an integral part of the treating team, it might constitute an unnecessary duplication of services to require comprehensive occupational therapy vision screening first. In such an ideal situation, the occupational therapy evaluation would emphasize the functional impact of visual system problems.

Over the years, my clinical experience suggests that rarely can nonoptometric vision screenings be relied on to rule out visual problems. In Gianutsos et al. (1988), mentioned earlier, approximately half of the cases screened were determined to have some problem warranting rehabilitative optometric services. All but one of those sent for rehabilitation optometric services were determined to have visual system problems, most of which were ameliorated by treatment. Our high hit rate probably made the administrators happy: Few unnecessary consultations for rehabilitation optometric services were made. What we must be concerned about, especially in view of the high hit rate, is the possibility that our screening misses someone who has visual problems. If any doubt exists that a rehabilitation optometric services consultation is in order; it is always preferable to have an optometrist rule out any need for treatment.

Information the Occupational Therapist Gathers to Be Helpful to the Optometrist

This information ranges from the practical (special methods of communication, toileting needs and ability to transfer, the reliability of the patient as an informant, medications) to the more interpretive (such as underlying visual problems being mistaken for patient inattention). Is a visual problem accounting for what appears to be an aphasic reading disorder? Are there visual problems that might interfere with this person's ability to drive safely? The therapist should describe the behaviors observed that indicate a possible vision problem, for example, Ms. X sits very close to the television; Mr. Y holds his head askew when reading. A behavioral observation record form, such as the one in Gianutsos and Ramsey (1988), might be useful and has been reproduced in Figure 8.2.

A clear list of medications and suspected side effects is helpful. For each medication the person is taking, the occupational therapist can use the Optometric Drug Information Summaries (ODIS) software database (Levine, 1993) to determine effects and side effects on the visual system. Several classes of medications taken by people who have survived brain injury have visual side effects, including anticonvulsant (antiseizure) and antispasticity medications, antipsychotics, and tranquilizers. Some of these can be substituted for and some cannot. It is important for the optometrist to know what medication is being taken and for what purpose. Ask the optometrist to review and comment on the list of medications. The occupational therapist can be helpful in facilitating the interdis-

CHECKLIST: Vision Problems

Name _____ Date _____ Therapist _____
(Adapted from *The Primary Visual Abilities Essential to Academic Achievement*,
Optometric Extension Program Foundation, Inc., Santa Ana CA, 1968.)

Rating Codes: Typ = typical pattern
               Obs = observed
               NO = not observed
               IO = insufficient opportunity to observe

	Typ	Obs	NO	IO
1. APPEARANCE OF EYES:				
One eye turns in or out at any time	—	—	—	—
Reddened eyes or lids	—	—	—	—
Eyes tear excessively	—	—	—	—
Encrusted eyelids	—	—	—	—
Frequent styes on lids	—	—	—	—
2. COMPLAINTS WHEN USING EYES FOR CLOSE WORK:				
Headaches in forehead or temples	—	—	—	—
Burning or itching after reading or close work	—	—	—	—
Nausea or dizziness	—	—	—	—
Print blurs after reading a short time	—	—	—	—
3. BEHAVIORAL SIGNS OF VISUAL PROBLEMS:				
A. *Eye Movement Abilities (Ocular Motility):*				
Head turns while scanning, e.g., as reads across page	—	—	—	—
Loses place often during reading	—	—	—	—
Needs finger or marker to keep place	—	—	—	—
Displays short attention span, e.g., in reading or copying	—	—	—	—
Too frequently omits words	—	—	—	—
Repeatedly omits "small" words	—	—	—	—
Writes up or down hill on paper	—	—	—	—
Rereads or skips lines unknowingly	—	—	—	—
Orients drawings poorly on page	—	—	—	—
B. *Eye Teaming Abilities (Binocularity):*				
Complains of seeing double (diplopia)	—	—	—	—
Repeats letters within words	—	—	—	—
Omits letters, numbers or phrases	—	—	—	—
Misaligns digits in number columns	—	—	—	—
Squints, closes, or covers one eye	—	—	—	—
Tilts head extremely while doing close work	—	—	—	—
Consistently shows gross postural deviations in close work activities	—	—	—	—

	Typ	Obs	NO	IO
C. *Eye-Hand Coordination Abilities:*				
Must feel things to assist in any interpretation required	—	—	—	—
Eyes not used to "steer" hand movements (extreme lack of orientation, placement of words or drawings on page)	—	—	—	—
Writes crookedly, poorly spaced, cannot stay on ruled lines	—	—	—	—
Misaligns both horizontal and vertical series of numbers	—	—	—	—
Uses his hand or fingers to keep his place on the page	—	—	—	—
Uses other hand as "spacer" to control spacing or alignment on page	—	—	—	—
Repeatedly confuses left-right directions	—	—	—	—

Figure 8.2 Behavioral checklist of symptoms of visual system dysfunction.

Figure 8.2 *Continued.*

	Typ	Obs	NO	IO
D. *Visual Form Perception (Visual Comparison, Visual Imagery, Visualization):*				
Mistakes words with same or similar beginnings	—	—	—	—
Fails to recognize same word in next sentence	—	—	—	—
Reverses letters and/or words in writing and copying	—	—	—	—
Confuses likenesses and minor differences	—	—	—	—
Confuses same word in same sentence	—	—	—	—
Repeatedly confuses similar beginnings and endings of words	—	—	—	—
Fails to visualize what is read either silently or orally	—	—	—	—
Whispers to self for reinforcement while reading silently	—	—	—	—
Returns to "drawing with fingers" to decide likes and differences	—	—	—	—
E. *Refractive Status (Nearsightedness, Farsightedness, Focus Problems, etc.):*				
Comprehension reduces as reading continues; loses interest too quickly	—	—	—	—
Mispronounces similar words as reading continues	—	—	—	—
Blinks excessively at near vision tasks (i.e. reading) and not elsewhere	—	—	—	—
Holds book too closely; face too close to desk surface/ computer screen	—	—	—	—
Avoids near-point tasks or close-up work	—	—	—	—
Complains of discomfort in tasks that demand visual interpretation	—	—	—	—
Closes, covers, or squints one eye while reading or doing close work	—	—	—	—
Makes errors in copying information from the distance to paper (e.g. copying a sign from the wall)	—	—	—	—
Makes errors copying from reference book to notebook	—	—	—	—
Squints (e.g. to read signs on the wall) or requests to move nearer	—	—	—	—
Rubs eyes during or after short periods of visual activity	—	—	—	—
Fatigues easily; after doing close work blinks to clarify distance information (e.g., sign on the wall)	—	—	—	—

OBSERVER'S COMMENTS:

ciplinary process by communicating to other team members the visual side effects of a person's medications.

The occupational therapist is often able to obtain historical information regarding the patient's vision. A good place to begin is with the eyeglasses the patient wore before the injury. Look around. Ask the family to bring in the patient's glasses from home. If you cannot find the glasses, you can often find the relevant records with a phone call to the former eye doctor. These records contain useful information that will be appreciated by the current eye doctor. If available, the old lenses are probably a better interim solution (pending an optometric consultation) than no lenses. Unless the patient appears to reject the lenses, the glasses belong on the patient, not in the bedside table.

Eye doctors have a device that allows them to determine the prescribed correction in a pair of eyeglasses. Pending optometric consultation, the ability to infer what conditions a given pair of lenses was intended to treat is helpful when looking at the glasses last worn by a comatose patient.

The following techniques are useful for reading a pair of eyeglasses:

• If the lenses magnify the image, they correct for farsightedness (hyperopia) or are reading lenses for a person over 40 years old, perhaps with presbyopia.

• If the lenses minify, they correct for nearsightedness (myopia). If you are not sure, try moving the lenses from side to side. If the image moves with the lenses, the lenses are minifying—they are minus lens power and are meant to correct for nearsightedness. Conversely, if the image moves against the lens, the lenses are magnifying—they are plus lenses and probably correct for hyperopia or presbyopia. This basic magnification or minification is the spherical correction in the lens.

• In some cases, the correction may be cylindrical or, loosely speaking, correcting for a warped (or astigmatic) eye. Correction for astigmatism appears as distortion when you rotate the lens one at a time. Subjectively, astigmatism may not produce any obvious impairment, although an astigmat who is accustomed to corrective lenses may feel out of sorts and experience eye fatigue.

• Older people often need a different correction for near- and far-point activities. Bifocal lenses are the traditional approach. In recent years, progressive lenses have become common in which the near-point correction (or add) is incremental in the lower portion of the lens. This can complicate the techniques described above for reading lenses. A good idea is to practice on lenses that have a known correction, for example, over-the-counter reading glasses are plus spheres with no astigmatic correction.

• Lenses that have prisms ground in are more complicated. If you look at the lens sideways, you will see that the lens is thicker on one side and thinner on the other. The thick side is the base of the prism, and the effect is to displace the image toward the thin side, away from the base.

The Optometric Consultation

It is especially helpful for the occupational therapist to accompany the patient to the optometrist. This experience is often an excellent learning opportunity, as well as a good way to develop lines of communication with the eye doctor. The occupational therapist sometimes has to serve as an interpreter, both for the patient to the optometrist and for the optometrist to the patient and concerned others. While often receptive to rehabilitation needs, optometrists may have little experience. They usually are very interested and feel rewarded by the opportunity to learn and to be helpful. However, they may need to be alerted to the special problems of the person who has experienced ABI (e.g., poor memory), so always back up oral recommendations with written ones.

During the session, the accompanying occupational therapist should make notes and be available for clarification and assistance if the optometrist and the patient have a communication problem. Remember that the patient is the one getting the consultation. Sometimes the eye doctor forgets this; you should encourage direct communication with the patient. Be a facilitator and a scribe. Even patients who do not have memory problems are likely to appreciate having someone to make notes on their behalf.

The occupational therapist can be helpful in discussing the implications of proposed treatment options. For example, it may not be a good time to introduce bifocals when the person is becoming ambulatory again. The near-point correction in the lower portion of the lens may interfere with monitoring the path ahead. It takes time to adjust to bifocals; following a brain injury this adjustment may be difficult. In some cases, two pairs of glasses (one for reading and one for distance) may be recommended—unless the patient's memory is very poor or the patient cannot change glasses easily. Progressive lenses can be of special value when the patient's medical condition warrants, and when the amount of near-point lens power varies.

Whatever decisions are made, the occupational therapist should make clear notes including who is responsible for what. In collaboration with the optometrist, the occupational therapist can assist by explaining (in writing as well as orally) the findings and recommendations to family and concerned others (e.g., the treating team, the school). When the occupational therapist has made notes regarding the evaluation and recommendations, it is a good idea to have the optometrist review the notes for accuracy and emphasis.

Optometric Interventions After the Optometric Consultation

In rehabilitation, interventions generally fall into one of three categories: (a) restorative exercises, (b) compensatory devices and techniques, and (c) environmental redesign. The discussion below concerns interventions for visual system dysfunction. For other areas you should consult textual material in those areas. For example, in the field of cognitive rehabilitation an excellent text by Sohlberg and Mateer (1989) contains innumerable practical suggestions for interventions.

Restorative Exercises

Within optometry, restorative approaches are usually subsumed under the title, vision therapy. It is important to appreciate that these exercises are often not designed to strengthen weak muscles; rather they are techniques or activities that are used to maximize coordination in the visual system through speed and automaticity. Many of these exercises use simple devices, the most elegant of which is the Brock String. This "device" is a piece of string from 3 to 20 feet long with three colored beads. Several tasks can be devised, including fixating on one bead and monitoring to see if the patient sees two lines that appear to cross at the bead itself. Your patient may need a little extra reminding about the purpose of this exercise (focusing and maintaining an image with both eyes). The optometrist may ask the patient to move the bead closer, while maintaining images in both eyes (both lines remain visible) and crossed at the bead (otherwise the eyes are not focusing on the bead). Advanced Brock String exercises involve shifting focus from one bead to another, while simultaneously maintaining vision in both eyes.

People who have survived brain injury may need to be guided through these exercises with careful monitoring because they may lapse into bad habits, such as suppressing vision in one eye so that only one line is seen. Structure is often helpful, such as a checklist to keep count of how many times the exercise is done. If one is supposed to hold a fixation on a target, the therapist may suggest counting out loud.

The Brock String needs to be adapted for use with hemiparetics, who cannot hold the string to the bridge of their nose and move the bead at the same time. Here, a baseball cap put on backwards can be helpful. Tie the string around the plastic fastener and wear the hat pulled down to the bridge of the nose.

As with any exercise program, it is helpful to show interest. Keeping scores helps in this regard; the score sheet is something the therapist can examine with great interest. Bear in mind that exercises sometimes do not produce instantaneous or substantial results. All, however, is not lost: The process of doing exercises with feedback should at least improve the individual's metavision. Perhaps the best example of this is in the case of training visual field awareness using REACT (Reaction Time Measure of Visual Field; Gianutsos, 1988). In this task the individual monitors the computer screen for numbers that can appear suddenly on any part of the screen. The numbers are actually counters; so when a response is finally made, the response time is displayed, offering immediate feedback. Patients find it useful to practice with this task, attempting to compensate for delayed processing on their affected side. Often they discover the limits of their ability to compensate. Although this exercise does not solve the underlying visual field problem, it does give information necessary to manage the problem. (Remember, visual field losses are often not experienced as such.)

The occupational therapist can help with many vision exercises. Some exercises require special equipment, although computers are used increasingly for exercises, for example, those listed in the Resources at the end of this chapter. As the relationship with the optometrist grows, the occupational therapist may become increasingly active. Susan Arnsten, an occupational therapist specializing in vision, illustrates this occupational therapy role in her article "Vision Therapy Within Occupational Therapy" (1994). It is even possible for an occupational therapist to become a vision therapist, working under the direction of an optometrist (see chapter 4, COVTT).

If the software is available in the occupational therapist's clinic, offer the patient an opportunity to do the exercises during therapy sessions, enabling more frequent practice in a location where the patient is already going to be. Many exercises within occupational therapy address visual perception. Some of these will bear a close similarity to the optometric exercises, especially those that emphasize visual perception.

In their zeal to be helpful, therapists need to recognize that the optometrist has overall responsibility and authority for the vision therapy program. Much as the occupational therapist operates under prescription from a physician, in the area of vision the optometrist prescribes. In most states an optometric practice act legally defines the activities that are the responsibility of optometry. A key feature of optometric practice is placing lenses in front of a patient's eyes. Strictly speaking, this would include anaglyph (red-green/blue) glasses used to dissociate images to each eye, use of a stereoscopic vision screener, and over-the-counter reading glasses (useful in the clinic for testing, especially when patients forget to bring their glasses). Some optometrists are comfortable with therapists using these devices on a temporary basis; however, the occupational therapist should always work closely with the optometrist.

Compensatory Devices

The compensatory device that we are all familiar with is eyeglasses, or spectacle correction for refractive (optical) error. This treatment is commonplace, but the occupational therapist can still be helpful. When spectacles have been prescribed, the occupational therapist can contribute to further decisions. For example, if more than one pair of glasses is to be made, each pair should be distinctly different, and the purpose indicated clearly on the lens case if not on the frames themselves. The occupational therapist can assist in obtaining a spectacle case that can be placed in an accessible and secure location. For a hemiplegic, spring loaded frames can be of special benefit. Otherwise, frames will easily get pulled out of alignment by being donned and doffed with only one hand.

Sometimes lenses do not produce an immediate sense of satisfaction. This may be an indication that the glasses were not filled or fitted properly. The doctor may also advise that it is to be expected and to use the glasses for a designated period of time and to observe performance. In either situation, the occupational therapist should monitor the situation and communicate with the optometrist so corrective action is not unnecessarily delayed. In general, the occupational therapist should monitor adherence to the treatment plan and encourage optometric follow-up sooner than originally planned, if needed.

Prisms

Prismatic correction refers to the use of optical correction to displace the image. This approach can be done (a) to treat an eye turn or deviation, (b) to bring an unseen portion of the visual field into a seeing area, or (c) to induce postural improvements. We shall discuss each of these.

When the eyes do not align on a particular target at the same time (strabismus) or do not converge and aim outward (exophoria or exotropia), or when they turn in (esophoria or esotropia), prismatic lenses can help bring the eyes close enough so that they can complete the alignment process. Here the prism in one eye is going the opposite direction from the prism in the other eye. Occasionally, a small amount of magnification will accomplish the same thing. The point here is that prisms are being used to facilitate the coordinated use of both eyes, or to achieve binocularity. This use of prisms is fairly standard.

Other uses of prisms are not so conventional, including the use of prisms for increased visual field awareness. Here prisms are yoked, that is, both eyes have prisms directed in the same way. So if a person has a left *homonymous hemianopia* (lost vision in the left half of each eye), base left prisms might be used to bring the image from the left into the right field. It is important for the therapist to check this out: it would not be the first time that an occupational therapist discovered a prismatic correction going in the opposite direction.

Another use for yoked prisms is for postural adjustment. This is a creative application pioneered by optometrist William Padula, which takes advantage of the primacy of vision over other senses (see chapter 9). The idea is to modify vision in such a way as to induce a postural correction. For example, if lenses make it look as if you are tilting to one side, you will adjust yourself accordingly. A patient who slouches can be induced to sit up in this manner. We had a patient who was a long-term head injury survivor. For a variety of reasons, he tended to lurch backwards on his heels and had fallen backwards on several occasions. Because of a severe memory, frontal lobe, and attentional disorder, he was unable to learn to compensate by leaning forward without constant prompting. Base-up prisms (which gave him the sensation of walking downhill) required that he pitch his head forward in order to look where he was stepping and indirectly enhanced his stability. The dilemma was that within 2 weeks this benefit had vanished. He did somewhat better alternating between his prismatic lenses and his old glasses—an alteration introduced to prevent a chronic adjustment to the prisms. Occupational therapists should be aware that prisms do not always have an enduring effect. Observation of the temporary nature of the prisms' effects is more likely to take place by an occupational therapist, who may see the patient more frequently, than by the optometrist. If this is the case, the occupational therapist should encourage the patient to return to the optometrist or inform the optometrist directly of any problem encountered.

Prismatic correction can be implemented in two ways: (a) ground prismatic lenses and (b) Fresnel prisms. Ground prismatic lenses are a customized optical correction that usually requires extra time and expense. When the magnitude of the deviation is large, these lenses can be heavy and cosmetically unappealing. Fresnel prisms are used for temporary prismatic correction. They are made of plastic that is overlaid, so if one runs a fingernail across, serrations are obvious. The smooth side is pressed onto the individual's eyeglasses. They cling to the lenses with a good, clean bond. Fresnel prisms are instantaneous and relatively inexpensive; however, they get dirty easily and then the clarity of transmission of light is reduced. Furthermore, they are not subtle: other people will definitely notice, which becomes a problem for patients who are very self-conscious.

What can the occupational therapist do to be helpful when a patient has Fresnel prisms? Probably the most useful thing is to help the patient keep them clean. Also, if the Fresnel prism does not cover the lens, it may slip out of position: the occupational therapist can monitor and rectify slippage. Because they are easily shaped, Fresnel lenses have been used to create a kind of spot viewer to compensate for hemianopic field losses (Perlin & Dziadul, 1991). Here the positioning is especially important. Finally, the occupational therapist can reinforce the Fresnel prisms' advantages and help the patient persevere, or help the patient recognize the options, for example, time and expense versus clarity and appearance.

Reversing Mirror

An optical approach to dealing with visual field loss is a wedge-like mirror mounted on the inside of the lens (Cohen & Waiss, 1993a; Cohen & Waiss, 1993b). Not unlike a rearview mirror, this allows information from the nonseeing field to be brought into view. Reports describe clinical test cases with some enthusiasm; however, some patients reject the approach because of appearances. It is possible that the reversing mirror might be reserved for certain special circumstances, such as driving. This approach has not been proven, but it is certainly worth further investigation. In fact, no intervention for visual field loss has proven to be a spectacular success. Often, interventions are not appreciated because the individual fails to recognize that a problem exists.

Environmental Redesign

The final intervention strategy is to design the individual's environment to improve function. Here, the most basic issues apply, such as checking the home environment to be sure it is well illuminated and that things are located where they can be seen. Consider installing lighting that is activated by motion detectors. Good contrast is important in the home environment. Steps should be clearly delineated, particularly when binocular depth perception is poor. Large-print labels and color coding are helpful. Iconic (nonverbal) symbols are also more easily visible than verbal signs. However, the downside is that the individual has to remember what the symbols mean.

For profound homonymous hemianopic visual field impairments, one might consider placing important objects on the side where the person does see, as suggested by Zoltan (1983). This solution is simplistic but quite common. It is probably best when used to accomplish a specific end, such as rotating the dinner plate when the person has finished the right half of the meal to allow a view of the other half. This approach might be more promising from the standpoint of therapy if the patient learned to rotate his or her own plate.

Summary

Because of the occupational therapist's ability to determine how underlying deficits affect functional performance, the occupational therapist has an important role to play in assuring that persons who have survived brain injury receive appropriate diagnosis and treatment for the visual system dysfunction that often follows central nervous system injury. This is an opportunity to be active and interdisciplinary. The occupational therapist's unique emphasis on ADL is an important contribution to the overall process.

Acknowledgments

I am grateful to the following colleagues for reading and offering input on the manuscript: occupational therapists Susan Arnsten and Michele Gentile and optometrists Irwin Suchoff, Neera Kapoor, and Marie Marrone.

I remain inspired by the pioneering work of the late Mary Jane Bouska, OTR/L, who forged some of the earliest links between optometry and occupational therapy.

REFERENCES

Arnsten, S. (1994, December 9). Vision therapy within occupational therapy. *Occupational Therapy Forum, 411.*

Bouska, M. J., Kauffman, N., & Marcus, S. (1990). Disorders of the visual perceptual system. In D. Umphred (Ed.), *Neurological rehabilitation.* St. Louis, MO: Mosby.

Bouska, M. J., & Gallaway, M. (1991). Primary visual deficits in adults with brain damage: Management in occupational therapy. *Occupational Therapy Practice, 3,* 111.

Cohen, A. H., & Rein, L. D. (1992). The effect of head trauma on the visual system: The doctor of optometry as a member of the rehabilitation team. *Journal of the American Optometric Association, 63,* 530–536.

Cohen, J. M., & Waiss, B. (1993a). An overview of enhancement techniques for peripheral field loss. *Journal of the American Optometric Association, 64,* 60–70.

Cohen, J. M., & Waiss, B. (1993b). An overview of visual rehabilitation for stroke and head trauma patients. *Aging and Vision, 6,* 311.

Diller, L., & Weinberg, J. (1970). Evidence for accident-prone behavior in hemiplegic patients. *Archives of Physical Medicine and Rehabilitation, 51,* 358–363.

Gianutsos, R. (1988). Computer programs for cognitive rehabilitation (Vol. 5): Software tools for use with persons emerging from coma into consciousness [Computer software]. Bayport, NY: Life Science Associates.

Gianutsos, R., & Ramsey, G. (1988). Enabling the survivors of brain injury to receive rehabilitative optometric services. *Journal of Vision Rehabilitation, 2,* 37–58.

Gianutsos, R., Ramsey, G., & Perlin, G. (1988). Rehabilitative optometric services for survivors of acquired brain injury. *Archives of Physical Medicine and Rehabilitation, 69,* 573–578.

Gianutsos, R., Perlin, R., Mazerolle, K., & Trem, N. (1989). Rehabilitative optometric services for persons emerging from coma. *Journal of Head Trauma Rehabilitation, 4,* 1725.

Hellerstein, L. F., & Freed, S. (1994). Rehabilitative optometric management of a traumatic brain injury patient. *Journal of Behavioral Optometry, 5,* 143–148.

Levine, L. (1993). Optometric Drug Information Summaries [Computer software]. Forest Grove, OR: Pacific University.

Perlin, R. R., & Dziadul, J. (1991). Fresnel prisms for field enhancement of patients with constricted or hemianopic visual fields. *Journal of the American Optometric Association, 62,* 58–64.

Sohlberg, M. M., & Mateer, C. A. (1989). *Introduction to cognitive rehabilitation.* New York: Guilford Press.

Suter, P. (1995). Rehabilitation and management of visual dysfunction following traumatic brain injury. In M. J. Ashley & D. K. Krych (Eds.), *Traumatic brain injury rehabilitation* (pp. 187–219). Boca Raton, FL: CRC Press.

Warren, M. (1990). Identification of visual scanning deficits in adults after cerebrovascular accident. *American Journal of Occupational Therapy, 44,* 391–399.

Warren, M. (1993a). A hierarchical model for evaluation and treatment of visual perceptual dysfunction in adult acquired brain injury, Part 1. *American Journal of Occupational Therapy, 47,* 42–54.

Warren, M. (1993b). A hierarchical model for evaluation and treatment of visual perceptual dysfunction in adult acquired brain injury, Part 2. *American Journal of Occupational Therapy, 47,* 55–66.

Warren, M. (1994). *Visuospatial skills: Assessment and intervention strategies.* Bethesda, MD: American Occupational Therapy Association.

Zoltan, B. (1983). Remediation of visual-perceptual and perceptual-motor deficits. In M. Rosenthal, M. R. Bond, E. R. Griffith, & J. D. Miller (Eds.), *Rehabilitation of the adult and child with traumatic brain injury* (pp. 351–365). Philadelphia: F. A. Davis.

RESOURCES

American Vision Therapy, PO Box 197, Cicero, IN 46034, (800) 346-4925, Fax and local phone (317) 984-9400. [Groffman's Vision Therapy Programs; Cooper's Automated Vision Therapy Instruments]

Bernell Corporation, 750 Lincolnway East, PO Box 4637, South Bend, IN 46634-4637, (800) 348-2225. [Vogel's Computer Aided Vision Therapy]

Learning Frontiers, 175 Admiral Cochran Drive, Suite 103, Annapolis, MD 21401, (410) 266-8244. [Ludlum's OPTI-MUM System]

Dr. Leonard Levine, Pacific University, Forest Grove, OR 97116, (503) 357-6151. [ODIS Software]

Life Science Associates, 1 Fenimore Road, Bayport, NY 11705, (516) 472-2111. [Gianutsos' Computer Programs for Cognitive Rehabilitation/ PERFIELD, CENFIELD and PERCEPT]

Optometric Extension Program Foundation, Inc., 2912 South Daimler Street, Santa Ana, CA 92705, (714) 250-8070.

OPTOMETRIC ASSOCIATIONS

American Optometric Association (AOA), 243 N. Lindbergh Blvd., St. Louis, MO 63141.

American Academy of Optometry (AAO), 4330 East-West Highway, Suite 1117, Bethesda, MD 20814-4408.

Optometric Extension Program Foundation, Inc. (OEP), 2912 S. Daimler St., Santa Ana, CA 92705.

College of Optometrists in Vision Development (COVD), PO Box 285, Chula Vista, CA 92012.

Neuro-Optometric Rehabilitation Association (NORA), PO Box 1408, Guilford, CT 06437.

9 Visual Rehabilitation of the Neurologically Involved Person

Maureen Connor, OTR/L, and
William Padula, OD, FAAO

Introduction

The underlying theme of occupational therapy, frequently reinforced during the schooling of therapists, is one of *holism*. Holism is the process of treating the whole person and choosing therapeutic activities that have specific personal meaning to the patient. This approach to treatment is the cornerstone of the profession. Yet it has been the observation of the authors that in the face of the ever-changing, rapid-paced, and time-limited health care system, some clinicians resort to reductionistic views that limit seeing the patient as a whole person.

Health care clinicians in general have felt the need to reduce their focus and define specialties specifically to accommodate the complexity of the human body. The need for reductionism for detailed study and scientific understanding is evident. However, it is essential to continue to view the human system or systems as wholes, as the complexity of physiology gives us reason to believe that systems are somehow greater than their parts.

It is this perspective that requires the visual-perceptual function of the neurologically impaired patient be viewed in light of all the other systems with which it interacts. The observation of the authors is that therapists frequently do not focus enough on the profound relationship of vision and function. In general, optometrists and ophthalmologists tend to concentrate exclusively on oculomotor function and the health of the eyeball, optic nerve, and visual cortex. Both of these views demonstrate inherent limitations when attempting to assess the functional behavioral impairments of patients with posthead injury.

It is the purpose of this chapter to present the following: a working model of the visual process, a brief definition of neuro-optometric rehabilitation, the symptomatology of posttrauma vision syndrome (PTVS) and visual midline shift syndrome (VMSS), treatment approaches of both optometrists and therapists, some case examples, and some conclusions.

Central and Ambient Visual Processes: A Working Model of Vision

A model of vision as divided into two processes—the central and the ambient—will help qualify the further discussion of the interaction between vision and function. This model is described by Trevarthen (1968) and Leibowitz and Post (1982). The central or focal visual process involves that which we classically think of as seeing in both the real and anatomical senses. Through this focal system, the object of focalization, that is, the object being attended to, is seen in detail with acuity and color perception. Neurologically, the central processing begins at the macula, which is composed of cone cells responsible for high resolution and color detection, and progresses to the central areas of the visual cortex through the optic nerve. In contrast, spatial awareness and detection of movement are the primary purposes of the ambient system. The ambient process interrelates with the central visual process by providing the peripheral awareness required for a reference environment or background. This will spatially orient both the object of focus and the perceiver's body in space.

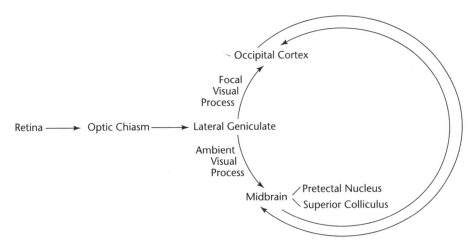

Figure 9.1 Neurological relationship of vision to occipital cortex and midbrain.

Many nerve cells originating from the eye send collateral fibers to other areas of the brain before reaching the highly organized seeing area in the cortex (see Figure 9.1). Trevarthen (1968) and Bishop et al. (1953) have concluded that the dorsal ganglion of the lateral geniculate body may function as an integrating center in addition to its role as a relay and distribution center. This means that the lateral geniculate is important for the relay of visual information to portions of the brain other than the visual cortex. The lateral geniculate body actively responds to diffuse illumination and any movement of light across the retina. Cortical cells respond to detail as well as specific axes of illumination on the retina. Ganglion cells emanate from the retina through the optic nerve and optic chiasm to the optic tract, where all the fibers synapse at the lateral geniculate body. At this point, axons are directed to the pretectal nucleus (pupillary constriction) and the superior colliculus, which importantly becomes related to posture, movement, and orientation to position in space (Wolfe, 1968). The superior colliculus receives fibers from the optic tract via the superior brachium and occipital cortex via the optic radiations through the lateral geniculate and from the spinotectal tract connecting it with sensorimotor information from the spinal cord and medulla.

The Ambient Visual System and the Sensorimotor Feedback Loop

The ambient visual process links with and becomes part of the sensorimotor feedback loop at the level of the midbrain. The matching of information that occurs between the ambient visual process and the kinesthetic, proprioceptive, vestibular, and tactile systems sets up a spatial framework that becomes the basis of higher sensory interpretation. The sensorimotor feedback loop involving the midbrain provides a feed forward system to areas of higher cortical function through receiving as well as sending fiber tracts to the occipital, temporal, parietal, and frontal cortexes (Nelson & Benabib, 1992). The superior colliculus receives a large quantity of axons in relationship to vision. Without the matching of information that occurs between the ambient process (including the vestibular ocular reflex) and the other portions of the sensorimotor feedback system, we would actually perceive an image as jumping and moving about each time we made a shift of our eyes or our body (Padula, 1996). The midbrain is responsible for providing information to the visual cortex about aligning and developing integration of the central images from both eyes.

Post Trauma Vision Syndrome (PTVS)

This working model for vision provides us with a perspective through which we can begin to assess and treat the functional deficits observed in patients with traumatic brain injury, CVA, or other neurological disorders. Those optometrists who have observed the functional behaviors of these patients and are treating the visual process with techniques that have been specifically found to be beneficial to this population have developed a specialty termed neuro-optometric rehabilitation. Optometrists practicing this specialty and other clinicians working in the field of neurologic rehabilitation have observed consistencies in the visual and motoric symptomatology of this population. Posttrauma vision syndrome as defined by Padula, Argyris, and Ray (1994) presents with consistent characteristics and symptoms.

Common Characteristics:

- Exotropia or high exophoria
- Low blink rate
- Convergence insufficiency
- Poor fixations and pursuits

- Accommodative dysfunction
- Unstable ambient vision
- Spatial disorientation
- Increased myopia.

Common Symptoms:

- Possible diplopia
- Staring behavior
- Poor visual memory
- Perceived movement of print or stationary objects
- Asthenopia
- Photophobia
- Poor concentration and attention.

The introduction of a theory postulating an explanation for the above characteristics of PTVS is relevant here as a prerequisite to further discussion of observed functional behaviors and appropriate treatments. Dysfunction in the ambient visual process at the level of the midbrain (mechanism described above) following a traumatic brain injury may contribute to the observable visual as well as perceptual, cognitive, and motoric deficits. The ambient process normally provides stabilization and orientation of the external visual world. Neurological damage disrupts spatial awareness, causing distortion of temporal and spatial concepts.

Exophoria As a Characteristic of PTVS

To understand the effect of a perceptually based spatial dysfunction on eye posture, we will first review normal eye postures. *Convergence* is the turning in of the eyes to view a near object. *Divergence* is the turning out of the eyes to observe an image further away. *Exophoria* is the tendency for both eyes to align on a point in space further than the object of intended focus or the tendency for one or both eyes to drift outward on a cover test (see chapter 4). A cover test requires that one eye of the patient be covered by the examiner during the act of having the patient look at an object with both eyes. Normally, the covered eye maintains posture toward the object of regard. In the case of an exophoria, the eyes deviate outward upon being covered. The difference between exophoria and exotropia is that in the latter an actual deviation of one eye outward is exhibited. As described earlier, the balance between the focal and ambient processes is mediated by sensorimotor feedback. Eye posture can be used as a barometer of this balance. An imbalance between those processes causes the spatial distortion of an expansion of central space with a relative compression of peripheral space. This spatial distortion promotes objects appearing to the perceiver to be farther away with a concurrent exophoria or exotropia noted. It is, therefore, postulated that this spatial distortion mediates the behavior of exophoria and other difficulties with binocularity, rather than the other way around.

A further description of the concept of spatial distortion may assist the reader here. Think of a three-dimensional face with the closest point to you being the tip of a big nose. Notice all the contours of the face spatially, what is further away and what is closer, what is more central to the face and what is more lateral. Now imagine the face made of putty in your hands. If peripheral space were expanded equally on either side of the head, with a relative compression of central space and with only so much space that the face can occupy, this would cause the face to flatten from the sides as if you were pressing in the putty ears. Notice what this does to the face, moving the tip of the nose closer to you and flattening the face in the lateral to medial plane. Now try expanding space centrally, with a relative compression of peripheral space, causing the face to flatten front to back, as if you are pressing in at the nose and the back of the head. Relatively speaking, if the nose were your point of regard again, it would move farther away from you and the face would eventually appear flat, or more two-dimensional, taking up more space centrally and appearing wider. This is a simplification; however, it begins to ground the concept of spatial distortion.

As previously stated, exophoria is a common characteristic of PTVS. It is easier now to appreciate how an expansion of central space is concurrent with an exophoria or exotropia. To simplify, central space flattens and expands, while peripheral space becomes relatively compressed. The exophoria, in this case, is a result of the mismatch of information caused by this distortion and not a cause in itself.

*Convergence Insufficiency, Accommodative Spasm, and
Time-Space Dysfunction as Characteristics of PTVS*

Convergence is the ability of the eyes to come together to fuse the image
of objects at near. According to this theory, convergence insufficiency is
noted as a by-product of spatial distortion, originating from the imbalance
between the ambient and focal visual processing systems, not as an
oculomotor deficit in and of itself. Again, the perceptual mismatch causing the eyes to deviate outward will be concurrent with a convergence
insufficiency or difficulty with bringing eyes inward to focalize at near.

Because of a flattening of space on the near to far axis, as described
above, depth perception is impaired and temporal relationships are disturbed. As an example, a ball coming toward the person will appear to
become larger but not necessarily moving through an accurate representation of space. Suddenly, the ball will appear to speed up when it reaches
the zone of space that the person perceives more accurately (i.e., that
which has not been perceptually flattened). Secondary to this perceptual
mismatch, far space tends to be conceptually lost and an overfocalization
at near occurs, causing the patient to present with an accommodative
spasm, that is stuck at near, or an ability to accommodate or focus on
far images and a tendency, therefore, toward myopia or nearsightedness.
On the face of it, this may appear to the reader to be a contradiction to
the above-described exophoria when viewed in traditional oculomotor
terms. However, myopia as described here can be thought of as an
overfocalization as compensation for a high exophoria or exotropia to
prevent diplopia (see below). In other words, in working hard to fuse
the image, a compensatory near focus causes accommodative spasm at
near and myopia. Again, the problems of binocularity are not the place
of origin of the perceptual motor mismatching, but the result of the
process of spatial distortion related to dysfunction in the ambient system
as described above.

Double Vision as a Characteristic of PTVS

Diplopia (blurred or double vision) often results from the deviated eye
posture and convergence insufficiency described above. Where in space
the object of regard is when diplopia is experienced depends on the

severity of spatial distortion and subsequent degree of convergence and fusion insufficiency. When the ambient visual process, which normally assists in organizing and orienting the images from both eyes (through the information it receives from kinesthetic, proprioceptive, and vestibular centers), is disrupted by neurological damage, diplopia can occur related to visual spatial disorientation.

Attention and Cognitive Deficits as Related to PTVS

Highly intense focalization or an overattention to objects of detail tends to be the compensation for a highly confusing perceptual world. It is also the natural result of an expansion of central space with a relative disregard for peripheral spatial awareness. A relationship has been observed, not only between these perceptual distortions and visual motor mismatching (causing changes in muscle tonus, coordination, balance, and posture) but between vision and cognition.

To assist in concretizing the relationship between the visual-perceptual process and cognition, it may be helpful for the reader to think of how one internalizes visual space (i.e., in the mind's eye) to think about and understand concepts. It has been demonstrated through repeated observation and interview that people encode their experiences or memories through specific, predictable visual parameters or submodalities (Bandler, 1985) such as quality or amount of light, amount of movement, or size of the picture (the picture in one's head as the experience is being recalled). In other words, one person might prioritize the importance of past experiences by the amount of light in the picture when remembered, and another might do this through the size or panoramic quality of it. This is a process the mind does without conscious awareness but can be retrieved consciously when intended.

This concept is introduced only to assist the reader in understanding cognition in visual terms. It is from this perspective that various measures of cognition, for example, attention, memory, and mental flexibility, can be discussed.

The reader may note how one attends to one object, concept, or picture in internal visual space by arranging or knowing where that object fits spatially or in relationship to other objects or concepts, that is, when thinking about the object of attention, it may tend to be placed more centrally for immediate attention, while related concepts may be placed peripherally. Other unrelated concepts are off the screen entirely, so to speak. An analogy for those who have used computers is the program Windows®; one can call many related documents to the screen at one time with some made smaller, others larger, depending on present focus. Another way of demonstrating this is that people who talk with their hands are frequently showing their internal representation of ideas in space (again, in the mind's eye) by where they place that idea in space with their hands.

Given this model, the reader may begin to predict what may occur in the case of a patient who has experienced a traumatic brain injury (TBI). If external spatial concepts are distorted (as described above under the beginning description of PTVS), an amplification of central space with a flattening of depth may conceptually correlate with all objects of regard (objects of present cognitive attention) having equal rate with little control over placing objects of intended focus in an internal spatial place of importance or priority. This visual-cognitive correlation or parallel relates to the behavior initially observed with those coming out of coma at Ranchos level 4 or 5, as an example. Many clinicians have observed that external stimulation at this point in recovery must be reduced and introduced in a graded manner to promote understanding and reduce agitated behavior. It is as if all information is equal with no filtering mechanism. In visual terms, this attention disorder is similar to having all external stimuli overlapping in the central field in the same place, with little ability to sort or prioritize for attentional strategies.

One can only assume that this individual would begin to attempt to cope with this experience. Because the perceptual cognitive distortions still coexist, one barometer clinicians can observe regarding this coping is the overfocalization process. Objects are conceptually spread out, and then space is pulled in from a panorama of objects or concepts that appear to have no relationship to each other to a single object of focus that is singled out at any given time with a required relative disregard for the periphery of objects around it. Attention deficits noted in those who have had TBI, stem from both the former and latter mechanisms, that is, first, no filtering mechanism and second, overfocalization as a coping strategy. The former promotes confusion regarding where to attend, while the latter causes an overattention to one object of regard with a relative inattention to others. Clinicians may note this transition as behavioral change from the agitated, confused behavior of RLA Scale Level 4 to the cognitive inflexibility of RLA Scale Levels 5–7.

Overfocalization correlates to concrete thinking as one idea or concept is overemphasized without adequate comparison to those ideas related to or affecting that concept. Many people may relate to a time when under stress they thought they knew a solution to a problem and sped down the trajectory of that one solution analogous to a super highway, disregarding contradictory information or better solutions popping up in the periphery in the form of exit signs. This is a very mild example of what patients with TBI experience and why they are often noted to be adverse to change. Too much movement literally and figuratively is quite challenging to the accompanying strategy of overfocalization.

This tendency toward overattention to one object or concept visually and cognitively also relates to a cognitive behavior often demonstrated by patients with TBI termed *perseveration*. Frequently, verbal clients will state the same worry or idea repeatedly saying, "I can't get it off my mind." Those around them often say, "Why can't you just put that in the back of your mind?" Notice the words used and remember the analogy of the computer screen. Another fear of patients with TBI is that once they let it go, the idea will not be able to be retrieved from memory, a result of overattention to a new concept.

Impaired memory post-TBI correlates to aforementioned attentional deficits, as memory requires adequate attention for the encoding process. Also, neurologically the mechanism to encode memories (as described above) may be disrupted.

Other Symptoms of PTVS

Observable staring behavior is related to the symptoms reviewed thus far: staring can be related to either general inattention or the locking in process of overattention to one idea or object.

Overfocalization represents another attempt at stabilizing a visual world that may appear to move. As described above, the ambient system is believed to be responsible for stabilizing an image so that it does not appear to move when the eyes, head, or body move. Frequently, those who have suffered a TBI experience their external world as moving or print as jumping around as they attempt to read. Those whose cognition is too impaired to make sense of the movement often make sense of it in other ways, which may be somewhat inaccurately termed as hallucinations, such as seeing snakes, or bugs crawling on the walls. Smooth pursuits and saccades are interrupted both by the instability of the visual world and the compensatory overfocalization. This overfocalization while reading is like reading with tunnel vision or with a magnifying glass. Overattention or "locking in" on one word or set of words without the overall reference picture of the other words limits the ability to find the next word to read and, most notably, to connect the words to make meaning, reducing reading comprehension.

Visual instability and spatial distortion, as described, very much affect and interrelate with gross and fine motor coordination, balance, posture, and imbalances in muscle tonus. Muscle tonus may be increased around the head, neck, and thoracic regions when the visual system is stressed. The example of the ball given earlier to demonstrate disturbed temporal spatial relationships helps to explain observed incoordination and perceptual motor mismatching. During the complete evaluation, the effect of disturbances of the visual process as well as of motor components requires consideration. Table 9.1 serves as a summary and an overview for use with a thorough assessment of a neurologically impaired patient. Please note that these are generalizations only, and many exceptions may exist.

Interventions for PTVS

Now that the reader has become familiar with the behavioral symptoms of PTVS and the authors' theory of the cause of these symptoms, it is satisfying to present treatment ideas that appear to be consistently helpful with this visual syndrome. Two of these treatments are base-in prism and binasal occlusion. Two diopters base-in prism ground into prescription lenses have been observed to effectively decrease the visual stress

Table 9.1 Parallel between functional systems. Table created by M. Connor.

Visual	Severe imbalance between focal and ambient processes	→		Balance between focal and ambient processes, allowing normal attention to objects of regard within a spatially referenced environment
	Exophoric posture →	Exophoric posture →		Aligned posture
	Severe convergence deficit →	Convergence insufficiency noted only at near →		Normal convergence near point
	Diplopia all the time →	Diplopia only at near →	Blurriness	Fusion
	All visual space appearing to move →	Larger objects →	"Jumping" words when reading →	Stable visual world
Motor	Gross motor incoordination or ataxias →	Fine motor incoordination or tremors →	Coordination within functional limits	
	Proximal tonus and postural changes →	Distal tonus and postural changes →	Balanced muscle tone	
	Rancho Los Amigos Scale level 1-3 →	Level 4-5 →	Level 6-8	
Cognitive	No apparent visual attention or tracking →	Limited visual attention for short periods and highly distractible limited memory →	Overfocalization to one object of regard and limited memory →	Balanced attention and memory
	Little awareness of external environment with a need for stimulation →	Too much stimulation from external environment and highly distractible with no filtering mechanism →	Overattention with mental inflexibility →	High level of reasoning and flexibility

*Arrows indicate continuum from severe deficits or just post-injury through recovery.

and therefore the symptomatology described above. The base side of prisms compress space, therefore, both prisms base-in will compress central space and relatively amplify peripheral space to assist in remediating the spatial distortion described above. The base-in prism counters the expansion of central space and the compression of peripheral space. It creates a relative balance between the focal and ambient processes, in turn affecting visual, motor, and cognitive function.

Binasal occlusion is a treatment technique whereby translucent tape is placed over a person's lenses, partially occluding the nasal portion of the visual field. This technique may further reduce stress in the ambient system both by filtering out some of the visual information and by providing a vertical line by which visual space can be organized, much the same way one might grab a pole on the subway to stabilize oneself. Research (Padula, Argyris, & Ray, 1994) using base-in prism and binasal occlusion on persons with TBI demonstrated with *visual evoked potentials* (VEP) that the binocular symptoms observed following TBI are not oculomotor in origin but are a result of interference in the ambient visual process at the level of the midbrain. This research showed a correlation between an increase in the VEP amplitudes and the use of binasal occluders on those with TBI. The control group showed a decrease in amplitude. The amplitudes of VEP (brain waves produced by the occipital cortex) appear to be highly influenced by the ambient visual process. Dysfunction of the ambient visual process such as found after a TBI reduces the amplitude of the VEP for persons with PTVS. As proposed earlier, the ambient visual process is an integrative process involving vision, kinesthetic, proprioceptive, and vestibular feedback. Therefore, in addition to incorporating neuro-optometric interventions, such as base-in prism and binasal occlusion, therapists and optometrists alike should incorporate such integrative approaches as neurodevelopmental treatment, proprioceptive neuromuscular facilitation, and sensory integration to assist in concurrently influencing the motor and ambient visual systems. The information relayed to the ambient visual system through weight bearing, challenging righting reflexes, vestibular activities, reaching activities, and tactile activities is essential to the remediation of the visual spatial awareness required for effective focalization. Because focalization is the system most immediately understood as traditional seeing, the focus in evaluation and treatment of vision all too often is the mechanism of focalization in the eyeball and the immediate visual cortex. Therefore, the authors propose that neuromuscular reeducation in combination with optometric intervention is the most effective treatment approach.

Hemianopsia and Visual Inattention

Evaluation and treatment will be further addressed after the following discussion of other types of perceptual and spatial distortions observed in patients who are post-CVA, head trauma, and so forth. Once the reader has a complete perspective of the theories presented here, a discussion of treatment will be more relevant.

Any clinician who has worked with patients post-CVA or other neurological event has observed that these patients frequently present with some form of visual perceptual deficit; some are immediately observable in any context, others only while functioning in certain distracting environments. However, the common link is that these deficits are quite influential in the patients functioning, often disturbing activities of daily living (ADL), coordination, posture, attention, reading, and figure–ground tasks.

Visual-perceptual neglect or inattention and visual field deficits (most commonly homonymous hemianopsia) are common deficits noted post-CVA. The former presents as an inattention or decreased perceptual awareness of a portion of visual space, the latter as an actual visual field loss, that is, not being able to see a portion of visual space. A homonymous hemianopsia occurs when vision is lost in the nasal portion of one eye and the temporal portion of the other, causing an inability to see in half of the visual field. These deficits may be observed by therapists in a more formal screening or in behavioral assessment. If a patient is able to verbalize and attend adequately, visual fields may be generally assessed by sitting in front of the patient with his or her eyes focused on the practitioner's face, holding long dowels with colored tips at arm's length behind the patient's head. Bringing the dowels into different quadrants of the periphery, the practitioner asks the patient to report when he or she sees the dowels come into view in the periphery. This should be performed both binocularly and monocularly (by covering one eye). Any test like this may make apparent other deficits like decreased visual attention, dysfunctional level of distractibility, and impaired immediate memory. A perceptual neglect may be observed by standing behind the patient with one dowel positioned on each side of the head, quickly placing and removing one dowel into the periphery on the right or left side or both sides, and asking the patient to indicate seeing on the left, right, or both. If the patient consistently misses one side when one or both are introduced, an inattention to that side is possible.

Patients can present with one or both of these deficits (i.e., visual field loss or visual field neglect). The distinction between the two can often be noted behaviorally when objective measures are difficult to complete because of cognitive-linguistic dysfunction. With a visual field loss, frequently searching behavior is noted when the patient is attempting to locate an object of intended focus. In the case of an inattention or neglect, the object of focus is found more quickly when using other senses as reinforcing anchors to the image, such as a person's voice or having the patient touch the object of regard. Behaviors such as running into the wall while walking or propelling a wheelchair, reading or writing on only one side of the page, and not locating objects on one side when performing functional tasks can be indicative of one or both of these deficits. It is important to note that patients with milder deficits may only demonstrate them under personal stress or in stressful environments. For example, a patient may demonstrate a high level neglect while in a grocery store by being unable to locate certain objects on the left side of the aisle.

These deficits have thus far been presented primarily from a visual perspective. It is instructive now to return to the model that shows motor and sensory to be inseparable, requiring that visual and motor components be assessed together and addressed as very much interrelated. It is postulated that as inaccurate information is being received from the proprioceptive centers (because of the sensory and motor deficits related to neurological damage), the perception of the body in space will change, and as the perception of the body in space changes, motor components, such as motor control, posture, balance, and coordination will be affected. This interrelationship is important to reinforce, as treating the motor side of the loop will affect visual perception and treating visual perception will affect motor functioning. For example, visual-perceptual neglect, impaired motor function, and decreased sensation in the affected side are frequently noted as simultaneous symptoms that affect one another. It has been the observation of some clinicians that in some cases visual field loss has been partially resolved with the return of other neurological mechanisms, such as motor or sensory (tactile), to reinforce the re-instatement of perception of that visual space, which corresponds motori-cally (e.g., as sensation and motor return are noted in the left extremities, concurrent opening of the visual field to the left is also noted). This has been an observation only, but serves to reinforce the model of the ambient visual processing system and the sensorimotor feedback loop as a possible or partial explanation for such events.

Hemiplegia and Visual Midline Shift Syndrome

In addition to or in combination with the perceptual deficits just de-scribed, a shift in perceptual midline is frequently noted both perceptually and behaviorally in those patients who are post-CVA or head trauma. Visual Midline Shift Syndrome (VMSS) (as defined by Padula, 1996) is theorized to be caused by the ambient visual process dysfunction changing orientation to the concept of midline through spatial distortion. Given a neurological event such as a CVA causing hemiparesis or hemiplegia, sensorimotor input from one side of the body is disrupted at the same time that integration of these systems may be disturbed centrally, causing a breakdown in the integration and the accurate perception of the body itself and its location in space.

The ambient process is a relative processing system, and it attempts to create a relative balance on the basis of the information established. Given the interference in the information received from one side of the body relative to the other, the ambient visual process attempts to recreate a spatial relationship that corresponds to the mismatch of information received from the sensorimotor feedback loop. This phenomenon causes a shift in the concept of midline, usually shifting away from the involved side: a midline shift to the right with a left hemiplegia, for example (see Figures 9.2 and 9.3). Midline concepts can shift in the anterior-posterior axis, causing the midline to be shifted forward or backward (see Figures 9.4 and 9.5). When a midline shift exists, the person will relate on testing when a wand or other object is moved across the visual field that the object is in front of his or her nose when it is in fact lateral, above, or below the nose. Combinations of the anterior-posterior and lateral shifts are also common. VMSS frequently causes the person to lean toward where midline is perceived to be while resisting weight bearing into the involved or hemiplegic side. The opposite is also noted, though, in behavior that has been termed the *pusher syndrome* by some neurodevelopmental therapists. This behavior entails the person pushing their weight into the hemiplegic, often visually neglected side, while avoiding weight bearing into the uninvolved side. The mechanism for this is not fully understood, but it is the experience of the authors that this behavior is most commonly noted in those with more severe or dense infarcts or bleeds. When a midline shift occurs in the near-far axis, the person will be observed to be leaning into an extensor or flexor pattern while resisting weight shifting in the opposite direction. Any therapist who has experience with this type of case has observed that this resistance to weight bearing can be extreme, as the patients feel they are falling because they perceive

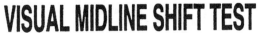

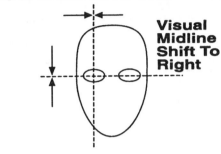

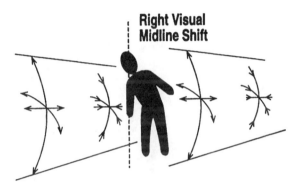

Figure 9.2 Visual midline shift to the right. From *Neuro-Optometric Rehabilitation*. Copyright Optometric Extension Program. Reprinted with permission.

the therapist is pushing them way beyond their midline. In the example of a person with a posterior midline shift, leaning forward for a normal sit-to-stand position can be frightening and the person's extensor tone will increase. Another way to understand this concept of the distortion of space through the coupling of an amplification and relative compression of different portions of space is to think of the person's perception as being as if the floor is tilted either laterally, up- or downhill, or a combination. Some people who are cognitively able may say the floor appears tilted. This spatial distortion causes the corresponding appropriate posture; for example, if one were walking uphill, one would lean forward (see Figures 9.2–9.5).

Yoked Prisms

A neuro-optometric approach that has worked effectively in trials with MSS is the use of yoked prisms placed before both eyes with the base

VISUAL MIDLINE SHIFT TEST

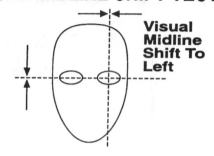

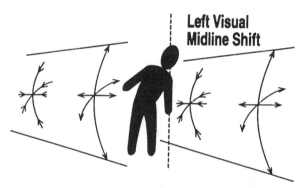

Figure 9.3 Visual midline shift to the left. From *Neuro-Optometric Rehabilitation.* Copyright Optometric Extension Program. Reprinted with permission.

pointing in the same direction. It is important to state here that the traditional use of prisms has been from a sensory or sight only perspective, which is also beneficial. When used in this manner, the prisms are placed with the base away from the affected hemiplegic side to affect a neglect by moving objects in space toward that side to move the eyes more in the direction of the neglect, attempting to increase awareness of the neglected field.

However, the authors and other clinicians have observed that applying the yoked prisms with the base toward the hemiplegic side (frequently the side the person is leaning away from) is noted to be more consistently effective with VMSS. The theory is that the base of the prisms contracts space on the hemiplegic side so that concept of midline is shifted back to a more normal position. This approach is not used in a compensatory manner, rather in a remedial fashion with a regimen prescribed to be used usually a few hours a day specifically during therapy sessions when motor tasks such as balance, coordination, ambulation, and reaching are

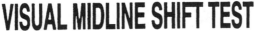

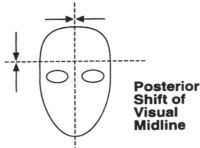

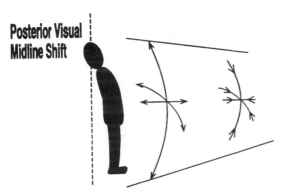

Figure 9.4 Posterior visual midline shift. From *Neuro-Optometric Rehabilitation*. Copyright Optometric Extension Program. Reprinted with permission.

being performed. The amount of diopter to be used depends on the severity, established through evaluation trials and with the lowest diopter that is effective. It is important to restate that the prisms are used in conjunction with motor tasks in an attempt to affect motor and functional outcomes. Yoked prisms should be used with the following guidance in mind:

Visual Midline Shift	Prism Orientation
Right	Base left
Left	Base right
Anterior	Base down
Posterior	Base up

Other Focuses of Treatment

Areas of potential focus in the rehabilitation of the neurologically impaired patient with corresponding treatment ideas are given. It is import-

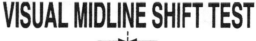

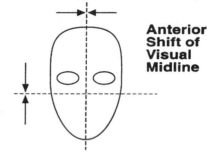

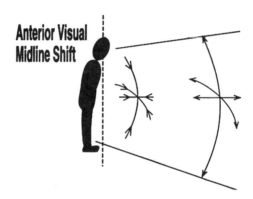

Figure 9.5 Anterior visual midline shift. From *Neuro-Optometric Rehabilitation.* Copyright Optometric Extension Program. Reprinted with permission.

ant to remember that these ideas need to be used simultaneously or in a graded manner to create treatment activities that promote the individual patient's needs and goals.

Wheelchair Positioning

Wheelchair positioning problems arise not only from muscle weakness and abnormal muscle tone, but also are compounded and accentuated by perceptual deficits. Positioning can frequently be a problem with those at Ranchos Los Amigos Scale 1–3, that is, the stages of coma. In addition to muscle control issues, abnormal muscle tone, especially in the head, neck, and trunk, contributes to the challenge of positioning to prevent contracture and skin breakdown. Optometrically, base-in prism and nasal occlusion may be helpful even at this early stage in reducing high tone. Also, if behaviorally a midline shift is apparent that is causing significant leaning or asymmetrical tone, yoked prisms may reduce leaning behaviors. This is also true for positioning of higher-level patients. The authors have found in cases of severe leaning that may cause a falling or hanging of the affected upper extremity, difficulty in feeding, and orthopedic changes promoting pain, the use of yoked prisms to remediate misperception of the body in space has been quite helpful. In addition to these optometric interventions, multisensory feedback experiences, including moving the patient in many positions, allowing vestibular feedback, and providing weight-bearing experiences through the trunk and extremities, will continue to assist and integrate any changes in spatial perception.

Sitting and Standing Balance and Ambulation

Standard therapeutic approaches to remediating deficits in posture and balance, in addition to improving muscle control and strength, are handling activities that reinforce normalization of tone and righting reactions on which to superimpose functional movement, for example, facilitating equal weight shifting side to side with elongation of the trunk on the weight-bearing side during balance activities. In addition, if balance deficits appear to have a more apparent vestibular component, such as complaints of vertigo, specific vestibular programs with graded movement to desensitize or retrain vestibular mechanisms are implemented. As mentioned previously, PTVS or VMSS from disruption of the ambient visual process often affect perception of the body in space and therefore impede balance, normalized posture, and functional mobility. Therefore, in addition to and in conjunction with the above modalities, use of base-in prism and binasal occlusion may reduce the stress on the ambient system, reducing symptoms and assisting the patient with orientation in space. Also, use of yoked prisms to remediate midline shift can be essential in promoting equalized weight shifting for balance and ambulation. Again, the important behaviors to note that are indicative of a shift in midline are a resistance to weight bearing to one side or the other or shifting weight forward into flexion or backward into extension with potentially increased tone toward the direction of the shift. A commonly observed example among patients with posterior midline shift, is a resistance is noted to leaning forward in preparation for sit-to-stand with concurrently increased extensor tone that is aggravated by resistance when the therapist pushes the person forward. The person may resist placing his or her feet flat and will instead push the feet into plantar flexion. All these symptoms make perfect sense when one thinks the floor is tilted downward or downhill. Would you lean forward into a downhill slope? In addition, if that same person were ambulating, he or she would be leaning backward with potentially increased extensor tone. In contrast, with anterior midline shift, the therapist might note a flexed, shuffling gait.

Visual Attention, Pursuits, and Saccades

Visual attentional deficits are sometimes evidenced by such behaviors as distractibility, decreased ability to read without assistive techniques such as the use of a finger to scan the page, decreased ability to read for a length of time, scanning a visual acuity chart, and impaired processing of the visual environment as a whole, especially in crowded or busy places. The important idea to reinforce here is that poor scanning abilities and poor visual attention are not best remediated through oculomotor exercises to start (even functional ones such as graded forms of near reading or scanning tasks), but through integration of the ambient processing system through base-in prism, nasal occlusion, and visual tasks requiring an overlap with the motor systems to integrate spatial-temporal concepts, such as a balance activity at the same time that the patient is requested to touch different objects of focus. The tasks and level of skills required can be modified and graded to fit the specific needs of the patient, as long as they incorporate as many of the following systems as can be tolerated: *visual*, including visual attention, convergence, accommodation, pursuits, and saccades; these are used preferably in *functional* activities incorporating tactile, proprioceptive, kinesthetic, and vestibular components. This provides the basis for many therapy activities such as graded sports activities, both gross and fine motor, crafts, and ADLs graded or modified to encompass the above. A few specific examples are:

• A patient with a dense left neglect should be guided verbally, tactilely, or both to place his or her hand on the sink while brushing the teeth. To visually locate the toothpaste just beyond midline to the left, the patient is instructed to glide his or her hand slowly toward that side of the sink while following the hand with his or her eyes until the tube is located both visually and tactilely. At first, the task should be easy to accomplish, including putting the tube just beyond visual awareness and perhaps giving the patient therapist assistance with a hand-over-hand technique.

- The patient should maintain focus on an object in space that he or she is touching while on a balance board. Focusing on a point in space while ambulating assists the patient in stabilizing peripheral spatial awareness.

- The patient is requested to visually track toward and attend to the cone being manipulated with neurodevelopment theory techniques that incorporate trunk rotation and weight bearing into the affected side in such activities as cone stacking. This needs to be graded in the beginning so the patient can easily access the cone.

Documentation of Services

Information has been presented to provide the therapist with a framework both for complete assessment and remediation of common visual motor deficits observed in neurologically involved patients. A clear statement of methods used in assessment and treatment will assist in documentation to facilitate reimbursement. Visual-spatial deficits very much impede progress in many potential areas of rehabilitation focus, including but not limited to the following:

- wheelchair positioning to prevent orthopedic changes, promote posture for ADL such as feeding, and facilitate equal weight bearing for normalized motor return

- normalizing posture and weight bearing during transfers, standing balance training, and ambulation to promote improved functioning in these areas

- promoting awareness of the affected extremities to improve the probability of motor return and to promote awareness of body scheme for use in all self-care tasks

- improving attention to all quadrants of visual space for localizing functional objects in space (including reading and writing)

- improving overall attention, memory, and cognitive flexibility for improved independence with functional tasks.

The theoretical information in this chapter provides a basis to relate visual-perceptual remedial intervention to these rehabilitation goals and in fact more than implies an incorporation of a visual-perceptual focus into other rehabilitation tasks such as balance, postural work, ADL, and so forth. Each will improve most effectively when combined with the other. Therefore, documentation of rehabilitation time spent in this way can be stated in specific functional terms as part of the treatment plan as any modality such as neuromuscular reeducation is part of a treatment plan to improve transfers, ambulation, and functional motor return.

REFERENCES

Bandler, R. (1985). *Using your brain for a change.* Moab, UT: Real People Press.
Nelson & Benabib. (1992). 1992 Conference on Head-Neck Treatment Issues, Cuernavaca, Mexico.
Padula, W. V. (1996). *Neuro-optometric rehabilitation.* Optometric Extension Program Foundation, Inc., 1921 East Carnegie Avenue, Suite 3L, Santa Ana, CA 92705.
Padula, W. V., Argyris, S., & Ray, J. (1994). Visual evoked potentials (VEP) evaluating treatment for post-trauma vision syndrome (PTVS) in patients with traumatic brain injuries (TBI). *Brain Injury, 8*(2), 125–133.
Trevarthen. (1968). In C. B., & Speery, R. (1973). Perceptual unity of the ambient visual field in human commissurotomy patients. *Brain,* 564–570.
Wolfe. (1968). *Anatomy of the Eye and Orbit.* Philadelphia, PA: W. B. Saunders.

SELECTED READINGS

Ayres, A. J. (1973). *Sensory integration and learning disorders.* Los Angeles: Western Psychological Services.
Ayres, A. J. (1979). *Sensory integration and the child.* Los Angeles: Western Psychological Services.
Buktenica, N. (1968). *Visual learning.* Sioux Falls, SD: Adapt Press.
Corbin, C. B. (1980). *A textbook of motor development.* Dubuque, IA: Wm. C. Brown.
Held, R. (1965). Plasticity in sensory-motor systems. *Scientific American, 213*(5), 84–95.
Ilg, F., & Ames, L. (1995). *Child behavior.* New York: Harper & Row.

Langley, B., & Dubrose, R. (1976). Functional vision screening for severely handicapped children. *New Outlook for Blind, 70*(8), 346–350.

Liebowitz, H. W., & Post, R. B. (in press). The two modes of processing concept and some implications. In J. J. Beck (Ed.), *Organization and representation in perception.* Hillsdale, NJ: Erlbaum.

Trevarthan, C. B., & Speery, R. (1973). Perceptual unity of the ambient visual field in human commissurotomy patients. *Brain, 96,* 547–570.

10 Driving and Visual Information Processing in Cognitively At-Risk and Older Individuals

Rosamond Gianutsos, PhD, FAAO, CDRS

Although few people question the importance of visual information processing for the safe operation of a motor vehicle, the relationship between vision and driving is surprisingly controversial (Nouri, Tinson, & Lincoln, 1992). While virtually all states in the United States and most countries have a minimum standard for acuity (usually 20/40 or 6/12), many researchers and driver rehabilitation specialists (Ramsey, 1990) question the importance of acuity per se, citing examples of persons who have driven safely with poor acuity. These experts believe that a much more critical, if not the most critical, factor is the integrity of the visual fields. Their evidence, however, is based largely on clinical experience rather than formal research: a study by Johnson and Keltner (1983) is one of the few available reports. The controversy sometimes emphasizes the relative importance of other functions, most notably attention (Owsley & Ball, 1993). This relationship between driving and vision comes into focus in individuals who are cognitively at risk, for example, from brain injury or advanced age.

Before examining the specifics of the relationship between vision and driving in cognitively at-risk individuals, it is important to consider some general issues about human abilities and safe driving. Nobody would dispute the fact that driving is an extremely complex form of human behavior for which many competencies are either required or helpful (Colsher & Wallace, 1993; van Zomeren, Brouwer, & Minderhoud, 1987). While there may not be a consensus regarding the "required" category, there is more agreement on what is "helpful." For instance, binocular vision is not required for operation of an ordinary motor vehicle; however, it is helpful in that it affords an appreciation of space, especially at night when texture gradient information (an important monocular cue for depth) is lost. Monocular drivers usually develop other techniques for evaluating spatial information.

Significantly, when multiple impairments are present, the combined effect may be considerably greater than the sum of the individual parts (Colsher & Wallace, 1993). In research, the components are called *main effects* and the combined effect is called the *interaction effect.* Impairments of two helpful competencies may produce an interaction that is deadly. For example, my experience with profoundly amnestic survivors of herpes simplex encephalitis—none of whom stopped driving—convinces me that it is possible to drive safely despite extremely poor recent memory; such amnesia combined with impulsivity, however, can lead to dangerous lane changes and last-minute turns to cope with a forgotten route.

On the other hand, cognitively intact individuals may indeed be able to deal with substantial but isolated and well-recognized impairments. A psychologist (Chapman, 1995) who had been struggling for 25 years with progressive loss of visual acuity due to Stargardt's disease described his own experience driving with field constriction associated with the use of special bioptic (telescope-like) lenses. He drove over 650,000 miles with the bioptic lenses and has only recently begun to limit his driving. In his experience, it was only when his acuity worsened to 20/240 correctable to 20/40 and fields narrowed to below 6.5 degrees that he began to question his ability to drive safely. Most jurisdictions that have standards for visual fields and driving specify well over 100 degrees in the horizontal meridian; it is astounding that this man could drive safely with such narrow fields.

However, it would be a mistake to conclude that peripheral vision is unimportant for driving. The logical error is failing to take into account the interaction effects: the effects of disabilities tend to combine multiplicatively, not additively. While a well-functioning person might be able to compensate for constriction of the visual fields, with cognitive impairment such compensation may require attentional and other mental resources that are unavailable or required for other tasks.

A positive view of interaction effects is to appreciate that there is much to gain from fixing a relatively small impairment that serves to multiply the impairment caused by another condition. If, for instance, reduced distance visual acuity (a minor impediment to safe driving) is corrected, the benefit may be a disproportionate gain of attentional resources previously needed to compensate for the poor acuity.

Wood (1993) and Szlyk, Brigell, and Seiple (1993) consider the combined effects of visual and cognitive impairment on driving. Many conditions that cause cognitive impairment also cause visual impairment, so this combination is, unfortunately, not rare. The good news is that many visual problems can be treated and some can be rectified without unusual expense, technology, or effort.

What conditions put a driver in the category "cognitively at risk"? Anything that affects the brain can compromise cognitive function. In this chapter the emphasis will be on the individuals with acquired brain injury—persons who developed normally until some event or condition affected brain function. Usually such people are seeking to resume or to continue driving. Persons with developmental disabilities, especially cerebral palsy and spina bifida, present a complex challenge for driver rehabilitation specialists, which will not be addressed here specifically. Another more common, but less widely recognized, etiology at risk for unsafe driving is attention deficit disorder, with or without hyperactivity. This condition usually does not combine with physical or visual disability.

The major etiologies to be considered include acquired brain injury (with cerebrovascular accident and traumatic brain injury the most common) and age-associated cognitive decline. Persons with progressive neurological conditions such as multiple sclerosis and Alzheimer's. Other forms of dementia present similar issues, together with some specialized considerations (e.g., the visual problems specific to multiple sclerosis) that are beyond the scope of this chapter. In cases where progression, variability in symptom expression, or recurrence is anticipated, there must be guidelines for reevaluating driving risk. If the initial evaluation is done early in the disease process, it can be used to establish a personal baseline and indicators for reviewing the situation. Planning can be started for mobility alternatives.

Age-associated cognitive impairment, though not universal and sometimes caused by correctable but undiagnosed problems, is a reality, especially as advances in medical treatment keep people living longer in better physical health. In some sense, the issues are similar to progressive conditions.

Stroke is the most common form of acquired brain injury, with older persons at increased risk. The most likely physical impairment following stroke is hemiplegia. Visually, the most common problem is hemi-field impairment, with or without hemi-inattention. Traumatic brain injury often strikes the younger, and sometimes inexperienced, risk-prone driver. Physical impairment, while similar to stroke, can be more severe, especially following prolonged loss of consciousness and immobility. Problems with motor coordination, balance, and vestibular function are not unusual after brain trauma. Not only may there be visual hemi-field impairment, but there is also a high incidence of accommodative and binocular dysfunction.

Driver Rehabilitation

Driver rehabilitation has advanced considerably in the last decade, especially under the auspices of the Association of Driver Educators for the Disabled, an interdisciplinary organization of occupational therapists, driver educators, and others. This organization has established a certification process leading to the title Certified Driver Rehabilitation Specialist (CDRS). While adaptation to accommodate physical disabilities is an important part of this specialty, addressing cognitive and sensory impairment is often the greater challenge. This latter enterprise, which includes evaluation, counseling, and intervention, may be called *driving advisement.*

The essential purpose of driving advisement is to enable the individual to make appropriate decisions about driving. Regardless of the legal context (i.e., some jurisdictions have mandatory reporting by professionals of drivers with certain diagnoses), the would-be driver is the ultimate licensor. On every trip, an implicit self-authorization is given; conversely, from time to time most drivers make conscious decisions to refrain from driving or to allow others to drive. These decisions are usually to accommodate some condition, such as fatigue, intoxication, or a broken bone. Older drivers frequently refrain from driving at night because they are sensitive to glare. Significantly, they recognize this problem and perceive it as interfering with their ability to drive safely. Little assessment of this problem (glare sensitivity) is needed: the problem is recognized by the driver, and steps are taken either to correct or to avoid it.

In the assessment part of driving advisement, the priority is on those conditions for which awareness may be compromised. The most striking example of such a condition is visual field impairment. Clinicians will frequently encounter persons who have dramatically constricted fields who insist that they are seeing everything. Hemianopic field losses are often unappreciated or underappreciated. The most convincing illustration for the neurologically intact individual is a demonstration in which an object is made to disappear in the area subtended by the physiological blind spot. (See Figure 8.1)

Sensory impairment needs to be evaluated because, unlike motor impairment, it can be inferred only indirectly from behavior and often the impairment does not lend itself to self-evaluation. It seems that the human organism is not built to monitor some sensory functions well. For instance, people with hearing problems may think others are mumbling. Another example is the loss of spatial vision following binocular dysfunction. It is not uncommon for persons with dramatic losses of acuity to present themselves for an eye exam with little or no complaint.

The driving advisement process usually includes an in-clinic and an on-the-road, behind-the-wheel component, typically (for obvious safety reasons) in that order. The on-road component can be deferred, based on severely deficient performance on the in-clinic component. Less often, a condition will be identified in the in-clinic component that disqualifies the person from licensure. A committee on which I served, charged with making recommendations regarding what should be included in driver rehabilitation assessment, concluded that no one should be recommended for driving without first demonstrating satisfactory performance on the road (Subcommittee on Driver Evaluation and Training for Individuals with Disabilities, 1993). Some functionally oriented driver rehabilitation specialists discount or minimize in-clinic findings, placing total reliance on the outcome of the road test.

The in-clinic assessment needs to address medical, sensory, motor, and cognitive functions. The medical consideration is the presence of conditions that could produce a rapid change in the person's abilities, including consciousness, vision, debilitating pain, or contact with reality. Included here is the effect of substances, prescribed and otherwise, that might affect the individual's performance. The sensory assessment emphasizes vision, although joint and position sense are important, especially for reliable and efficient pedal control. Motor function is particularly important in relation to the need for adaptive equipment, including mirrors.

It is in the areas of cognition and vision that the in-clinic assessment can have unique value because in these domains are hidden problems that may not be safely or intentionally tested in an ordinary road test. Recommendations for the vision screening will be discussed later. Table 10.1 summarizes features of procedures for evaluating cognition in relationship to driving.

Critical features include apparent (face) validity, psychometric properties (demonstrated standardization, reliability, and validity), and clinical practicality. Apparent, or face, validity (the test looks like it measures

Table 10.1 Features of procedures used for pre-driving advisement.

Comparative Summary of Major Driving Assessment Procedures

ISSUE	Porta Clinic/Glare	Driver Performance Test	Doron Simulator	Driving Advisement System	Elemental Driving Simulator	Neuropsych. Testing	On-road Testing	Cog Behav Driver Inventory	Visual Attention Analyzer—Useful Field of View	Atari
FACE VALIDITY	Mod. Low	Mod. High	High	Mod. High	Mod. High	Low	Highest	Mod. Low	Mod. Low	Mod. High
SCOPE	Focused	Focused	Focused	Broad	Broad	Test dependent	Broad	Broad	Focused	?
PROTOCOL	Standard	Standard	Select proc.	Standard	Standard	Select proc.	No standard	Standard?	Standard	No standard
NORMS	Marines	Yes	Non-empirical	Yes	Yes	Usually	?	Yes	Yes	No
RELIABILITY	not reported	not reported	not reported	Yes	Yes	Usually	?	Yes?	Yes	No
VALIDITY	not reported	not reported	not reported	Yes	Yes	Not for driv.	?	Yes	Yes	No
TIME (MIN)	15 min.	45 min.	60+ min.	60+ min.	20 min.	15–60 min.	60 min.	60 min.	30 min (?)	60 min.
SPACE/EQUIP.	Tabletop+20 VCR	Room	Room	Computer	Computer	Tests	Vehicle+	Computer+Test	Console	Console
COST (EST.)	$1,200.	$200.	$30,000.	$1,800.+	$1,800.+	<$500.	Direct + ind.	$120.++	$20,000	$15,000.
SOURCE	DTE	ADSI	Doron	LSA	LSA	Test	self	PSS	VRI	Atari

ADSI = Advanced Driving Skills Institute, 4660 Brayton Terrace South, Palm Harbor, FL 34685 (813) 785-0034
Atari = Atari Games Corp., 675 Sycamore Dr., Milpitas, CA 95035
Doron = Doron Precision Systems, PO Box 400, Binghamton, NY 13902 (607) 772-1610—Jane Townsend
DTE = Driver Testing Equipment, Inc., 1020 S. Main Ave., Scranton, PA 18504, (717) 347-7772
LSA = Life Science Associates, 1 Fenimore Rd., Bayport, NY 11705, (516) 472-2111
PSS = Psychological Software Services, 6555 Carrollton Ave, Indianapolis, IN 46220, (317) 257-9672
++ CBDI also requires Brake Pedal RT, Keystone Driver Vis. Test, WAIS PC & DS, Trailmaking Test (time, cost addit'l)
VRI = Visual Resources Inc., Kristina K. Berg, 216 S. Jefferson, Suite 600, Chicago, IL 60661 (312) 454-0603

what it is supposed to measure) is important if the examinee is to be convinced of the relevance of the findings. It is central to the driving advisement process and must not be discounted as "mere cosmesis." The appeal of the on-road assessment is its face validity. Simulation attempts to maximize face validity, although procedures vary in what is simulated and range from hardware simulations (e.g., the Doron Simulator®) to task simulations (e.g., the Elemental Driving Simulator®).

Driving advisement procedures vary in their scope. For example, none, other than the on-road test, addresses binocular depth perception. In addition, they vary in whether they include a defined assessment protocol. Some (e.g., Doron Simulator®, neuropsychological assessment) consist of a large collection of potentially useful scenarios or tasks. With regard to psychometric development, it is amazing how often this crucial ingredient is lacking. Until recently the most widely used device, the Porto-Clinic Glare®, had norms derived from 18- and 19-year-old Marine recruits—a fact not generally known. No reliability and validity data were offered. Clinical practicality starts with cost of materials, but also includes space and therapist time.

Because most existing procedures did not possess all these features, in the late 1980s I developed the Driving Advisement System (Gianutsos, 1988; Gianutsos, Campbell, Beattie, & Mandriota, 1992) and subsequently the *Elemental Driving Simulator* (EDS) (Gianutsos, 1994; Gianutsos & Beattie, 1992). Research on the validity of the EDS is ongoing and includes significant correlations with an independent on-road assessment (A. Campbell, personal communication, 1995), at-fault crashes (Brown, Greaney, Mitchel, & Lee, 1993), and limitation of driving by older drivers (DeLibero, 1995). In the DeLibero study a group of older drivers (free of neurological diagnoses) were compared with a young adult group of drivers. EDS performance correlated strongly ($r = .68$) with reported driving pattern: specifically, the older drivers struggled with the EDS, but also reported that they limited their driving (e.g., avoided driving in bad weather, at night, long distances, and in congested or unfamiliar places). Interestingly enough, these drivers felt they were still above average in their basic abilities! Generally, their self-appraisals bore no relationship to their performance; however, they were making appropriate decisions about driving.

The EDS is experienced as difficult by most persons who are cognitively at risk. Licensed drivers who were tested for the purpose of collecting normative information, however, performed consistently and efficiently. Still, most feedback suggests that the EDS is more difficult than ordinary driving. That is as it should be. Most of the time driving calls for relaxed vigilance. However, in a heartbeat the task can require complex decisions implemented with precise and rapid timing. Driving advisement requires an aggressive and challenging exploration of all the potential areas of difficulty. It is far better to err in the direction of making the assessment too stringent than too lax.

The EDS is a physically elemental simulator protocol designed to address simple and complex reaction time, impulse control, response consistency, lateral responsivity, and steering steadiness. Individuals are asked to predict how well they will do compared to other licensed drivers and are later given norm-referenced performance ratings. Because the predictions and performance are anchored to the same numeric scale, the report affords a direct comparison of the two. If there is a high disparity, indicating that the person has unrealistic expectations, the clinician has a good foundation to address issues of judgment and driving beyond one's capabilities.

Performance on the road test is often regarded as the ultimate indicator of driving ability—much as it is in the licensure process. Yet the road tests used in most rehabilitation contexts fail to meet psychometric standards, including reliability and validity. Driving environments vary, courses vary, and so does the behavior of other drivers. Standardization of procedure, much less of scoring, is not possible in on-road tests. Most on-road assessment protocols (in the author's informal survey) emphasize the operational level of driving—the basic skills needed for keeping the vehicle on the road. Little attention is paid to the more proactive tactical (van Zomeren, Brouwer, & Minderhoud, 1987) level of driving, including, for example, route selection, anticipation of erratic behavior based on such clues as out-of-state plates, and even the decision of whether and when to make a trip. This tactical level of driving calls for precisely the kind of "frontal" abilities that are often compromised by traumatic brain injury. Typically, the road test evaluator assumes full responsibility for the route, which may or may not be a familiar driving environment for the examinee. Also, it can be impractical to evaluate comparative performance when tests are given at different times of day and in different weather conditions.

The bottom line is that the evaluation process is an evolving clinical art and far from perfect. Important as the on-road test is, especially to the would-be driver, it should not be the only or ultimate test. If a person does poorly on the in-clinic procedures, but does well on the on-road test, it does not mean that the in-clinic procedures should be discounted or overridden. The road test is not the ultimate measure of success; rather, the ultimate successful outcome is the accumulation of safe miles.

Visual Processing and Impact on Driving

Based on years of clinical experience, in a masterful application of an understanding of basic processes to an important activity of daily living, occupational therapist Carmella Strano (1989) analyzed the specific visual problems associated with brain injury and their impact on specific aspects of the driving task. Complementing Strano's analysis is the review by Shinar and Schieber (1991) of empirical research on this topic.

In clinical practice, static acuity is addressed first. Static distance acuity is almost universally included in licensure standards, where it tends to be overemphasized. However, it can be important in unfamiliar situations, where information must be derived from signs. Good distance acuity can permit early recognition of potential hazards, such as misdirection of gaze by another driver.

Contrast sensitivity, often reduced in older persons, can affect safety in night driving and in conditions where visibility is compromised by bad weather (Schiff, Arnone, & Cross, 1994). Some investigators (Shinar & Schieber, 1991) emphasize the importance of *dynamic acuity*—the ability to discriminate information in moving stimuli in driving. Dynamic acuity is most likely mediated by different neurological systems for vision and by receptors for motion as opposed to light intensity, what Suter (1995) calls the magnocellular or "where" pathway, together with a midbrain ambient system. Clinically, the distinction between conventional static and dynamic acuity has helped explain the mobility of some persons with apparently poor vision. Unfortunately, clinically practical methods for evaluating dynamic acuity are not yet available.

Format (iconic vs. verbal), size of letters, width, color, and composition of roadway markings are all parameters that can be used by highway planners and engineers to overcome problems with acuity. Individuals can make changes in the routes they drive, but they are usually unable to change the roadways. A personally unforgettable exception is the writer's own father, who sought her assistance in finding a good source of reflectors. Later she discovered that he had installed them at a difficult, otherwise unmarked turn he frequently had to navigate.

Near-point acuity is unlikely to be important for most aspects of driving, other than reading maps and certain gauges on the dashboard.

The dynamic functions of the visual system—those that depend on coordinated use of the musculature in the eyes—support binocularity, accommodation, and eye movements. Each of these can be helpful to the driver. For example, *stereopsis* (a product of binocular function) affords a three-dimensional appreciation of space. Loss of binocular function, and hence stereopsis, is common after traumatic brain injury. Also, if a person uses an eye patch to manage diplopia, or has lost an eye, stereopsis is lost. Less well appreciated, but possibly more frequent, is the loss of stereopsis in early stages of conditions that affect the elderly (cataracts, macular degeneration) where one eye is impaired first. Drivers use stereopsis in parking and making judgments about following distance and gaps in the traffic flow for merges and turns. Stopping too soon or too late at intersections is a symptom of poor stereopsis.

There is a fairly high incidence of impaired stereopsis in the general population, and a patient may never have had stereopsis. History is the best way to evaluate this possibility: Persons in certain occupations (e.g., pilots, police officers, and truck drivers) are required to have binocular vision and probably always had stereopsis. On the other hand, persons who had an eye turn when young or were given patching or eye exercises in childhood may never have had stereopsis. Under these circumstances, there was nothing to lose and in all likelihood such persons still use the monocular spatial analysis cues they used before the injury. It is the *loss* of stereopsis, not simply the *lack* of stereopsis, that is significant for driver rehabilitation. Other than for commercial drivers (who require binocular vision for licensure), this loss usually can be addressed through patient education and supervised practice.

Eye movement disorders are often difficult to treat, especially those characterized by spontaneous eye movements. If there is a restricted range of motion, mirrors and explicit head turns may enable safe driving.

Accommodative function may be helpful in allowing the driver to adjust focus from road to console. To address the loss of accommodation, which is almost universal in older drivers, automotive engineers have designed "heads up" displays in which important dashboard information appears on the windshield. Bi-, multi-, or variable-focus lenses also serve to compensate for loss of accommodation. In most cases this problem is easily and routinely addressed.

At the opposite end of the spectrum, neither easily nor routinely addressed, are visual field impairments. These have been alluded to throughout, and the reader is referred to other works by the present author and others on the subject (Gianutsos & Suchoff, 1997; Parisi, Bell, & Yassein, 1991). Visual field loss is compounded by a total or partial lack of awareness of that loss. If *homonymous hemianopia* (loss of visual responsivity in corresponding halves of the field of view) were experienced as a black stage curtain covering the field, it is unlikely that the individual would consider driving. When hemianopics attempt to drive, or perform dynamic visual search tasks, they often display a "robbing Peter to pay Paul" effect. They are so busy compensating that they fail to notice something on the intact side. This effect is also seen in steering, in which they have difficulty maintaining a central position in their lane. At one time they may drift too far into their missing field; at other times they drift into the intact field.

Since visual field impairment disqualifies one for licensure in many jurisdictions, and is regarded by many as incompatible with safe driving, there is little opportunity to evaluate its effects. For that reason it is perhaps appropriate to share my own clinical experiences in this regard. The EDS affords an extremely sensitive measure of responsivity to peripheral stimuli on the left and right sides while performing a preview tracking (steering) task. In 95% of the normative sample the difference in median response time is less than 0.10 second. If a person is 0.5 second slower on one side, the result will be flagged as extremely abnormal. Nonetheless, in more than one such case, driving performance was acceptable to an experienced road test examiner instructed to address this potential problem rigorously. Another individual with a dense left homonymous hemianopia from a stroke 6 months earlier continued to drive against advice. He bumped into furniture in the examiner's office, got lost, and could not fill out a paper and pencil form. On the EDS he was 1.5 seconds slower on the left side, and he missed some targets altogether. Apart from questionable judgment on this particular issue, he did well on other assessments, was well aware of the visual loss, and explicitly attempted to compensate. He was urged to pursue optical compensation using a reversing spectacle mounted mirror, and eventually did so. In New York State his field loss would have come to the attention of the licensing authorities only if his best corrected visual acuity were marginal, and he would have been required to submit a visual evaluation report. Unfortunately, New York does not afford immunity from a lawsuit for violation of confidentiality to concerned professionals who would report such cases.

I am aware of at least two cases in which persons with right homonymous hemianopia drove for several years, one with a reversing mirror. Both eventually stopped driving. In each case the final mishap was a crash in which the field problem was likely contributory, although in neither case did this information come to the attention of the authorities. One of these individuals, shortly after turning left onto a busy two-way commercial street, hit a parked delivery van on his right side. Another survivor of a severe stroke that left him with profound expressive aphasia, right hemiplegia, and a reduced visual responsivity in the lower right quadrant amassed over 100,000 safe miles. He actively denied any visual field impairment, although there were consistent reductions in response on functional visual field tasks (Gianutsos, 1991). For a month or two during which he was given a medication that made him drowsy, he had three minor scrapes on his right side. After stopping the medication, however, he once again drove safely.

My opinion is that it is very difficult for a person with homonymous hemianopia to maintain a safe driving record. In some cases where the problem is isolated and awareness is good, it may be possible to drive safely with mirrors and optical aids such as oversize, wide-angle, center-mounted rearview mirrors, reversing mirrors, and yoked prisms (Cohen & Waiss, 1993). Further, the amount and kind of driving may make a difference. Optometrist Daniel Gottlieb has reported favorably on this approach (Gottlieb, 1993; Gottlieb, Freeman, & Williams, 1992). My own approach is to demonstrate the problem to the patient by offering speeded visual processing tasks with feedback based on stimulus position. If the person can compensate on one task, switch to another. Let the person determine if he or she can generalize compensation to the new task. Increase the information density (visual complexity) of the display or the task complexity. Does the problem reemerge when the task is difficult or when the individual is tired? Have the person analyze and tabulate his or her performance separately for each side of the display. If the person does well on these off-road tasks and qualifies for driving lessons, be sure the driving instructor observes carefully for problems symptomatic of lateralized differential response and brings them quickly and bluntly to the individual's attention. Even with an optical device, the hemianopic driver must maintain an extraordinary level of vigilance. Such drivers should be monitored over an extended period and encouraged to keep a driving log and to discuss their experiences, including near misses.

Visual attention and visual perception have a significant cognitive aspect; however, they are built on a foundation of visual sensory processing, which logically and practically should be addressed first. The practical reason is that visual sensory function can often be treated, if not fixed, more easily than attention and perception can. Logically, attention can mean different things, including

- arousal
- sustained focus of effort
- resistance to distraction
- selection of relevant and filtering out of irrelevant information
- simultaneous or divided information processing
- mental flexibility or switching from one level or aspect to another efficiently.

Instead of "attention," it would be preferable to use terms that differentiate these aspects of information processing. Because of these many different meanings, attention (together with "motivation") is often used as a scapegoat, or explanation for variability that is not understood (an example of the nominal fallacy: naming something is not explaining it). A person responds inconsistently to stimuli presented to the field of vision contralateral to their brain injury: it is explained as "hemi-inattention." A boy is erratic about completing his schoolwork: his motivation is questioned, or he may be suspected of having attention deficit disorder.

With that caveat in mind, there are very real attentional problems associated with cognitive impairment that profoundly affect driving (Brouwer, Waterink, van Wolffelagr, & Rothengatter, 1993). It is possible to identify specific aspects of driving that require each of the six types of attention cited above (Mitchell, 1994). The best clinical research on this subject addresses the constriction in the *useful field of view* (UFOV) among older drivers (Ball & Owsley, 1991; Owsley & Ball, 1993; Owsley, Ball, Sloane, Roenker, & Bruni, 1991). Owsley, Ball, and their collaborators have demonstrated that recent driving records correlate with UFOV performance, that UFOV can predict driving, and that training can be used to counter these effects. The UFOV is a field of visual attention. One way to understand it is to consider the constriction of awareness that people experience when they are working hard on a specific task, such as being engrossed in a book or a movie. UFOV research has been used to account for the fact that older drivers have a disproportionate number of crashes making left turns at intersections where they need to deal with multiple issues in real time, for example, judging the gap in oncoming traffic, monitoring pedestrians, being aware of other drivers who may also be turning, and controlling their vehicle.

The field of visual attention can be assessed in several ways. A straightforward approach is to evaluate the functional visual fields using increasingly complex displays. While all people need more time to process informationally dense displays, some are more affected by the increase in information density than others. Using this approach, detailed in chapter 8 (Gianutsos, 1997) and in Gianutsos and Suchoff (1997), one can differentiate the contribution of sensory and attentional field impairment. Older drivers have more difficulty, relative to younger drivers, on the informationally complex tasks (Hall, 1995).

Finally, visual perception includes the interpretation of visual information. Recognition of objects (visual gnosis) may be delayed or impaired. Knowing that something constitutes a hazard is critical to dealing with it appropriately. The old saw that a driver must "expect the unexpected," is an implicit acknowledgment of the importance of efficient visual perception in driving. Clearly, visual perception is important in finding one's way (route finding).

Vision Screening for Driving

What then is recommended as a visual screening procedure in conjunction with driving advisement? A comprehensive examination by an eye care practitioner has clear advantages. Occupational therapists should address their efforts toward making this happen and assisting in appropriate understanding of and follow-through on recommendations. Usually, the eye care practitioner appreciates the therapist's help in working with patients who have known or suspected cognitive problems.

That said, a stereoscopic vision test can efficiently assess most of the aspects of vision cited earlier, especially in individuals sufficiently able to be candidates for driving advisement.

The one area that should be investigated further is the peripheral visual field. For this purpose, I use a collection of computerized tasks (REACT, SDSST, SOSH, and SEARCH) in which the attentional demands are progressively increased. These tasks (Gianutsos & Suchoff, 1997), which are together called PERFIELD, are very practical in that they may be conducted with most IBM-compatible computers. Normative data for younger and older adults accompany the programs. A summary sheet (Table 10.2) is useful to guide this part of the evaluation.

REACT is always used first. The task, which takes about 2.5 minutes, is repeated several times with varying conditions. Initially, it is conducted binocularly with eyes free to move and normal contrast. The examiner encourages response speed, especially on the central trials, which come first. Attention is drawn to the fact that the numbers that appear measure reaction time and that the goal is to get as low a score as possible. To

Table 10.2 Form for organizing data from functional visual field tasks.

Peripheral Visual Field: Functional Assessment

Patient: _____ ID# _____

Examiner: _____ Date: _____

Procedures:

---------- *REACT (Reaction Time Measure of Visual Field)* ----------

	Eye Tested	Fixate /Move	Dynamic /Stable	Contrast	Distraction	Mean Left	Mean Cntr	Mean Right	Median Left	Median Cntr	Median Right	Comment
1	Both	M	D	full	N	—	—	—	—	—	—	—
2	Both	M	D	full	Y	—	—	—	—	—	—	—
3	R	F	D	full	N	—	—	—	—	—	—	—
4	L	F	D	full	N	—	—	—	—	—	—	—
5	R	F	D	1%	N	—	—	—	—	—	—	—
6	L	F	D	1%	N	—	—	—	—	—	—	—
7			S	—	—	—	—	—	—	—	—	—
8			—	—	—	—	—	—	—	—	—	—
9			—	—	—	—	—	—	—	—	—	—
10			—	—	—	—	—	—	—	—	—	—

Variables addressed:

___ Eyes free to move vs. Eyes fixated

___ Binocular / Monocular

___ Normal vs. reduced contrast

___ Without vs. with distraction

___ Dynamic / Stable

Interpretation:

Field problems?:

Compensation?:

Prismatic assist: Effect:

Table 10.2 *Continued*

-------- *SDSST (Single & Double Simultaneous Simulation)* --------

Administration

	1: __/__		2: __/__	

Overall correct / N of trials:

Errors

		Left	Right	Left	Right
Single	Confusions	—	—	—	—
	Omissions	—	—	—	—
	Intrusions	—	—	—	—
Double	Confusions	—	—	—	—
	Omissions	—	—	—	—

Pattern of impairment:

Left or right side

Confusion vs. omission

'Extinction' (Double << Single)

Prismatic assist: Effect:

-------- *Visual Search—SOSH (Search for the Odd Shape) & SEARCH (Search for Shapes)* --------

Search Times

		Left	Right	Both
SOSH	Median	—	—	—
	Mean	—	—	—
SEARCH	Median	—	—	—
	Mean	—	—	—
	Error %	—	—	—

Interpretation:

explore the effect of distraction, the examiner can tell the patient, "We need to do this again, but you can answer some questions for me." Similarly, one can investigate the effects of fixation versus eyes free to move, and high and low contrast. The latter is most conveniently accomplished by testing the individual with special dark glasses that filter all but 1% of the light; that is, 1% transmission, gray-green wraparound lenses (very dark sunglasses) for implementing REACT low-contrast conditions, available from NoIR Medical Technologies, PO Box 159, South Lyon, MI 48178 (313-769-5565 or 800-521-9746). These can be placed over existing glasses. The patient often interprets the procedure as addressing night driving, although no claims are made in that regard. REACT conducted monocularly with fixation is most comparable to perimetric visual field testing. With eyes free to move, the individual is given the opportunity to demonstrate compensation for field loss. When hemianopic impairment is observed only with dark glasses, it is likely that there is a relative, but not absolute, loss.

SDSST is a computerized version of the Single and Double Simultaneous Stimulation Test, where stimuli are flashed on one or both sides in discrete trials. The computer tabulates omissions and confusions for each side of the display for single and double presentations. The classic "extinction" pattern, which is rather rare, is for errors on the affected side that occur only on double trials.

The SOSH (Search for the Odd Shape) task involves scanning an array of shapes ("Martian faces") for one that is different (the Martian that "fell asleep"), and poking him to "wake him up," the faster the better. This task is easy to understand and perform; however, some brain injury survivors encounter difficulty on this task. This pattern suggests reduced attentional capacity. This effect may be even more pronounced on SEARCH (Searching for Shapes). On both tasks the search times are displayed in the target location and summarized by quadrant and side.

One helpful feature of the PERFIELD procedures is that the results are displayed immediately in a format that the patient can understand. This feedback is of special value because it helps the individual become aware of visual field impairment.

In summary, these procedures clearly go well beyond the minimal standards for licensure. After all, driving advisement is for the purpose of giving the individual all the relevant information. While it is appropriate to address the issue of whether the person meets the minimal standard for licensure, it is not sufficient. The decisionmaking is the responsibility of the licensing authorities and, in a deeper sense, the prospective driver and concerned others. In driver rehabilitation the therapist is charged with identifying problems in functions that ordinarily are helpful for safe driving. In weighing the information and formulating recommendations, one must keep in mind the potential for interaction effects—compounding of impairments.

Acknowledgment

This chapter was made possible through the kind support and tranquility of Timbercreek.

REFERENCES

Ball, K., & Owsley, C. (1991). Identifying correlates of accident involvement for the older driver. *Human Factors, 33*(5), 583–595.

Brouwer, W. H., Waterink, W., van Wolffelaar, P. C., & Rothengatter, T. (1991). Divided attention in experienced young and older drivers: Lane tracking and visual analysis in a dynamic driving simulator. *Human Factors, 33*(5), 573–582.

Brown, J., Greaney, K., Mitchel, J., & Lee, W. S. (1993). *Predicting accidents and insurance claims among older drivers.* Southington, CT: ITT Hartford Insurance Group.

Chapman, B. G. (1995). Driving with the bioptic. *Journal of Vision Rehabilitation, 9*(4), 19–22.

Cohen, J., & Waiss, B. (1993). An overview of enhancement techniques for peripheral field loss. *Journal of American Optometric Association, 64,* 60–70.

Colsher, P. L., & Wallace, R. B. (1993). Geriatric assessment and driver functioning. *Clinics in Geriatric Medicine, 9*(2), 365–376.

DeLibero, V. (1995). *Self-appraisal and driving simulator performance in younger and older drivers.* Dix Hills, NY: Touro College School of Health Sciences, Department of Occupational Therapy.

Gianutsos, R. (1988). Computer programs for cognitive rehabilitation (Vol. 6): Driving Advisement System [Computer software]. Bayport, NY: Life Science Associates.

Gianutsos, R. (1991). Visual field deficits after brain injury: Computerized screening. *Journal of Behavioral Optometry, 2,* 143–150.

Gianutsos, R. (1994). Driving advisement with the Elemental Driving Simulator (EDS): When less suffices. *Behavior Research Methods, Instruments, & Computers, 26*(2), 183–186.

Gianutsos, R. (1997). Vision rehabilitation after brain injury. In M. Gentile & S. Schiff (Eds.), *A therapist's guide to the evaluation and treatment of vision dysfunction and low vision.* Bethesda, MD: American Occupational Therapy Association.

Gianutsos, R., & Beattie, A. (1992). Elemental driving simulator. *Proceedings of the Johns Hopkins National Search for Computing Applications to Assist Persons with Disabilities* (pp. 117–120). Los Alamitos, CA: IEEE Computer Society Press.

Gianutsos, R., Campbell, A., Beattie, A., & Mandriota, F. J. (1992). A computer-augmented quasi-simulation of the cognitive prerequisites for resumption of driving after brain injury. *Assistive Technology, 4,* 70–86.

Gianutsos, R., & Suchoff, I. B. (1997). Visual fields after brain injury: Management issues for the occupational therapist. In M. Scheiman (Ed.), *Vision: Screening and intervention techniques for occupational therapists.* Thorofare, NJ: Slack.

Gottlieb, D. D. (1993). *Enhancing awareness, increasing safety, and returning to driving for patients with visual field loss and neglect.* Paper presented at the meeting of the Neuro-Optometric Rehabilitation Association, International, Washington, D.C.

Gottlieb, D. D., Freeman, P., & Williams, M. (1992). Clinical research and statistical analysis of a visual field awareness system. *Journal of American Optometric Association, 63*(8), 581–588.

Hall, C. (1995). *Functional visual fields: Norms for younger and older viewers.* Dix Hills, NY: Touro College, School of Health Sciences, Department of Occupational Therapy.

Johnson, C. A., & Keltner, J. L. (1983). Incidence of visual field loss in 20,000 eyes and its relationship to driving performance. *Archives of Ophthalmology, 101,* 371–375.

Mitchell, S. (1994, October 20). *Brain injury and memory deficits in driver rehabilitation.* Paper presented at the meeting of ADED Northeast, Albany, NY.

Nouri, F. M., Tinson, D. J., & Lincoln, N. B. (1992). Cognitive ability and driving after stroke. *International Disability Studies, 9*(3), 111–115.

Owsley, C., & Ball, K. (1993). Assessing visual function in the older driver. *Clinics in Geriatric Medicine, 9*(2), 389–401.

Owsley, C., Ball, K., Sloane, M. E., Roenker, D. L., & Bruni, J. R. (1991). Visual/cognitive correlates of vehicle accidents in older drivers. *Psychology and Aging, 6,* 403–415.

Parasuraman, R., & Nestor, P. (1993). Attention and driving: Assessment in elderly individuals with dementia. *Clinics in Geriatric Medicine, 9*(2), 377–388.

Parisi, J. L., Bell, R. A., & Yassein, H. (1991). Homonymous hemianopic field defects and driving in Canada. *Canadian Journal of Ophthalmology,* *26*(5), 252–256.

Ramsey, W. E. (1990). *Low vision and driving.* Presented at AAA Driving Instruction Course: Focus on the Handicapped, College Park, MD.

Schiff, W., Arnone, W., & Cross, S. (1994). Driving assessment with computer-video scenarios: More is sometimes better. *Behavior Research Methods, Instruments, & Computers, 26*(2), 192–194.

Shinar, D., & Schieber, F. (1991). Visual requirements for safety and mobility of older drivers. *Human Factors, 33,* 507–519.

Strano, C. M. (1989). Effects of visual deficits on ability to drive in traumatically brain-injured population. *Journal of Head Trauma Rehabilitation, 4*(2), 35–43.

Subcommittee on Driver Evaluation and Training for Individuals with Disabilities. (1993). *Final report.* Albany, NY: New York State Vocational and Educational Services for Individuals with Disabilities (VESID).

Suter, P. S. (1995). Rehabilitation and management of visual dysfunction following traumatic brain injury. In M. J. Ashley & D. K. Krych (Eds.), *Traumatic brain injury rehabilitation* (pp. 198–220). Boca Raton, FL: CRC Press.

Szlyk, J. P., Brigell, M., & Seiple, W. (1993). Effects of age and hemianopic visual field loss on driving. *Optometry and Vision Science, 70*(12), 1031–1037.

van Zomeren, A. H., Brouwer, W. H., & Minderhoud, J. M. (1987). Acquired brain damage and driving: A review. *Archives of Physical Medicine and Rehabilitation, 68,* 697–705.

Wood, J. M. (1993). Can driving performance be predicted by vision testing? [Abstract]. *Optometry and Vision Science, 134.*

Part III.   Low Vision

11 Optometric Assessment of Low Vision

Bruce P. Rosenthal, OD, FAAO, and
Michael L. Fischer, OD, FAAO

Definitions

Many terms have been employed over the last 65 years to define low vision. One of the first definitions of low vision was given by Faye (1984), who described low vision as bilateral subnormal visual acuity or abnormal visual field resulting from a disorder in the visual system. The vision loss in low vision cannot be corrected to a normal visual acuity level with standard corrective lenses (including contact or intraocular lenses) or by medical or surgical intervention. In 1975 Mehr and Freid described *low vision* or *partial sight* as reduced central acuity or visual field loss that, even with the best optical correction provided by regular lenses, still results in visual impairment from a performance standpoint. Mehr and Freid pointed out that this definition assumes that the loss is bilateral, that some form vision remains, and that regular lenses do not include reading aids over +4.00 diopter, telescopes, pinholes, visors, or other unusual devices which will be categorized as low vision aids.

Arditi and Rosenthal (1996) introduced a new definition of *functional visual impairment* as a significant limitation of visual capability resulting from disease, trauma, or congenital condition that cannot be fully ameliorated by standard refractive correction, medication, or surgery and that is manifested by one or more of the following:

- insufficient visual resolution (worse than 20/60 in the better eye with best correction of ametropia)
- inadequate field of vision (worse that 20 degrees along the widest meridian in the eye with the more intact central field; or homonymous bilateral hemianopsia or quadranopsia)
- reduced peak contrast sensitivity (0.3 log unit loss in the better eye).

This definition addresses some of the primary visual disorders that may be encountered by the occupational therapist. That is, the definition specifically includes *hemianopsia*, which is a loss of one-half of the visual field owing to a stroke, a tumor, or other damage in the cortical visual pathway. This definition also tries to quantify a loss in contrast, which may affect mobility, activities of daily living, and reading.

Colenbrander (1976) was the first to introduce the following terms, commonly used in rehabilitative medicine, to the field of low vision: disorder, impairment, disability, and handicap.

Colenbrander defined visual *disorder* as any deviation from normal structure or function of the body or parts thereof (e.g., cataract, cornea, or scar on the retina). A disorder leads to an *impairment*, which is a disorder interfering with an organ function (e.g., reduced visual acuity, decreased contrast sensitivity, reduced visual field, or color vision deficits). An impairment can then lead to a *disability*, which is the lack, loss, or reduction of an individual's ability to perform certain tasks (e.g., a person cannot read a newspaper or travel safely in the environment). Note that impairment refers to the basic functions performed by a part of the body; disability refers to tasks performed by a person. A visual *handicap* is the societal and economic consequences of a disability. A person could be considered handicapped if reading the newspaper is an important activity in the person's life.

Colenbrander (1976) described visual acuity impairment, visual field impairment, and contrast sensitivity impairment as a progression of loss from none to slight to moderate to severe to profound to near-total to total visual loss.

Colenbrander assessed visual disability and visual handicap in the same terms. Under the visual disability classification, a person with near-normal vision can perform all visual tasks, while an individual with a moderate to severe visual loss needs optical appliances for detailed visual tasks. An individual with a severe visual disability needs optical appliances and other senses for gross visual tasks. With respect to visual handicap, an individual with normal or near-normal vision can meet societal expectations, while a person with a moderate to total visual handicap cannot meet societal expectations visually.

Colenbrander also noted that clinicians and researchers should use accurate universal terminology that will maximize communication and team work and foster further development of rehabilitation techniques.

During the last 25 years, the expression *low vision* has taken on various connotations. It has not only come to define a person with a bilateral vision loss but also has become synonymous with an area of expertise dealing with persons who have visual impairments. Vision rehabilitation has come generally to imply a team approach in the remediation process.

It should be noted that amblyopia is sometimes confused with or substituted for low vision. However, by definition *amblyopia* is a monocular loss in vision rather than a loss in both eyes.

Legal Blindness

Being diagnosed with low vision does not necessarily mean that a person is legally blind. *Legal blindness* is a term that was introduced in the United States in the 1930s for state and federal aid to the blind (Nowakowski, 1994), and it is still used today as a measure of a person's eligibility for such benefits. Legal blindness is used to identify those individuals who have a visual acuity of 20/200 or less in the better eye or a visual field of 20 degrees or less in the better eye. It should also be noted that by international standards an individual may be considered to have low vision when visual acuity is as good as 20/40 or 20/50 (6/12 or 6/15 [the numerator in the test distance being expressed in meters]) or the visual field is anywhere from 100 to 20 degrees (Johnston, 1991).

Epidemiology

Four classic studies, the Framingham Eye Study (Kahn et al., 1977), the Beaver Dam Eye Study (Klein, Klein, Linton, & Demets, 1991), the Baltimore Eye Survey (Tielsch, Sommer, Witt, Katz, & Royall, 1990), and the Mud Creek Valley Study (Dana et al., 1990), concluded that visual impairment and blindness increase significantly with age. Greater life expectancy translates into more and more people with significant visual impairments. In fact, it has been estimated that by 2030, 65.6 million persons will be over the age of 65 (U.S. Bureau of the Census, 1989). With increasing numbers of older people comes increased prevalence in conditions associated with an aging population. These include macular degeneration, glaucoma, diabetic retinopathy, and optic atrophy.

However, some populations have a greater prevalence of ocular disease with aging. For example, the Baltimore Eye Survey (Tielsch et al., 1990) pointed out that the prevalence of visual impairment and blindness is twice as high in the Black population compared with the White population owing to the incidence of glaucoma and diabetic retinopathy.

Many conditions have a hereditary basis, including optic atrophy, cataract and macular degeneration. A careful case history will often detail the incidence of the condition in immediate family members as well as in past generations. Some diseases, if present during pregnancy (such as rubella or syphilis), may be passed on to the fetus and can have ocular complications that are manifested at birth. Other causative factors resulting in congenital low vision include prematurity, low-birth-weight babies, fetal alcohol syndrome, and drug abuse during pregnancy.

The Low Vision Team

Remediation of visual impairment involves more than just treating the eyes. Many individuals may take part in the vision rehabilitation of persons with low vision. These individuals may include a(n)

- optometrist or ophthalmologist
- optician
- social worker
- orientation and mobility instructor
- rehabilitation teacher
- educator
- low vision instructor
- vision rehabilitation therapist
- nurse
- physical therapist
- occupational therapist
- psychologist
- medical specialists
- internist
- neurologist
- diabetologist
- psychiatrist.

A low vision evaluation is generally recommended or is provided by the ophthalmologist or optometrist. Some situations that require medical intervention may warrant attention prior to the low vision evaluation. These can include

- removal of a cataract
- laser treatment of the retina for hemorrhaging or leakage of fluid in conditions such as macular degeneration or diabetic retinopathy
- surgery for a detached retina that can be associated with high myopia or trauma
- corneal transplant
- determination of the type of or combination of eye drops, systemic medications, laser treatment, and surgery to reduce the eye pressure in glaucoma therapy

• *vitrectomy* (a procedure involving removal of the vitreous, a jellylike fluid occupying the center of the eye) when there is, for example, hemorrhage, debris from trauma, or fibrous bands that cloud the vitreous

• lid problems such as *ectropion* (lid turning out) or *entropion* (lid turning in).

The Low Vision Evaluation

The referral for a low vision evaluation is usually made to a low vision service in a rehabilitation agency, a private group or individual practice with an optometrist or ophthalmologist specializing in low vision, or a vision service at a university. (Some of the many programs for advanced study in low vision include low vision residencies and internships as well as The Lighthouse Low Vision Continuing Education Program.) Institutions offering low vision services often have additional services that may be of benefit in the evaluation or rehabilitation of the patient with low vision. For example, an agency that specializes in vision rehabilitation may also offer

- training in the use of low vision devices
- orientation and mobility training
- social service and counseling
- techniques or training in daily living activities
- technology and computer centers
- reader service
- art, music, and dance classes
- children's services
- adult and children recreation services.

A university clinic may offer other specialties, as well as specialized testing procedures not generally available in a private practice. Some examples of these special procedures, which may be integral in the diagnosis or prognosis of the individual with low vision, will be discussed.

Electrodiagnostic Procedures

Electroretinogram (ERG)

The *ERG* is an objective test that reflects overall retinal function. It is the summed electrical response from the retina resulting from stimulation of the rods and cones by light energy. It is the test most frequently used to confirm or deny the diagnosis of retinitis pigmentosa (Sherman & Bass, 1995).

Visual Evoked Potential (VEP)

The *VEP* is another objective test of visual function. The electrical activity of the brain is monitored at the occipital cortex by scalp electrodes while the patient views a visual stimulus. The electrical response at the occipital cortex is measured and recorded. Because the response is evoked by a visual stimulus, it is called an evoked potential (Sherman & Bass, 1995). The VEP is used in certain situations as an objective measurement of visual acuity, and retinal and optic nerve dysfunction in the absence of observable pathology. The test is also used in objectively estimating binocular fusion and stereopsis, in the prognostic assessment of amblyopia, as well as with nonverbal patients having autism, Down's syndrome, Alzheimer's, or cerebral palsy (Sherman & Sutija, 1991).

The most common types of visual evoked potential tests include the flash and the pattern VEP. *Flash VEP* is a method of obtaining the visual evoked potential using a bright flashing stimulus. It may be used in predicting the integrity of the visual system in a patient with a scarred cornea or cataracts. *Pattern VEP* is a response to checkerboard patterns stimulation. The checkerboard squares appear on a monitor in various sizes and rapidly alternate from black to white to black squares. The pattern VEP is the one test that allows objective measurement of visual acuity. Pattern VEP results can be influenced by uncorrected refractive error or lack of attention on the stimulus.

Electro-Oculogram (EOG)

The *EOG* is another electrodiagnostic test that assesses the integrity of the pigment epithelium layer in the retina. (Sherman & Bass, 1984). The EOG is not used as frequently as the ERG or VEP but is used as a differential diagnostic test for such unusual conditions as Leber's congenital amaurosis or retinitis pigmentosa sine pigmento.

Ultrasound

Ultrasound (Bass & Sherman, 1991) is a test that uses the reflection of sound waves to provide a visual representation of the internal ocular structures. This is especially useful when media opacities make it difficult or impossible to see inside the eye. A-scan is frequently used to determine the axial length of the eye for the determination of the power of an intraocular lens used in cataract surgery. B-scan is used in many clinical applications including determining the existence of a detached retina, the detection of intraocular tumors, and the presence of lens dislocation.

Other Procedures

Fluorescein angiography (FA) (Fingeret, Casser, & Woodcome, 1990) is a diagnostic photography procedure used to detect vascular compromise to the retina, choroid, and optic nerve. FA allows evaluation of the presence of subretinal vasculature changes that may not be seen with the ophthalmoscope. It is frequently used in the assessment of certain forms of macular degeneration and diabetic retinopathy, among other conditions.

Magnetic resonance imaging (MRI) (Oshinskie, 1991) is a noninvasive method of examining an internal body structure including the orbit and its components. It has been shown to be effective in imaging many brain lesions and space occupying lesions. It is used, for example, in imaging lesions in multiple sclerosis and intraocular tumors.

Computer axial tomography (CAT) (Oshinskie, 1991) uses x rays like conventional tomography but produces a series of slices of the structure studied. The CAT scan is used in the diagnosis of ocular masses, tumors of the optic nerve, blowout fractures of the orbit, and bone erosion.

Evaluating Visual Impairment—The Case History

Low vision remediation begins with a functional low vision evaluation. As noted above, the low vision evaluation generally follows medical intervention. Concurrent medical treatment may take place during the low vision intervention since many conditions may be progressive in nature (including macular degeneration, diabetic retinopathy, or glaucoma).

A detailed case history is the first step in low vision rehabilitation. A common part of present routine medical care is to have the patient complete a preexamination written survey that includes a medical history and a systems analysis (e.g., heart, lungs, kidneys, integument, genitourinary, neuro, etc.). A similar survey, which includes functional problems, is helpful prior to low vision assessment but it may be difficult for the patient with low vision to fill out, because persons with impaired vision generally have difficulty filling out forms. In these cases, another option is to obtain the intake information over the telephone, prior to the evaluation. The optometrist or ophthalmologist can then review any problem areas and cover in detail the eye history as well as the medical history.

It is during the telephone intake or when the clinician reviews the history that problems other than vision may be manifested. It is normal for persons with vision loss to experience symptoms of anger, denial, or depression. Often, success in the vision rehabilitation process depends on the progress made in coming to terms with the vision loss.

The case history comprises patient observation, ocular history, general medical history, living situation, and task analysis of traveling, distance viewing, daily living activities, near tasks, lighting, and school-related tasks.

Patient objectives are established during the history. The ultimate goal of the evaluation, however, is to provide *prescriptive* optical, electronic, or other adaptive devices along with rehabilitative services, such as orientation and mobility, activities of daily living, or social service intervention when indicated. A prescriptive device may be a spectacle correction such as distance, near, bifocal, or trifocal lenses. Prescriptive devices may also be magnification systems, such as hand or stand magnifiers, telescopic systems, absorptive lenses, or electronic magnification systems.

The appropriate strength of a prescriptive device is determined from the low vision evaluation. A loss of ability to use a prescriptive lens that previously worked may indicate a serious change in the visual status owing to an active disease process (e.g., hemorrhage, retinal detachment, or increase in the intraocular pressure). These conditions warrant immediate attention.

In infants and children, the low vision history will include not only questions to the parents about the child's visual behavior but also questions about the child's overall development. Because physical, cognitive, and social development are all influenced by vision, a vision problem should be identified early so that, if necessary, other types of intervention might be instituted to assist the child as he or she grows.

The clinician should note any medications, either ocular or systemic, that may affect the functional vision of the patient with low vision. Some of the more common medications are

- antihistamines
- antidepressants
- carbonic anhydrase inhibitors
- corticosteroids
- mydriatic agents
- nonsteroidal anti-inflammatory drugs (NSAIDs)
- anti-infective agents
- glaucoma agents (including miotic agents).

Medications may affect the visual system as well as the patient's psychological status. Some of the areas that may be affected (Oliver, 1996) are

- color perception
- contrast sensitivity
- depth of focus
- depth of field
- extraocular muscle function (eye movements)
- lacrimation (tearing or dry eyes)
- lighting needs
- magnification requirement
- ocular surface integrity
- overall contrast
- patient's psychological status
- perceived brightness
- pupil size
- rate of blinking
- spherical aberration
- tear film quality
- visual acuity measurement
- visual field.

Oliver (1996) noted that the low vision evaluation should be performed prior to the instillation of any medications into the patient's eyes to eliminate the risk of adverse reactions that may affect the patient's visual performance. Oliver also noted that all patients using topical steroids need to be closely monitored for the development of elevated intraocular pressure, cataracts, or other complications that could have a detrimental effect on ocular health or efficient visual performance. Problems such as a loss in contrast sensitivity (to be discussed) and a decrease in visual acuity can result.

The history will provide information on the major areas of difficulty, and recommendations will be made at the conclusion of the evaluation for the appropriate low vision devices or additional services warranted.

Visual Acuity

Visual acuity is a measure of the smallest target an eye can recognize or detect at a specific distance. Visual acuity measurement follows the case history. For the patient with low vision, it is important to determine an *accurate* visual acuity and *not* to use other notations, such as counts fingers (CF) or hand motion (HM). These terms do little to describe the visual function.

To enable the accurate measurement of a functional visual acuity, specialized charts are used in the low vision evaluation. These charts take the place of the projector chart found in a typical examination room.

Distance visual acuity measures generally use single letters calibrated according to the distance at which the letters subtend 5' (minutes of arc) and each component of the letter subtends 1'. The Snellen fraction is given by the test distance in the numerator and standard distance of the smallest letter correctly identified in the denominator.

As noted above, the chart generally used in the primary eye examination room is a chart that is projected on the wall. This chart is often not the best way to measure low levels of visual acuity and, therefore, does not permit the most accurate measurement of acuities worse than 20/100.

A variety of other charts are preferred for use in the low vision examination. One in frequent use today is known as the ETDRS chart, which comes from Early Treatment of Diabetic Retinopathy Study (Figure 11.1). (This is also the standard eye chart used in research for all studies conducted by the National Eye Institute.) The chart's specific properties are

- an equal number of letters (5) on each line
- a logarithmic progression from line to line
- an equal level of difficulty on each line (in terms of recognizability of the letters)
- an equal spacing between the letters and the lines.

Using the ETDRS chart, visual acuity can be accurately measured from as low as 20/800 to as high as 20/20. However, notation of low vision acuity (both distance and near) with the ETDRS chart is done in metric (M) units.

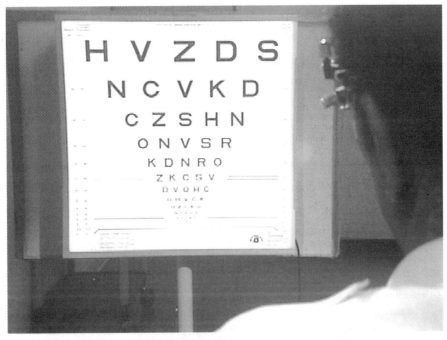

Figure 11.1 ETDRS chart. From *The Lighthouse Low Vision Examination Techniques,* "Function Tests." Copyright 1996 The Lighthouse, Inc. Reprinted with permission.

Acuity in metric notation is done the same way as traditional Snellen acuity (which is in foot notation). For example, if the testing is at 2 meters, the numerator of the fraction is 2. If the visual acuity is measured at 4 meters, the numerator is 4. The denominator, as noted previously, would be the size of the smallest letter read at the test distance.

Therefore, if the testing was at 2 meters and the smallest letter read was the top line of the ETDRS chart, the visual acuity would be 2/40. Conversion to Snellen acuity is easily accomplished. In this example, adding a 0 to the digits of the numerator and denominator would give an equivalent Snellen acuity of 20/400. If the smallest line read was the 20M-size letter at 2 meters, then the acuity would be 2/20 (equivalent to 20/200).

Another low vision chart in common usage is the Designs for Vision or Feinbloom number chart (Figure 11.2) that has numbers as large as 700 feet, allowing the doctor to measure visual acuities that are even lower than with the ETDRS chart. As an illustration, if the largest number read is the 700-foot number, and the patient can see it only at 1 foot away, then the visual acuity is 1/700, which is equivalent to 20/14,000. It is important to note that the testing distance and the letters used to take the acuity must be measured in the same units (i.e., both in meters or both in feet; you cannot mix the two units in a single fraction).

When taking acuity with these larger targets (whether by ETDRS, Designs for Vision, or some other acuity chart), patients may be encouraged to use the part of their vision that allows them to see more clearly. Patients with loss of central vision may need to intentionally look off to the side to make out the letters on the chart, a technique known as eccentric viewing. Persons with inherited vision loss frequently use these off-center points instinctively, while those with an acquired vision loss may need training or prisms to help them find the point that allows optimal visual performance.

Near visual acuity is taken at the habitual reading distance (where the patient normally reads). For instance, if the patient routinely holds the reading material 3 inches from the nose, the low vision doctor will begin taking near acuities at this distance. Near acuities will be taken at specific

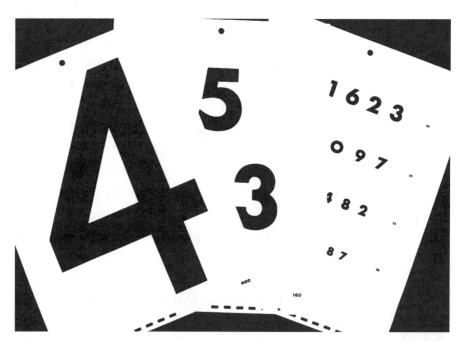

Figure 11.2 Designs for Vision number chart. Photo courtesy of Richard Feinbloom, President, Designs for Vision, Ronkonkoma, Long Island, N.Y. Reprinted with permission.

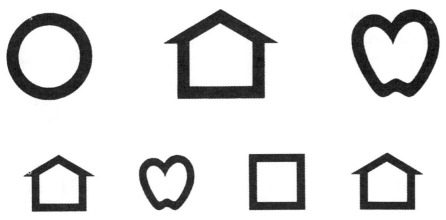

Figure 11.3 Lea symbols. Courtesy of Precision Vision, Chicago. Reprinted with permission.

distances later in the exam to help determine how much magnification the patient will need for various near tasks. The importance of lighting control may be initially addressed during this phase of the testing, as illumination can be critical to the patient's success with low vision devices.

Visual acuity can also be measured (or at least estimated) in infants and young children with low vision by using specialized testing procedures. The procedures used will depend on the child's age and responsiveness. One such test is preferential looking, in which cards with grating patterns (stripes) on one side only are presented in front of the child. The basis of the test is that if the child can see the stripes, he or she will prefer to look in that direction. If the child reacts positively to the cards with the smaller stripes, this suggests better visual acuity. The person performing the test must be trained to perform it properly and to interpret the child's responses. Other tests that use symbols (Figure 11.3), instead of letters or numbers, can be used with more responsive children to more accurately estimate visual acuity.

Refraction

Refraction is the procedure used to determine which lenses are needed to accurately focus light from distant objects on the retina. In simpler terms, it is the way the doctor determines whether the patient is farsighted or nearsighted, or has astigmatism (which can cause blurry vision at all distances).

A careful refraction is essential prior to any determination of the appropriate lens system. Significant changes in the refraction may occur owing to cataract formation or retinal changes. Specialized techniques are often used in the low vision exam in the determination of the refractive error, since these patients may be viewing eccentrically, have media interference from the cornea or the lens, or have high uncorrected refractive error.

In low vision, a trial frame is often used for the refraction instead of the standard *phoropter*, which is the instrument with many lenses used in the primary care evaluation. The subjective evaluation (where the doctor gives the patient a variety of lens choices to more accurately determine the appropriate lens prescription) may result in a prescription that is significantly different from the entering prescription. This difference may be due to physiologic changes in the eye or to the fact that the patient has not undergone an accurate refraction.

When a patient is too young to respond to lens choices or is noncommunicative for some other reason (as occurs sometimes after a stroke), a refractive evaluation can still be performed by the optometrist or ophthalmologist using a procedure called retinoscopy. By shining a light in the eye and using different lenses, the doctor can frequently get a very accurate, objective determination of the refractive error.

Predicting the Magnification

Following the refraction, the clinician will use specialized charts to determine the appropriate magnification for achieving the patient's objectives. These objectives may include everyday tasks like reading the daily newspaper, looking at prices or labels, reading the mail, or even loading a syringe (if the patient is a diabetic).

As noted earlier, low vision clinicians use M notation to record near visual acuity. A 1M letter is a letter subtending 5 minutes of arc when held at a 1-meter distance. A 1M letter, which is generally considered to be the size of newspaper print, is comparable to a 20/50 Snellen letter or 9-point type when it is viewed at 16″ (40 cm). A 2M letter is twice the size of a 1M letter.

Other Tests of Visual Function

Amsler Grid and Contrast Sensitivity

The Amsler Grid (Figure 11.4) and contrast sensitivity evaluation (Figure 11.5) follow the refraction. The Amsler Grid is a standard diagnostic test used to help identify early macular changes. However, the Amsler Grid has a different function in the low vision evaluation than the primary care examination. It is used as a prognostic indicator of a patient's success with low vision devices.

The grid, when viewed at 33 cm (13 in.), reflects the integrity of the central 20 degrees of vision. It is an important test that demonstrates

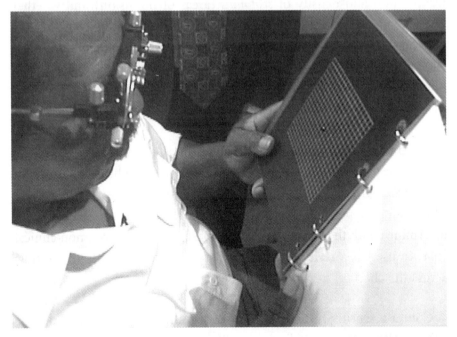

Figure 11.4 A patient being tested with an Amsler grid. From *The Lighthouse Low Vision Examination Techniques*, "Function Tests." Copyright 1996, The Lighthouse, Inc. Reprinted with permission.

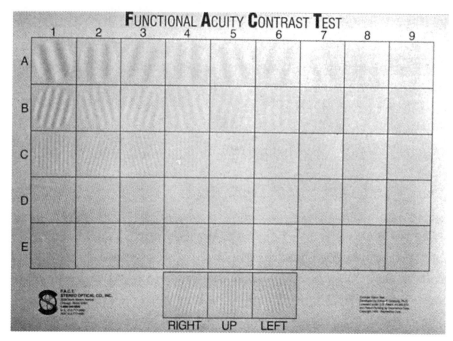

Figure 11.5 Contrast sensitivity. Developed by Arthur P. Ginsburg, PhD. Licensed under U.S. Patent # 4,365,873 and 5,414,479 by Visometrics Corp. Manufactured by Stereo Optical Company, Inc., Chicago, IL.

the position and density of *scotomas* (areas of no vision) and whether the patient should be using the right eye, left eye, or both eyes. Patients who have experienced changes in the macula from hemorrhaging, scarring, edema, or laser treatment may exhibit such scotomas. Damage to other structures in the visual pathway (like the optic nerve) can also lead to scotomas.

Contrast sensitivity function (CSF) testing is also important in determining the patient's visual function. CSF is similar to a hearing test where a person's high, middle, and low hearing frequencies are determined. In CSF testing, a person's high, middle, and low visual frequencies are determined with the use of specialized charts. The most common clinical chart in use has a series of sine wave gratings that decrease in contrast across the chart.

Contrast sensitivity tests may provide valuable information on the effect of lighting for reading, as well as determine whether increased magnification is necessary for near visual tasks. CSF has also been beneficial in predicting whether an individual may perform better with white letters on a black background (reverse polarity).

Visual Field Assessment

Visual field analysis provides subjective information on the extent of the loss of peripheral or central visual field (Figure 11.6). Some of the primary uses of the visual field analysis are to

- establish whether an individual is legally blind
- determine whether the visual field is large enough to drive legally
- establish a baseline for monitoring future change
- serve as an aid in the selection of low vision devices
- identify the need for orientation and mobility training (Nowakowski, 1994).

A variety of techniques are employed to determine the extent of a person's visual field loss. The Amsler Grid, previously described, provides information on the central 20 degrees of the visual field. The tangent screen is another central field technique that evaluates the central 30 degrees of the visual field. More sophisticated equipment is used to determine the visual field for driving or the progression of a visual field loss. The most commonly used visual field plotters are the Goldmann perimeter and the automated visual field units.

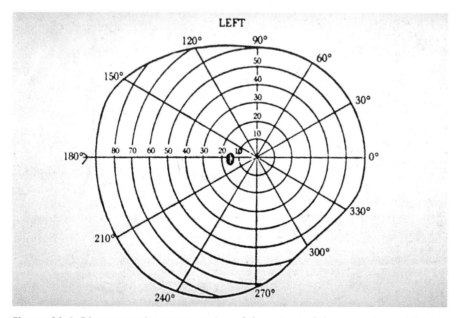

Figure 11.6 Diagrammatic representation of the extent of the normal visual field in the left eye.

Bass and Sherman (1996) stated that automated perimetry has paved the way for more standardized and accurate visual field testing in all types of patients, including those with low vision. They also point out that, although automated perimetry makes it relatively easy to perform visual field testing, the interpretation still lies with the practitioner.

A visual field screening in infants and young children is possible. Evaluation may involve the use of colored objects or lights. While the test in young children is often less accurate and more qualitative than quantitative, it is still possible to get a sense of whether a child has a significant visual field loss.

Color Vision Testing

Fischer (1996) noted two reasons for considering color vision testing in the patient with low vision:

• Diagnosis—color test results, in conjunction with other examination findings, can sometimes be an invaluable part of a diagnostic profile, where the etiology of a patient's vision loss is uncertain. For example, hereditary (congenital) defects are usually found in males, are red-green in nature, and show predictable and repeatable results; while acquired color deficiencies may be found in males or females, are blue-yellow or red-green, are unpredictable, and are often not repeatable.
• Function—some patients may depend on color vision for certain tasks in their daily lives.

Most commercially available color vision tests were designed to detect and classify hereditary color vision deficiencies; as such, they may have limited value for the patient with low vision. One of the more commonly used and beneficial color vision tests in the assessment of the patient with low vision is the Farnsworth Panel D-15 test, in which the patient is asked to put colored caps in a specific order. A similar but more extensive and time-consuming test of color perception is the Farnsworth-Munsell 100-Hue test, also a color-ordering task.

Individuals may experience color vision loss when a specific part of the visual system is affected. For example, persons with macular degeneration, glaucoma, and diabetic retinopathy may demonstrate a blue-yellow defect while those with optic nerve disease may reveal a red-green defect. Pharmaceutical agents may also cause a change on the color vision tests. For example, persons on medication for cardiovascular problems may demonstrate either a blue-yellow or a red-green defect and may report yellow vision.

As with the other portions of the low vision assessment, tests are available with simpler tasks that children can perform. An example is the PV-16 Precision Vision Quantitative Color Vision test by Hyvärinen (1995), which uses a matching task instead of an ordering task. In more responsive children, these tests can provide the same type of information as the tests used with teenagers and adults. Hyvärinen stated that evaluation of color vision is important in children because colors are critical to the recognition of certain objects. Further, in children with color vision defects colors may present problems if used as a coding system, necessitating other techniques for object identification.

Ocular Health Assessment

An ocular health assessment is done to determine the type and extent of disease present in the eyes and associated structures. A gross assessment is often performed early in the low vision evaluation (after visual acuities) to identify any obvious abnormalities that might impact on the functional portions of the exam. This external evaluation will include the pupillary reactions; ocular motility; evaluation of strabismus; the presence of nystagmus; and the appearance of the lids, cornea, and iris. More detailed testing, including ophthalmoscopy (used to look at the structures inside the eye), is generally performed at the end of the low vision evaluation to evaluate the lens, vitreous, retina, and optic nerve.

Supplementary Procedures

Additional tests, such as those mentioned earlier, may be ordered in particular cases where additional diagnostic information is required to help manage the patient. One such test, the visual evoked potential (VEP), can provide data about the type of information reaching the visual cortex in the brain and can sometimes estimate a person's visual acuity. The test can be useful with patients who are noncommunicative or uncooperative and with very young children.

Selecting the Appropriate Low Vision Device

Once the history, refraction, and functional assessment are complete, the clinician takes *all* the information and uses it to select the appropriate optical or adaptive device that will allow the patient to achieve his or her objectives. First, the doctor must determine whether a standard distance correction, bifocals, or reading glasses should be prescribed. This is followed by an assessment of the patient's performance with various low vision devices and the ultimate selection of the appropriate low vision device(s) to help the patient.

Low vision devices are grouped into the following categories:

- high plus spectacle lenses
- hand magnifiers
- stand magnifiers
- telescopes
- absorptive lenses
- electronic systems
- adaptive (nonoptical) devices.

Because low vision optical devices frequently require training to use them successfully, it is common to let patients have a trial period with the device(s) at home before making a final decision on the device to be prescribed. The doctor and patient, along with the low vision instructor, will work together to arrive at the most appropriate devices to address the patient's different needs.

Basic Optics

Some very basic concepts must be understood when working with lenses that are used for close work.

- Lenses are designated in plus and minus power (e.g., +5.00 or −5.00). Plus (+) lenses are prescribed over the distance refraction to focus the person for near. The lenses primarily used in low vision remediation are strong plus (+) lenses.

- The standard unit of measurement to describe the power of a lens, whether it is prescribed for distance vision or near vision, is the *diopter*. One diopter of lens power will focus parallel light 1 meter away. The larger the number of diopters, the stronger the lens. For example, a +5.00 diopter lens is twice as strong as a +2.50 diopter lens. A +10.00 lens is twice as strong as a +5.00. Exceptionally strong lenses may be used in low vision remediation (e.g., +10.00 diopters to +80.00 diopters).

- Another concept is the focal length of the lens. The stronger the lens, the shorter the focal length and the closer the reading material must be held to get it in focus. An easy way to visualize the focal length of a plus lens is to think of a leaf being burned by a magnifier. The stronger the magnifier, the closer it has to be held to the leaf.

Following are some illustrations of the focal length of lenses:

- A +2.50 diopter lens will focus at 40 cm (16 in.) to burn the leaf.
- A +5.00 diopter lens will focus at 20 cm (8 in.).
- A +10.00 diopter lens will focus at 10 cm (4 in.).
- A +20.00 diopter lens will focus at 5 cm (2 in.).
- A +40.00 diopter lens will focus at 2.5 cm (1 in.).

Some rules of thumb can generally be applied when working with patients with low vision.

- The poorer the vision, the stronger the lens prescribed.
- The stronger the lens, the closer to the page that one has to work.
- The stronger the lens, the more critical the lighting will be while reading.
- The stronger the lens, the smaller the area that one can see while reading. That is, an individual with normal vision can scan a line, while a person with a severe visual impairment might be able to read only a few letters at one time.
- Reading becomes progressively more difficult as the strength of the lens increases.

High Plus Spectacles, Hand Magnifiers, and Stand Magnifiers

The plus lens is prescribed in three forms that have equivalent power (strength). Specifically, the lens may be put into a pair of glasses known as a high plus or microscopic lenses; it may be placed into a more traditional hand magnifier; or it may be put in a rigid housing, known as a stand magnifier, that is placed on the reading material.

High plus lenses or microscopic spectacles are the most commonly prescribed low vision devices for close work. They offer the benefit of looking like normal glasses, and they allow the hands to be free for holding material. Depending on the findings of the function tests, they may be prescribed for binocular (two-eyes) or monocular (one-eye) use. Generally, binocular corrections are given to persons with vision better than 20/200. The most frequently prescribed binocular reading lenses used in low vision are the prism half-eye glasses (Figure 11.7), which can be prescribed up to +12.00 diopters.

High plus spectacles (Figure 11.8) may also be prescribed monocularly, especially when vision is significantly decreased. The most commonly prescribed microscopic lens is known as the *aspheric lens* (a lens with special curves to correct for aberrations in its periphery). Up to 12×

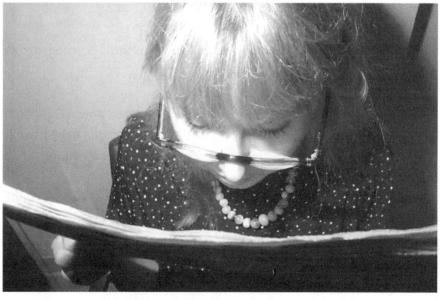

Figure 11.7 Half-eye prism glasses. Copyright 1996 by The Lighthouse, Inc. Reprinted with permission.

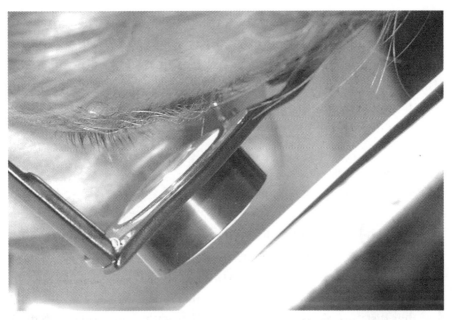

Figure 11.8 High plus microscopic lens. Copyright 1996 by The Lighthouse, Inc. Reprinted with permission.

magnification (+48 diopters) is prescribed. In addition to the aspheric lens, more sophisticated systems known as the *doublet lenses* (lenses composed of two plus lenses separated by an air space) are used. Doublet lenses (shown in Figure 11.8) have better optics and a wider usable field for reading. The most common doublet lens which is prescribed is the Clear Image lens, manufactured by Designs for Vision.

Hand magnifiers are used for common short-term activities such as looking at prices, labels, recipes, oven temperature, bills, or telephone numbers. They come in powers ranging from 1.5× to 20× magnification (6 to 80 diopters).

A variety of hand magnifiers are available. They range from inexpensive spherical magnifiers that generally have poor optics to sophisticated aspheric and multiple lens systems with superior optics. Prescription of the hand magnifier is again dependent on the patient's needs and the findings from the functional evaluative tests.

Stand magnifiers are also handheld devices, but, unlike hand magnifiers that require focusing by the user, stand magnifiers sit directly on the reading material, eliminating the need for the patient to find the focal distance. They can be very useful for patients who have hand tremors and thus cannot hold a hand magnifier or reading material steady. The optics of stand magnifiers are more complex than some of the other low vision devices, and expertise is required in selecting the appropriate power magnifier and the appropriate prescription lenses to be used in conjunction with the magnifier.

Telescopes

Patients with low vision frequently need assistance in seeing things more clearly at distance. Unfortunately, these patients do not always receive sufficient improvement in distance vision from standard distance glasses, because it is not possible to magnify with standard spectacles. The only way that distant objects can be magnified is with a telescopic system.

Telescopes come in a variety of styles and powers. Many patients with low vision will use handheld telescopes for spotting tasks involved with mobility (such as reading street signs and seeing traffic lights and Walk/ Don't Walk signals). Spectacle-mounted telescopes are often used for tasks where the person needs to use the telescope for extended periods or for tasks where the hands need to be free, such as driving, computer work, seeing the blackboard in school, and reading music. As with other low vision devices, the patient often needs training to use a telescope successfully.

Absorptive Lenses

Many patients with low vision are photophobic or disabled by various lighting conditions. This light sensitivity may be the result of a number of eye conditions, such as a corneal dystrophy, cataract, *aniridia* (absence of the iris), irregular pupil, albinism, or achromatopsia. Light sensitivity may be caused also by medication or occur after extensive laser treatment to the retina.

Typical questions asked on a case history include ones on glare and light sensitivity. It is usual to ask whether the sun is tolerated, whether a cloudy day or a sunny day is better, whether sunglasses are worn and if they are effective, and whether seeing in dim light is a problem.

Absorptive lenses are filters that may be worn both indoors and outdoors to reduce the glare and increase contrast. Some of these lenses are specially made to transmit only certain wavelengths of light, thus eliminating glare without making things too dark. They may come as wraparounds or clip-ons, and may be polarizing lenses as well. Two companies that provide some of these more specialized absorptive lenses are NOIR and Corning Medical Optics.

Closed-Circuit Television

The closed-circuit television system consists of a camera (handheld or stationary mounted) that projects an image onto a television monitor or head mounted display. Closed-circuit televisions offer certain advantages over and above optical low vision devices.

- High amounts of magnification are possible; depending on the system, viewing distance, and monitor, magnification can be achieved to greater than 40×. Optical systems are generally available to 20× but are often difficult to use above 6× to 8×.
- Polarity can be reversed. Images can be projected on the screen that are white on black or black on white; this may be especially important to the patient with poor contrast.
- Brightness and contrast can be controlled.
- Monitors are available in color.
- Some closed-circuit televisions can be interfaced with a computer.

The system may work better for individuals who have poor levels of vision (e.g., less than 20/400). Some newer units are head-mounted (V-Max and LVES [Electronic Vision Enhancing System, and the Aurora]), and can be used in a library, store, or at school to see the blackboard.

Adaptive (Nonoptical) Devices

Many nonoptical aids may benefit an individual with a visual impairment (Lighthouse consumer catalog) such as large-print watches, clocks, and timers; cassette players; television accessories; large-print books; writing supplies; special calculators; measuring tools; money identifiers and wallets; temperature gauges; special telephones; lighting; large-print cooking books; games; and mobility aids. Among the many health care aids are blood glucose monitoring systems and other devices for diabetics; voice output thermometers and scales and other voice output devices; and pill dispensers. The low vision doctor or instructor will recommend these types of assistive devices, in addition to the prescriptive optical devices, to try to address the patient's needs.

REFERENCES

Arditi, A., & Rosenthal, B. P. (1996). Developing an objective definition of visual impairment. Paper presented at Vision 96, International Conference on Low Vision, Madrid, July 1996.

Bailey, I. L. (1988). Measurement of visual acuity—Towards standardization. In *Vision science symposium* (pp. 215–230). Bloomington: Indiana University.

Bass, S. J., & Sherman, J. (1991). Ophthalmic ultrasonography. In J. B. Eskridge, J. F. Amos, & J. D. Bartlett (Eds.), *Clinical procedures in optometry* (pp. 530–549). Philadelphia: J. B. Lippincott.

Bass, S. J. & Sherman, J. (1996). Visual field testing in the low vision patient. In B. P. Rosenthal & R. G. Cole (Eds.), *Functional assessment of low vision* (pp. 89–104). St. Louis, MO: Mosby.

Colenbrander, A. (1976). Low vision: Definition and classification. In E. E. Faye (Ed.), *Clinical low vision* (pp. 3–6). Boston: Little, Brown.

Colenbrander, A. (1977). Dimensions of visual performance. *Transactions of the American Academy of Ophthalmology and Otolaryngology, 83,* 322.

Colenbrander, A., & Fletcher, D. C. (1995). Basic concepts and terms for low vision rehabilitation. *American Journal of Occupational Therapy, 49,* 865–869.

Dana, M. R., Tielsch, J. M., Enger, C., Joyce, E., Santoli, J. M., & Taylor, H. R. (1990). Visual impairment in a rural Appalachian community. *JAMA, 264,* 2400–2405.

Faye, E. E. (1984). *Clinical low vision.* Boston: Little, Brown.

Fingeret, M., Casser, L., & Woodcome, H. T. (1990). *Atlas of primary eyecare procedures.* Norwalk, CT: Appleton and Lange.

Fischer, M. L. (1996). Clinical implications of color vision deficiencies. In B. P. Rosenthal & R. G. Cole (Eds.), *Functional assessment of low vision* (pp. 105–128). St. Louis, MO: Mosby.

Hyvarinen, L. (1995). Considerations in evaluation and treatment of the child with low vision. *American Journal of Occupational Therapy, 49,* 896.

Johnston, A. W. (1991). Making sense of the M, N, and logMAR systems of specifying visual acuity. In B. P. Rosenthal & R. G. Cole (Eds.), *Problems in optometry: A structured approach to low vision care* (vol. 3, no. 3). Philadelphia: J. B. Lippincott.

Kahn, H. A., Leibowitz, H. M., Ganley, J. P., Kini, M. M., Colton, T., Nickerson, R. S., & Dawber, T. R. (1977). The Framingham eye study: Vol. 1. Outline and major prevalence findings. *American Journal of Epidemiology, 106,* 17–32.

Klein, R., Klein, B. E. K., Linton, K. L. P., & De Mets, D. L. (1991). The Beaver Dam eye study: Visual acuity. *Ophthalmology, 98,* 1310–1315.

The Lighthouse, Inc. Lighthouse low vision products *consumer catalog:* 800-829-0500.

Mehr, E., & Freid, A. (1975). *Low vision care.* Chicago: Professional Press.

New York Lighthouse. (1974). *Low vision examination* [Low vision continuing education curriculum].

Nowakowski, R. W. (1994). Assessment of visual fields. In R. Nowakowski (Ed.), *Primary low vision care* (pp. 55–59). Norwalk, CT: Appleton and Lange.

Nowakowski, R. (1994). *Primary low vision care.* Norwalk, CT: Appleton and Lange.

Oliver, G. E. (1996). Pharmaceutical effects on the management of the low vision patient. In R. G. Cole & B. P. Rosenthal (Eds.), *Remediation and management of the low vision patient* (pp. 123–138). St. Louis, MO: Mosby.

Oshinskie, L. J. (1991). Radiology. In J. B. Eskridge, J. F. Amos, & J. D. Bartlett (Eds.), *Clinical procedures in optometry* (pp. 580–595). Philadelphia: J. B. Lippincott.

Rosenthal, B. P., & Cole, R. G. (1993). Visual impairments. In M. G. Eisenberg, R. L. Glueckauf, & H. Zaretsky (Eds.), *Medical aspects of disability* (pp. 391–403). New York: Springer.

Sherman, J., & Bass, S. J. (1984). Diagnostic procedures in low vision case management. In E. E. Faye (Ed.), *Clinical low vision* (pp. 226–227). Boston: Little, Brown.

Sherman, J., & Bass, S. J. (1996). Electrodiagnosis in evaluation and managing the low vision patient. In B. P. Rosenthal & R. G. Cole (Eds.), *Functional assessment of low vision* (pp. 140, 148–157). St. Louis, MO: Mosby.

Sherman, J., & Sutija, V. G. (1991). Visual-evoked potentials. In J. B. Eskridge, J. F. Amos, & J. D. Bartlett (Eds.), *Clinical procedures in optometry* (pp. 514–529). Philadelphia: J. B. Lippincott.

Tielsch, J. M., Sommer, A., Witt, K., Katz, J., & Royall, R. M. (1990). Blindness and visual impairment in an American urban population: The Baltimore eye study. *Archives of Ophthalmology, 108,* 286–290.

U.S. Bureau of the Census. (1989). *Population profile of the United States: 1989* (Current Population Reports, Series P-23, No. 159). Washington, DC: U.S. Government Printing Office.

12 Pediatric Low Vision

Ocular Pathology and

Cortical Visual Impairment

Linda Baker-Nobles, MS, OTR

Introduction

Researchers have theorized that much of what is learned by infants and children during the early years of development is reinforced through the visual system. Vision is the primary sensory component that allows humans to perceive simultaneously an object in its total form and to perceive that object's relationship to all other objects in the environment (Groenveld, 1990). Vision provides a critical role in the overall development of children who are sighted, because vision allows infants and children to develop skills through imitation (Jan, Freeman, & Scott, 1977). Through visual imitation, children are able to gain incidental information about themselves and about their environment. During these early years, the role of vision is to motivate, guide, and verify the interaction with the surrounding world. It allows the development of the ability to integrate information from the various sensory input systems in order to obtain information from one sensory modality (e.g., touch) and apply it to other systems (e.g., hearing) (Ferrell, 1986).

Because of the importance of vision in the learning process, visual impairments can result in significant developmental delays, particularly in the absence of early intervention services (Zambone, 1989). Developmental delay appears to be the greatest in those children with the most significant visual impairments (Cass, Sonksen, & McConachie, 1994). Scholl (1986) stated that limited vision may yield imperfect perceptions that become vague impressions which might be confusing in the educational process (p. 67). Infants and children with visual impairment require early intervention to ensure residual functional vision is maximized and to ensure that visual limitations do not interfere with sensorimotor development and learning (Zambone, 1989). Warren (1994) noted that many of these delays are a result of environmental variables that accompany visual impairment and can be avoided with the appropriate environment. Occupational therapists, as members of teams of professionals who work with these children, must be able to understand the nature of visual impairments and their impact on the developmental process to assist in the planning of appropriate intervention programs (Baker-Nobles, 1990).

Ocular Visual Impairment

The term *ocular visual impairments* refers to conditions of the eyeball or to lesions of the anterior visual pathway, which run from the retina to the lateral geniculate nucleus. They can include pathology that impacts any part of the eyeball as well as the optic nerves, optic chiasm, and optic tract. These conditions impact visual acuity (Jan & Groenveld, 1993). The leading known causes of ocular visual impairment in infants and children include congenital cataracts, optic nerve atrophy, and *retinopathy of prematurity* (a condition in premature infants associated with low birth weight, early gestational age, and duraction and administration of oxygen received through the respirator that can result in changes to the vascular system that supplies the retina and that can subsequently cause retinal detachment). Common prenatal ocular conditions are congenital anomalies and absence of part or all of the eye structure. These include colobomas of the iris, cataracts, glaucoma, and albinism (Ward, 1986). Approximately 50% of infants and children with these visual impairments may present with other disabilities, depending on the cause of the ocular condition (Jan & Wong, 1991).

Children with ocular impairments often have eyes that look abnormal. They present with sensory nystagmus that is associated with bilateral ocular lesions. These eye oscillations can be slowly drifting or jerky movements. The presence of sensory nystagmus indicates an instability of fixation. Children with ocular lesions and some residual vision generally have normal visual attention span and can maintain fixation. If they have ocular field loss, they can use their heads to scan the environment. They may bring objects close to their eyes for the purpose of magnification (Jan & Groenveld, 1993). Although infants and children with ocular visual impairments may be attracted to light, studies have indicated that these children do not perseverate on looking at light sources unless they also present with other central nervous system involvement (Jan, Groenveld, & Sykanda, 1993).

Ophthalmologists diagnose visual impairment through a variety of observations and tests. They note the appearance of the eyes, check for physical symptoms, measure acuity and contrast sensitivity, and measure visual fields. In addition, they may use *electroretinography* (ERG) and visual evoked potentials (VEP). The ERG measures electrical responses from the retina when flashing light is presented to both the light- and dark-adapted eye. This test is particularly helpful in diagnosing conditions of the retina. The VEP is used to detect lesions in the optic nerves as well as lesions in the pathways to the visual cortex (Ward, 1986).

The term *legal blindness* is defined as a visual acuity of 20/200 or less in the better eye with the best possible correction or a visual field of 20 degrees or less in the better eye with the best possible correction. Although the diagnosis of legal blindness may imply no vision, 90% of the legally blind population have some residual vision (Scholl, 1986).

Development of Infants and Children with Ocular Impairments

The Impact of Vision on Motor Development

When a sighted infant is born, vision is the sensory system that drives the infant to visually seek out light, movement, color, and pattern. Vision is the stimulus that reinforces neck righting in the prone position and thus establishes the development of the critical synergistic visual, vestibular, and cervical triad. The ability of the eyes, neck, and vestibular systems to work together in coordination builds the foundation for the development of the extension posture (Moore & Baker-Nobles, 1995). Infants with severe visual impairment do not tolerate the prone position because they lack the input to begin visual searching. The prone position becomes an impediment to breathing, freedom, and motion (Phillips & Hartley, 1988). Lack of experience in this position can inhibit the development of extensor tone and strength and the bilateral coordination of the upper extremities needed for reaching (Hart, 1983).

The preference for the supine position in the infant with visual impairment reinforces the asymmetrical tonic neck reflex position. Sighted infants in this position become aware of visual stimuli overhead and begin to rotate their heads to locate the visual source. The asymmetrical tonic neck reflex position also allows sighted infants to visually regard their hands and to begin the process of bringing the hands together for exploration (Moore & Baker-Nobles, 1995). Impaired vision prevents the infant from turning the head to visually locate at midline, which prevents the initiation of the rotational components of movement necessary for transitions from one position to another. Impaired vision also prevents the infant from discovering the hands and bringing them together at midline for exploration (Ferrell, 1986). Fraiberg (1968) found in her studies that midline fingering is rare in babies who are blind and they tend to remain in this asymmetrical posture for longer periods of time.

The lack of visual-manual exploration of the hands at midline and the nonawareness of visual cues in the environment can prevent the infant with visual impairment from reaching (Adelson & Fraiberg, 1976). When sighted children begin to reach, they receive constant visual feedback that enables continuous correction of the movement until they attain their goal (Bushnell, 1985). Without this visual feedback, infants with visual impairment are dependent on auditory cues to develop ear–hand coordination. However, studies indicate that most of these infants are not able to localize the source of sound in their surrounding space until late into the first year of life, long after sighted infants have mastered eye-hand coordination (Fraiberg, 1977; Troster & Brambring, 1993). Even when ear–hand coordination does develop, it does not provide the level of integration afforded by the visual system (Gleason, 1984).

The knowledge that an object exists in the environment and that the object can be reached for and engaged allows the sighted infant to develop the cognitive concept of cause and effect within the first 6 months of life. The awareness that the infant can cause something to happen is primary in initiating self-directed play and subsequent movement. When an infant has significant visual impairment and is unable to localize a sound source and does not reach, the concept of cause and effect can be delayed. Without this concept, these infants are unaware that they have any control over the environment and have no incentive to initiate movement.

Reaching is the precursor to all other movement (Adelson & Fraiberg, 1976). Adelson and Fraiberg found that, although infants with significant visual impairment generally attain postural stability skills such as sitting and standing within normal limits, when compared to the sighted population, they display delays in self-initiated mobility. Adelson and Fraiberg concluded that vision provides sighted infants an incentive to move, because early eye–hand coordination enables them to reach out for what is seen and wanted. Adelson and Fraiberg also hypothesized that a lack of smooth motor coordination in children with visual impairment results from a deficit in visual feedback because these children have few possibilities to imitate movement.

Because auditory cues do not substitute for visual cues in the visually impaired population, and because these infants do not have the benefits of watching and imitating the movements of other people, they have no incentive to move. In addition, the inadequate development of the rotational components of movement contribute to difficulty performing transitions from one position to another (Troster, Hecker, & Brambring, 1994). As a result, these infants frequently skip the crawling stage entirely and do not have the opportunity to practice weight shift, reciprocal balance, and hip and trunk rotation. This results in a lack of fluidity and grace when they do walk (Ferrell, 1986). In addition, the lack of visual monitoring of the body in relation to the surroundings during movement makes it difficult to reduce initial uncertainty and anxiety regarding self-initiated locomotion and can contribute to unstable dynamic balance during walking (Troster & Brambring, 1993; Troster et al., 1994).

The lack of weight bearing and crawling can also affect the development of hand skills. These positions provide both tactile and proprioceptive input to the hands and fingers and prepare them for manipulation of objects (Ayres, 1979). Sighted infants discover objects and toys, visually imitate actions of parents, and experiment with different qualities of objects, developing a repertoire of new movements that prepare the way for symbolic play (Dunlea, 1996). Infants with visual impairments do not have the same opportunity for these varied experiences and tend to engage in concrete, repetitive actions with objects (Pogrund, Fazzi, & Lampert, 1992). This can have long-reaching effects on self-feeding, fine motor development, and exploratory behavior (Ferrell, 1986).

When there is no reach for or movement toward sound cues, then opportunities to cognitively understand the world are limited. Without vision, these infants do not know that when they drop something from their hands, the object is still there and can be retrieved. They do not realize that parents may come and go from their immediate proximity, but, in fact, still exist. Vision is the sensory system that allows the concept of object permanence to develop, and without vision the acquisition of this concept is often delayed (Hyvarinen, 1988; Nielsen, 1991). Ferrell (1986) stated, "Visually handicapped infants do not begin to move around on their own until they understand that objects and people exist even when not in direct contact with the infants sensory experience."

Locomotion is necessary for exploration. During attainment of postural control, visual information is integrated with the underlying vestibular, proprioceptive, and tactile senses to assist the infant in providing an awareness of body position to space (Fisher, Murray, & Bundy, 1991). The external space that affects infant's and children's movements cannot be understood until they have organized their own internal space. This includes the concepts of identification of body parts, planes, movement, laterality, and directionality (Cratty & Sams, 1968). In addition, it is important that the infant understand the relationship of the body to objects in space (Sleeuwenhoek, Boter, & Vermeer, 1995). Because infants with visual impairment are relying on incomplete data from the environment and because their movement experiences are often limited, it is difficult for them to understand the relationship of their bodies to auditory and tactile cues in order to develop spatial abilities (Nielsen, 1991). This can have major implications for their success in later orientation and mobility training (Hill, Dodson-Burk, & Talor, 1992).

The development of movement and exploration is a continuous, spiral process that engages the infant in the world and motivates continued development (Fisher et al., 1991). When infants and children with visual impairment do not develop these abilities, they may resort to self-stimulatory behaviors such as rocking and eye poking, initially due to a lack of sensory stimulation to the vestibular and visual systems (Hyvarinen, 1988). These behaviors can become habituated and further contribute to lack of exploration. They may become more problematic in developing learning and social interactions than the visual impairment (Brambring & Troster, 1992; Hyvarinen, 1988).

The Relationship of Vision to the Development
of Communication, Play Social Interactions,
and Concept Formation

Mutual orientation between infants and mothers is one of the first co-occupations of parents and children and can be disrupted by visual impairment (Dunlea, 1996). The visual interchange is a primary component in the bonding process that is necessary for attachment to occur. When infants are visually impaired, they tend to be passive and withdrawn and do not possess an extended variety of facial expressions reflecting different emotions (Stengel, 1981). Sighted infants are regularly responding to parents' faces with smiling by 6 weeks, but no consistent smiling occurs in infants with visual impairment. The lack of eye-to-eye contact between the infant with visual impairment and the mother can contribute to maternal withdrawal and may impede the infant from transferring interest from self to the external environment (Burlingham, 1979).

Studies performed by Dunlea (1996) with infants who were visually impaired indicated that maternal vocalizations alone are not enough to sustain interaction. Without the turn-taking routines of visual attention and vocalizations, these infants attempts at indicating interest can be missed. She found that an important component in eliciting the mother-infant dyad is the presence of physical body stimulation (touch and movement) in combination with vocalizations.

During the second 6 months of life, sighted infants begin communicating by gestures, which are developed through visual imitation. This can be muted or absent in the infant with visual impairment (Stengel, 1981). As a result, communication between parent and infant consists primarily of physical games (e.g., pat-a-cake) and routines (e.g., singing) where the reference point is the infant (Preisler, 1995).

When infants with visual impairments do begin to speak, they often have a greater number of action words and fewer object words than the sighted population. This may be partially due to a lack of exploration of objects in the environment that prevents these infants from understanding that words have a symbolic function to represent objects (McConachie & Moore, 1994). Tactile, auditory, and proprioceptive sensory systems are less meaningful without visual reinforcement, and it is more difficult for the child to synthesize information about objects and the environment in order to develop the concepts that contribute to the development of language (Fraiberg, 1977). When infants have enough vision to demonstrate visually directed reach and can explore and play with objects, these delays in expressive language do not occur (McConachie, 1990).

During the second year of development, children begin to offer and show objects to others, thus broadening their self-directed social interactions. This is a repertoire of behaviors absent in children with visual impairment (Dunlea, 1996). Without visual feedback, it is often difficult for these children to know if and when they are being addressed and to participate in reciprocal social interactions (Erwin, 1994). During this time, sighted children begin the imitation of domestic life (e.g., feeding a doll), initiating the beginning of imaginative play. Children with visual impairment are delayed in these abilities. The emergence of the understanding of self and the subsequent use of the pronouns I and me are related to this type of play and, as a result, these children are slower in acquiring this language development (Fraiberg & Adelson, 1973).

Erin (1990) noted that children with visual impairments are at risk for language delays and deficits, including excessive use of questions, echolalic responses, and the instability of the use of the pronouns I and you. She felt that children with visual impairments use language primarily to gain information while sighted children do so to relate objects to familiar situations or to refer to past experiences. The differences in communication can affect interactions between sighted children and children with visual impairment and result in a breakdown of interactive play (Erwin, 1994).

Young sighted children frequently use eye contact to initiate and sustain social interactions with other children, while children with visual impairments tend to use more physical contact. This is often interpreted by sighted peers as inappropriate and can inhibit opportunities for social and play interactions. The opportunity for children with visual impairments to interact, negotiate, and play with other peers is an essential component for good social-emotional development (Erwin, 1994).

Inadequate vision may contribute to poor concept formation. Scholl (1986) stated that although limited research exists on the development of concept formation during the preschool years, it might be assumed that the child with visual impairment will have difficulties with assimilation and accommodation because of limited experiences with the environment. The child with visual impairment has less access to objects and restricted opportunities to expand language because of the experiential background. She further stated that because concepts develop out of perceptual processes, the child may have difficulty acquiring these concepts.

In conclusion, because visual loss interferes with incidental learning and the use of visual modeling for learning, early intervention services to address developmental skills and concept formation are critical for this population (Zambone, 1989).

Evaluation

Several developmental tests have been adapted for visually impaired infants and children that can be helpful in assessing these children. The

Maxfield Social Maturity Scale for Blind Preschool Children is an adapted version of the Vineland Social Maturity Scale and covers the domains of self-help general, self-help dressing, self-help eating, communication, socialization, locomotion, and occupation. It is designed for preschoolers to children of the 5- to 6-year age level. This assessment was standardized on children with visual impairments.

The Reynell-Zinkin Developmental Scales for Young Visually Handicapped Children is designed for children 0 to 5 years and has a section on mental development and a section on motor development. The mental development section covers social adaptation, sensorimotor understanding, exploration of the environment, response to sound and verbal comprehension, expressive language, and communication. The motor development section covers hand function, locomotion, and reflexes.

The Oregon Project Developmental Checklist is designed for children 0 to 6 years. It covers the areas of socialization, self-help, fine motor, gross motor, language, cognition, vision, and compensatory skills. This checklist also takes into account items that may be delayed or never acquired by a child with visual impairment.

In addition to these tests, occupational therapists can incorporate other commonly used evaluations, such as tests for sensory integration. However, it is important to remember that the standardized scores obtained from the evaluations cannot be interpreted and applied to the visually impaired population because their development is different from that of sighted children, and these tests were not standardized on this population. These tests should be used only to assist in developing strengths and weaknesses for the individual child. Areas of occupational therapy assessment should include

- reflex development
- muscle tone and strength
- balance, stability, postural security, and endurance
- bilateral integration and coordination
- praxis
- identification of body parts and planes
- laterality and directionality

- controlled and isolated movements
- tactile and auditory discrimination
- spatial orientation
- functional skills in play and self-care.

Children who will be cane travelers need to be referred to an orientation and mobility specialist for specific training in this area.

A functional visual assessment should also be performed by the most qualified member of the team before the implementation of services. Occupational therapists should perform these evaluations only if they have had continuing education in the evaluation of visual responses. Areas that need to be covered include awareness of and fixation on light, color, and objects; the presence of the blink reflex; pupillary responses; convergence; eye preference; central fields; peripheral fields; visual field preference; muscle imbalance; tracking; gaze shifting; scanning; and accuracy during reach and movement.

Because infants and children with visual impairments have a variety of needs, it is important that they also be evaluated by and receive the services of an early intervention vision specialist or vision teacher, orientation and mobility specialist, and speech and language pathologist. All goals for the child need to be collaboratively written as a team and must include the family to ensure continuity and consistency of learning across all environments.

Intervention

Young children with visual impairment are at risk for secondary developmental disabilities. These include gaps in skill and concept development, splintered skill attainment, and poor developmental progression. However, because visual impairment is a disability of sensory input, many of these disabilities can be prevented or minimized through early intervention services (Zambone, 1989).

The occupational therapist needs to address those performance components and subcomponents that affect the child's occupational behavior in work, play, and self-care as it affects the childs functioning in all environments. Although each infant and child presents with a unique set of strengths and weaknesses, some general goals apply to addressing issues associated with visual impairment. Some of these general goals include

- encouraging and providing opportunities for reach, manipulation of objects, movement, and exploration of the environment
- minimizing tactile defensiveness and developing tactile perception
- providing vestibular and proprioceptive activities to promote body awareness in space and decreasing self-stimulatory behaviors
- developing the childs use of remaining functional vision during movement and play
- developing self-feeding and self-care skills in activities of daily living
- constructing environments where the child can self-direct play
- providing family members with support, education, and strategies for integrating activities within the framework of their home structures, routines, and environment.

In addition to these goals, the occupational therapist must incorporate activities that address the development of cause-and-effect relationships and object permanence.

A frame of reference that is particularly beneficial when working with children with visual impairments is *sensory integration.* The theory of sensory integration emerges from neuroscience and was developed by Dr. A. J. Ayres (1979) to better explain the relationship between behavior and neural functioning. The theory of sensory integration is based on five assumptions. The first assumption is that each child possesses neural plasticity, or the ability of the brain structure to be changed or modified. The second assumption is that sensory integration occurs in a developmental sequence. The third assumption is that the brain functions as an integrated whole but is composed of systems that are hierarchically organized. The fourth assumption is that an adaptive behavior promotes sensory integration and that the ability to produce an adaptive behavior reflects sensory integration. The fifth assumption is that children have an inner drive to develop sensory integration through participation in sensorimotor activities. Sensory integration theory assumes that the brain is immature at birth. The goal of sensory integration is to provide stimulation that will address primarily subcortical levels in the brain, to enable them to mature, and to assist the brain to work as an integrated whole (Fisher et al., 1991).

Because children with visual impairment have a disruption to the sensory system that unifies and integrates all information received through the other sensory systems, and because vision acts as the motivator for movement (Ferrell, 1986), the theory of sensory integration is an appropriate one to incorporate into intervention. Barraga (1986) noted that the child with visual impairment must be able to use all the sensory systems to the optimal capacity to reach the maximum learning potential.

In addition to providing sensory integration therapy, it is important for the occupational therapist to adapt and construct play areas within the home that will promote the infant's and child's inner drive to seek out and independently engage the environment. Real-life objects that have meaning in the childs life should be incorporated into play and daily living skills. Toys should be selected for their tactile qualities rather than for their appearance (Rettig, 1994). Because objects disappear when the child drops them, it can be helpful to attach them to a board or to an overhead pole, so the child can relocate them. This helps in the development of the cause-and-effect and object permanence concepts. Play should be performed on hard surfaces, such as a wooden floor, so that the child receives auditory feedback when kicking and hitting. A piece of equipment that was developed by Dr. Lilli Nielsen (1991) that is helpful in providing this feedback is the resonance board (see Figure 12.1). This board is made of 4 mm plywood, constructed as a shallow box having 2-cm-high sides and when placed on that 2 cm rim, accentuates the sounds the infant and child make during movement. It also allows objects to roll back to the center of the board, where the child is located (Hyvarinen, 1988).

Nielsen has also developed a piece of equipment that is an environment that assists in self-directed play and exploration. She refers to this as the little room (see Figure 12.2). The little room is made of pipe, which can be put together to form a small frame. Several panels of plexiglas acrylic plastic are put on the top and three sides to serve as a ceiling and walls.

Play environments to encourage self-directed play

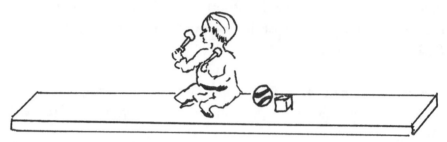

Figure 12.1 Resonance board.

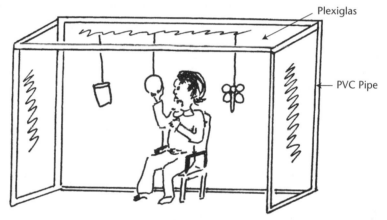

* Closed on all sides except floor & one wall

* Walls can be made of plexiglas or masonite

* Walls can be covered in textures or left smooth

* Objects hung from elastic cording from ceiling and if desired from walls

* Little room can be constructed in any dimensions to fit either seated child or child lying on floor

* Can also be placed on resonance board

Figure 12.2 Little room.

The walls can be covered in different textures and items can be attached from elastic cords from the ceiling. This environment creates a small space around the child and magnifies the sounds the child makes during play. It also provides a tangible awareness of space for the child because the child can reach out and touch the walls and ceiling (Nielsen, 1991). A catalog of Nielsen's equipment is available through LH-Verkstan, Ivarshyttevagen 14, 77633 Hedemora, Sweden. The concept of the little room can also be reproduced by materials available in the infant's and child's home environment.

It is critical to provide opportunities to develop the functional use of residual vision. Encouraging the use of residual vision can improve the development of children with significant visual impairments in all areas. It can increase the exploration of the environment, which influences the acquisition of appropriate movement and play (Baker-Nobles, 1990; Barraga, Collins, & Hollis, 1977). Use of different lighting and toys that have light can enrich the visual environment and should be incorporated into intervention. The light box (available through American Printing House for the Blind, 1-800-223-1839) is a piece of equipment that is very desirable. The use of black light and fluorescent toys is also a strategy for illuminating and isolating visual stimuli.

The necessity of incorporating visual sensory input into intervention is reinforced by Smith and Cote (1983) who stated,

> The area of the brain which is responsible for vision will remain underdeveloped unless stimulation and visual experiences are provided. How efficiently the child functions visually is a direct result of the quality of sequential presentation of visual stimulation experiences. For visually impaired children, vision is not an automatically learned process. (p. 11)

Cortical Visual Impairment

Characteristics of Infants and Children with Cortical Visual Impairment

Understanding visual impairment in children can be a complicated process. Traditionally, visual impairments have been associated with ocular impairments (Groenveld, Jan, & Leader, 1992). However, visual impairment can also refer to cortical visual impairment. *Cortical visual impairment* (CVI) refers to lesions in the posterior visual pathways that run from the lateral geniculate nucleus to the visual cortex and represents difficulty in processing and interpreting visual information in the visual cortex (Jan & Groenveld, 1993).

CVI is often referred to as *cortical blindness*, which is defined clinically as a bilateral loss of vision with normal pupillary response and an eye examination that indicates no other abnormalities (Whiting, Jan, Wong, Farrell, & McCormick, 1985). The term cortical blindness implies no sensory visual responsiveness. Since most children with a lesion in the visual pathways or visual cortex have some residual vision, the term cortical visual impairment is a more appropriate diagnosis (Good, et al., 1994).

Because CVI is a new area of study, the visual impairments of these children have often been overlooked by physicians, educators, and other professionals (Jan & Wong, 1991). The diagnosis of CVI has become more common in the last 5 years, and CVI is now considered to be one of the leading causes of visual impairment in infants and children in the developed countries (Good et al., 1994). Since CVI is associated with central nervous pathology, 100% of the children diagnosed with CVI present with other neurological impairments and disabilities (Jan & Wong, 1991). However, not all children with central nervous system dysfunction present with CVI (Groenveld, 1990).

The most probable cause of CVI in children is perinatal ischemic hypoxia (Flodmark, Jan, & Wong, 1990). The posterior visual pathways and the visual cortex seem to be most vulnerable to damage during the perinatal phase (Good, et al., 1994). Although the infant brain becomes more resistant to ischemic hypoxia episodes as it develops, CVI can still result and has been reported in children after cardiac arrest and open heart surgery. Other causes of CVI include trauma, epilepsy, cerebral angiography, infections, drugs or poisons, and metabolic disorders (Good et al.).

The diagnosis of CVI can be made through several medical tests that also can offer information in planning intervention strategies. However, these tests are expensive and difficult to access and some are invasive, so it may be better to interpret the visual behaviors of the infant or child and then decide whether these tests can offer essential information (Jan et al., 1993). Electroencephalography (EEG) provides general information about geniculocalcarine dysfunction and occipital responses to photic stimulation. Visual evoked potential (VEP) assesses the function of the visual pathways, although results vary with this test. Imaging techniques such as *computed tomography* (CT), *magnetic resonance imaging* (MRI), and *positron emission tomography* (PET) are also helpful in identifying where damage has occurred in the brain. *Visual evoked potential mapping* (VEPM) is a recent technique used for studying CVI. It examines larger areas of the brain in a dynamic manner rather than just measuring the electrical activity over the visual cortex (Good et al., 1994).

Infants and children with CVI present very different visual behaviors than do children with ocular impairments. Children with CVI have eyes that look normal, although they may present with a tropia (Moore & Baker-Nobles, 1995). Children with CVI do not present with a sensory nystagmus, unless they also have an ocular impairment. However, they often have a *motor nystagmus*, which is an unsteady, tremulous fixation of gaze that is due to impaired brain control and not due to an ocular impairment (Jan et al., 1993).

Children with CVI generally demonstrate a very short visual attention span (Jan et al., 1993). They often have a characteristic head turn when looking at or reaching for an object. They do not appear to look at objects with central vision, but instead seem to use peripheral or ambient fields (Baker-Nobles & Rutherford, 1995; Good et al., 1994; Jan et al.). They may also have a field loss and are not able to scan their environment to the side of the field loss. They generally turn their heads and look away from the side of the field loss (Jan et al.).

Like children with ocular disorders, children with CVI tend to bring objects close to their eyes, but they do so for very different reasons. In CVI, objects are brought close to the eyes to reduce the crowding affect (Jan et al., 1993). By bringing objects close to the eyes and filling the visual fields, these children are able to block out extraneous and nonessential background stimulation and focus attention on one visual stimulus. This allows them to better process the simpler visual information (Groenveld, 1990).

Compulsive light-gazing is common in infants and children with CVI, but eye poking and pressing is not seen in CVI unless an ocular impairment is also present (Jan et al., 1993). Color perception is generally intact because color perception has bilateral hemisphere representation and requires fewer functioning neurons than does form perception. Children with CVI are particularly attracted to bright colors such as red and yellow. Sensitivity to light is found in about one third of children with CVI (Jan et al.).

The prognosis for improvement in children with CVI depends on cause, age of onset, severity, and type of damage. Most children with CVI show some improvement in visual responses. To optimize visual responses in these children, modifying the visual environment is critical. Traditional methods of maximizing residual vision in children with ocular impairment rely on enriching and enhancing the visual environment. These methods of intervention may not help children with CVI because as the amount of visual input is increased, visual processing becomes more difficult. It is critical that the visual environment be simplified to expand opportunities for visual engagement (Groenveld, 1990).

Evaluation and Intervention

It is important to do a neuromuscular and motor evaluation of the infant or child initially and to decide the optimal position to reduce the effects of gravity. No visual expectations should exist during motor therapy because it is often too difficult for these children to visually engage while they are contending with gravity. When children with CVI have impaired motor skills, they appear to use a larger share of energy for posture and cannot maintain visual attention, so it is recommended that intervention plans for motor development and visual development not be carried out simultaneously (Baker-Nobles & Rutherford, 1995; Groenveld, 1990).

The evaluation of visual responses in these children needs to cover both the patterns of visual responses the child demonstrates as well as the complexity of visual information the child can handle without disengaging. Evaluation materials include the light box with overlays that range from single colors to more complex patterns, lighted wand toys and colored flashlights, and real-life objects and familiar toys. It is important to reduce the amount of extraneous visual clutter in the environment during the evaluation; when using the light box and lighted toys, the room should be as dark as possible. During the evaluation of visual responses the following factors should be observed and noted:

- the child's pattern of looking—central versus peripheral, length of fixation, length and frequency of pauses or looking away
  - presence of gaze shifting and following
  - field preferences
  - emotional and physical tone and responses when child is visually engaged.

When evaluating these responses the following questions need to be answered:

- Is the child aware of light?
- Is there a color preference?
- Does the child respond more to a moving visual stimulus or to a stationary stimulus? (Many children with CVI respond better to movement because they are using primarily peripheral or ambient fields of vision.)
- Is the child more attracted to a single color overlay than a three-dimensional object in normal lighting?
- Does the child recognize any familiar forms in the environment?
- When moving, how does the child navigate the environment?

Although visual goals should be individualized for each child, general goals for this population include

- improving awareness of light
- encouraging gaze shifting and following
- increasing ability to integrate more complex visual patterns
- improving abilities to move to and find familiar forms in the environment.

During intervention, it is critical that the environment is simplified. This also includes the infant's and child's home environment. It is important to assist parents in reducing the visual clutter in the infant's and child's room. One item should be presented against a solid, contrasting blanket or surface. Many infant blankets and bumper pads are visually busy, and when objects are placed on them the infants cannot find them against the background.

It is often easier for the infant and child to process two-dimensional forms (as on the light box) than it is to see the three-dimensional objects in the environments. The three-dimensional object is often very difficult to visually process because the child must deal with figure ground, depth, and changes in lighting and color over space. Bright, primary colors should be incorporated because the perception of color is a strength for these children. It is also helpful to always present the same color with the same visual form (e.g., a bottle) or symbol (e.g., a number) because the perception of color is a strength for the child with CVI and reinforces learning the form or symbol. Tactile cues should be provided to the hands with objects or toys when attempting to elicit visual fixation. The tactile input from the object helps to integrate and maintain visual fixation. The use of a color monitor computer and a switch is also beneficial. The color monitor screen is similar to the light box in that it is high-contrast and two-dimensional and employs color. This can be very helpful in eliciting visual engagement and promoting cause-and-effect concepts. Early computer software programs are provided by Apple Computer. Two easy programs include *Pictures and Music* and *The New Cause and Effect.*

Simplifying and modifying the visual environment is critical when working with these children. Occupational therapists frequently work with children with CVI and multiple disabilities. It is important to understand their strengths and weaknesses. Greater success with occupational therapy intervention may be achieved when the visual needs of infants and children with CVI are addressed (Baker-Nobles & Rutherford, 1995).

REFERENCES

Adelson, E., & Fraiberg, S. (1976). Sensory deficit and motor development in infants blind from birth. In Z. S. Jastrzembska (Ed.), *The effects of blindness and other impairments on early development* (pp.1–15). New York: American Foundation for the Blind.

Ayres, A. J. (1979). *Sensory integration and the child.* Los Angeles: Western Psychological Services.

Baker-Nobles, L. (1990). A multisensory approach to developing use of residual vision for quality movement. *Occupational Therapy Practice, 1,* 23–33.

Baker-Nobles, L., & Rutherford, A. (1995). Understanding cortical visual impairment in children. *American Journal of Occupational Therapy, 49,* 899–903.

Barraga, N. (1986). Sensory perceptual development. In G. Scholl (Ed.), *Foundations of education for blind and visually handicapped children and youth.* (pp. 83–98) New York: American Foundation for the Blind.

Barraga, N., Collins, M., & Hollis, J. (1977). Development of efficiency in visual functioning: A literature analysis. *Journal of Visual Impairment and Blindness, 71,* 387–391.

Burlingham, D. (1979). Psychoanalytic studies of the sighted and the blind. *Psychoanalytic Study of the Child, 34,* 6–49.

Bushnell, E. (1985). The decline of visually guided reaching during infancy. *Infant Behavior and Development, 8,* 139–155.

Cass, H., Sonksen, P., & McConachie, H. (1994). Developmental setback in severe visual impairment. *Archives of Disease in Childhood, 70,* 192–196.

Cratty, B., & Sams, T. (1968). *The body-image of blind children.* New York: American Foundation for the Blind.

Dunlea, A. (1996). "An opportunity for co-adaptation: The experience of mothers and their infants who are blind" In R. Zemke & F. Clark (Eds.), *Occupational science.* (pp. 229–241). Philadelphia: F. A. Davis.

Erin, J. (1990). Language samples from visually impaired four- and five-year-olds. *Journal of Childhood Communication Disorders, 13,* 181–191.

Erwin, E. (1994). Social competence in young children with visual impairments. *Infants and Young Children, 6,* 26–33.

Ferrell, K. (1986). Infancy and early childhood. In G. Scholl (Ed.), *Foundations of education for blind and visually handicapped children and youth.* (pp. 119–136). New York: American Foundation for the Blind.

Fisher, A., Murray, E., & Bundy, A. (1991). *Sensory integration: Theory and practice.* Philadelphia: F. A. Davis.

Flodmark, O., Jan, J., & Wong, P. (1990). Computed tomography of brains of children with cortical visual impairment. *Developmental Medicine and Child Neurology, 32,* 611–620.

Fraiberg, S. (1968). Parallel and divergent patterns in blind and sighted infants. *Psychoanalytic Study of the Child, 23,* 264–300.

Fraiberg, S. (1977). *Insights from the blind.* New York: Meridian Publishers.

Fraiberg, S., & Adelson, E. (1973). Self-representation in language and play: Observations of blind children. *Psychoanalytic Quarterly, 42,* 539–562.

Gleason, D. (1984). Auditory assessment of visually impaired preschoolers: A team effort. *Education of the Visually Impaired, 16,* 106–110.

Good, W., Jan, J., DeSa, L., Barkovich, A., Groenveld, M., & Hoyt, C. (1994). Cortical visual impairment in children. *Survey of Ophthalmology, 38,* 351–361.

Groenveld, M. (1990). The dilemma of assessing the visually impaired child. *Developmental Medicine and Child Neurology, 32,* 1105–1113.

Groenveld, M., Jan, J., & Leader, P. (1992, January). Observations on the habilitation of children with cortical visual impairment. *Journal of Visual Impairment and Blindness,* 11–15.

Hart, V. (1983). *Characteristics of young blind children.* Paper presented at the meeting of the Second International Symposium of Visually Handicapped Infants and Young Children—Birth to 7. Aruba, Lesser Antilles.

Hill, E., Dodson-Burk, B., & Talor, C. (1992). The development and evaluation of an orientation and mobility screening for preschool children with visual impairments. *RE:view, 22,* 165–176.

Hyvarinen, L. (1988). *Vision in children: Normal and abnormal.* Ontario, Canada: Canadian Deaf-Blind and Rubella Association.

Jan, J., Freeman, R., & Scott, E. (1977). *Visual impairment in children and adolescents.* New York: Grune & Stratton.

Jan, J., & Groenveld, M. (1993, April). Visual behaviors and adaptations associated with cortical and ocular impairment in children. *Journal of Visual Impairment and Blindness,* 101–105.

Jan, J., & Groenveld, M., & Sykanda, A. M. (1993). Light gazing by visually impaired children. *Developmental Medicine and Child Neurology, 32,* 755–759.

Jan, J., & Wong, P. (1991). The child with cortical visual impairment. *Seminars in Ophthalmology, 6,* 194–200.

McConachie, H. (1990). Early language development and severe visual impairment. *Child: Care, Health, and Development, 16,* 55–61.

McConachie, H., & Moore, V. (1994). Early expressive language of severely visually impaired children. *Developmental Medicine and Child Neurology, 36,* 230–240.

Moore, J., & Baker-Nobles, L. (1995, May). *Visual deficits in pediatrics, evaluation and treatment.* Workshop presented for occupational and physical therapists and speech pathologists, Baylor Medical Center, Dallas, TX.

Nielsen, L. (1991, January). Spatial relations in congenitally blind infants: A study. *Journal of Visual Impairment and Blindness,* 11–16.

Phillips, S., & Hartley, J. (1988). Developmental differences and interventions for blind children. *Pediatric Nursing, 14,* 201–204.

Pogrund, R., Fazzi, D., & Lampert, J. (1992). *Early focus: Working with young blind and visually impaired children and their families.* New York: American Foundation for the Blind.

Preisler, G. (1995). The development of communication in blind and in deaf infants—Similarities and differences. *Child: Care, Health, and Development, 21,* 79–110.

Rettig, M., (1994, September-October). The play of young children with visual impairments: Characteristics and interventions. *Journal of Visual Impairment and Blindness,* 410–420.

Scholl, G. (1986). *Foundations of education for blind and visually handicapped children and youth.* New York: American Foundation for the Blind.

Sleeuwenhoek, H., Boter, R., & Vermeer, A. (1995, July-August). Perceptual-motor performance and the social development of visually impaired children. *Journal of Visual Impairment and Blindness,* 359–367.

Smith, A., & Cote, K. (1983). *Look at me: A resource manual for the development of residual vision in multihandicapped children.* Philadelphia: Pennsylvania College of Optometry Press.

Stengel, T. J. (1981). Developmental and nondevelopmental obstacles to blind infant–sighted mother attachment. *Physical and Occupational Therapy in Pediatrics, 1(4),* 1–18.

Troster, H., & Brambring, M. (1993). Early motor development in blind infants. *Journal of Applied Developmental Psychology, 14,* 83–106.

Troster, H., & Brambring, M. (1994, September-October). The play behavior and play materials of blind and sighted infants and preschoolers. *Journal of Visual Impairment and Blindness,* 421–432.

Troster, H., Hecker, W., & Brambring, M. (1994). Longitudinal study of gross-motor development in blind infants and preschoolers. *Early Child Development and Care, 104,* 61–78.

Ward, M. (1986). Planning the Individualized Education Program in G. Scholl (Ed.), *Foundations of education for blind and visually handicapped children and youth.* (pp. 215–238) New York: American Foundation for the Blind.

Warren, D. (1994). *Blindness and children: An individual differences approach.* New York: Cambridge University Press.

Whiting, S., Jan, J., Wong, P., Farrell, K., & McCormick, A. (1985). Permanent cortical visual impairment in children. *Developmental Medicine and Child Neurology, 27,* 730–739.

Zambone, A. (1989). Serving the young child with visual impairments: An overview of disability impact and intervention needs. *Infants and Young Children, 2,* 11–23.

Analysis of common movement patterns observed in children with visual impairments

Area	Common Motor Problem Observed	Movement Component Impacted	Effect of Motor Problem
Postural tone	Low to normal postural tone base	Shoulder girdle stability Trunk stability Pelvic girdle stability	Due to low postural tone, there is a decrease in sensory information into muscles, joints and ligaments, therefore proprioception is impaired and child is less alert. Lack of good vision plus poor proprioception in turn impacts vestibular and tactile systems. Hypersensitivity and hyposensitivity to sensory input is sometimes seen. Low postural tone decreases stability in proximal points (shoulders, trunk and pelvis) which affects ability to control distal body parts (arms, hands, eyes, mouth, legs, feet). The child can compensate for this lack of stability by fixing at proximal joint, i.e., the child can elevate shoulders to help gain stability at shoulder girdle. This fixing then becomes a problem for free movement of that proximal joint. Also due to low postural tone, hypermobility can be seen at arms, shoulders and hips.
Muscle strength	1. Shoulder strength diminished	1. Shoulder girdle stability	1. Due to lack of shoulder strength and stability, it is common to see winged scapulae, shoulder elevation, shoulder protraction. Child has difficulty supporting weight in all-fours position, prone propping position. Upright against gravity, compensations to provide stability at shoulders are demonstrated, i.e., high guard position of arms during stance or gait.
	2. Upper extremity strength diminished	2. Co-contraction throughout range in upper extremities	2. Fluid, graded movement of upper extremities absent. Hyperextension of elbows sometimes seem to gain stability.
	3. Abdominal strength is poor	3. Abdominal strength Pelvic girdle stability Trunk stability Shoulder girdle stability	3. Lumbar lordosis is common; there is not good co-contraction of abdominals and back extensors to provide shoulder girdle, trunk and pelvic girdle stability.
	4. Hip adductors are weak	4. Pelvic girdle stability Hip joint stability; co-activation of hip abductors	4. A "frog-leg" position of lower extremities is common in sitting. A wide-base of support is seen in movement patterns, i.e., all-fours, standing, walking.
	5. Lower extremity strength is diminished	5. Co-contraction throughout range in lower extremities	5. There is a lack of fluid, graded movement of lower extremities that makes it difficult for child to maintain control in mid-range and end-range. Hyperextension of knees sometimes seen to provide stability.

Analysis of common movement patterns, *continued*

Area	Common Motor Problem Observed	Movement Component Impacted	Effect of Motor Problem
Sitting	1. Head stacking (head resting back on spine) or head down	1. Midline head alignment Cervical elongation with capitol flexion Shoulder girdle stability	1. Due to lack of shoulder girdle stability and the weakness of the neck muscles, the child finds it easier to passively rest his head either back or hang it forward. Lack of vision also reinforces head to be held down or rested back. This head placement interferes with the child's body alignment and center of gravity.
	2. Shoulder elevation	2. Cervical elongation with capitol flexion Shoulder girdle stability	2. By elevating his shoulders, the child can compensate for the lack of shoulder stability but this interferes with his ability to move his head separate from the shoulders, the eyes separate from the head, and one shoulder separate from another.
	3. Shoulder protraction (shoulders rounded forward)	3. Shoulder girdle stability	3. Having the shoulders rounded forward causes the arms to rotate inward. This along with the lack of stability at the shoulders interferes with the freedom of the top part of the arm to move the shoulder and with the outward rotation of forearms and wrist.
	4. Pelvis in posterior tilt - or - Pelvis in anterior tilt	4. Trunk stability Neutral pelvic alignment Pelvic mobility	4. Due to lack of trunk strength caused by weak back extensors and weak abdominals, the child compensates for lack of stability at the pelvis. The child can posteriorly tilt his pelvis sitting passively with rounded back or anteriorly tilt his pelvis providing a super-stable base with a hyperextended back. Both positions are static and interfere with the child's readiness to move at the pelvis. A lack of pelvis mobility hinders the child's freedom to shift weight forward, backward and to the sides.
	5. Wide base of lower extremities	5. Pelvic girdle stability Feet aligned with hips	5. Weak hip adductors cause a "frog-leg" position of legs. This provides a wide base of support in sitting to increase stability in this position but interferes with pelvic mobility and weight-shift off of midline.
Standing	1. Head stacking or head down	1. Midline head alignment Cervical elongation with capitol-flexion Shoulder girdle stability	1. With head down, child's center of gravity is in front of shoulders; with head rested back, center of gravity is behind shoulders.
	2. Shoulder elevation	2. Shoulder girdle stability	2. As in sitting posture, by elevating his shoulders, the child can compensate for the lack of shoulder stability but this interferes with his ability to move his head separate from the shoulders, the eyes separate from the head, and one shoulder from another.

Analysis of common movement patterns, *continued*

Area	Common Motor Problem Observed	Movement Component Impacted	Effect of Motor Problem
Standing (cont'd)	3. Lumbar lordosis Protruding abdominals	3. Trunk stability	3. Vertical alignment of body disrupted due to lack of back extensors and abdominals working together. At risk for scoliosis and lumber lordosis.
	4. Wide base of support Abduction and external rotation of legs Toe-out Weight-bearing on outside of feet	4. Pelvic girdle stability	4. These postures compensate for the lack of pelvic stability but prevent mobility at the pelvis which affects the child's ability to weight-shift.
	5. Hyperextension of knees or hip and knee flexion	5. Pelvic girdle stability Graded co-contraction (mid-range control)	5. Due to lack of proximal stability at the pelvis, the child provides stability by hyperextending the knees. This in turn interferes with the child's ability to grade movement of the lower extremities.
Movement	1. Patterns of movement not organized and graded	1. Graded movement; movement not controlled in all ranges	1. Child does not have control and stability to grade movement, i.e., cannot grade movement from stand to squat, usually see a collapse into gravity.
	2. Righting reactions and equilibrium are delayed	2. Righting and equilibrium reactions	2. Righting and equilibrium reactions are components of the body's postural reflex mechanism and provide a basis for balance. Inadequate development interferes with a child's ability to move in and out of positions and general ability to react to being moved.
	3. Movement occurs in straight planes	3. Rotation/counter-rotation	3. Adequate rotation and counter-rotation is absent in movement due to the inefficient development of antigravity extension and anti-gravity flexion working together. All transition movements (going from one position to another) involve rotation. A common example seen in the visually impaired child is coming from sitting on the floor to stand by pushing up to a hands and feet position in a straight plane movement instead of using rotation to come to a kneeling position to half-kneel to stand.
	4. Weight-shift inadequate	4. Shoulder girdle stability Pelvic girdle stability Righting/equilibrium Anti-gravity flexion and anti-gravity extension Elongation on weight-bearing side	4. Due to a super-stable position, the child may not be able to shift weight, or due to lack of movement components, there is lack of quality of the weight-shift. For example, when asked to stand one foot, a visually impaired child cannot keep the one foot up but falls into gravity on the weight-bearing side. Inadequate weight shift affects the child's gait, his ability to move from one position to another and all motor skills; crawling, knee-walking, climbing, running.

Analysis of common movement patterns, *continued*

Area	Common Motor Problem Observed	Movement Component Impacted	Effect of Motor Problem
Gait Pattern	1. Head stacking (head resting back on spine) or head down	1. Midline head alignment Cervical elongation with capitol flexion Shoulder girdle stability	1. As in sitting and standing postures, this head placement interferes with the child's body alignment and center of gravity.
	2. Shoulders elevated Shoulders protracted Occasional high-guard arm position with shoulders retracted	2. Shoulder girdle stability	2. As in sitting and standing, child compensates for lack of shoulder stability by elevating and protracting shoulders. Since he is moving against gravity, occasional high-guard arm position is seen which retracts the shoulders, pushing the scapulae toward the spine increasing stability in the shoulder girdle.
	3. Rotation and counter rotation absent in pelvis, shoulders and trunk	3. Rotation/counter-rotation	3. Due to lack of rotation and counter rotation in pelvis, shoulders and trunk, counterarm swing is absent during gait. (Counterarm swing is end result of shoulder rotation).
	4. Abduction and external rotation of legs Out-toeing	4. Pelvic girdle stability	4. Due to lack of stability at pelvis, child provides a wide base of support by abducting (moving legs away from body) and externally rotating legs. The feet follow in an out-toe position. This position of the legs and feet produce a waddle-like gait.
	5. Inadequate weight shift	5. Elongation of weight-bearing side with anti-gravity flexion on non-weight bearing side	5. Because the child cannot adequately shift weight, a side-to-side motion is apparent during gait. This causes a decreased stride length and an inadequate forward propulsion. This is evident when the child runs, often making many steps but not getting anywhere. Some children use a sideways shuffle to run that gives them propulsion without rotation.
	6. Knee hyper-extension	6. Abdominal strength Pelvic girdle stability Lower extremity strength	6. Due to lack of abdominal strength, pelvic girdle stability and lower extremity strength, child gives himself more stability by hyperextending his knees during both the stance and swing phase. This results in "back-kneeing" during gait.

Brown, C.J., & Bour, B. (1986). *Movement analysis and curriculum for visually impaired preschoolers.* Tallahassee, FL: State of Florida Department of Education. (Available from Educational Materials Distribution Center, Florida Department of Education (904) 488-6379).

13 The Treatment of the Child With Cerebral Palsy and Low Vision

by Tricia Geniale, BSc, Grad. Dip. OT, Dip. ACU, NDT

Introduction

In the population of children with cerebral palsy, the majority of diagnosed children are classified as having "cerebral palsy with spasticity" (McDonald, 1987). Children with spasticity or high tone are more likely to present with significant visual disorders than children with other types of cerebral palsy (Black, 1982; Duckman, 1987).

Many of the aetiological factors of cerebral palsy with spasticity produce deficits in the input, output, and processing of visual information (McDonald, 1987). Studies reveal high percentages of strabismus, refractive error, amblyopia, and accommodative insufficiency (Black, 1982; Duckman, 1987). In addition, it is common that there may be cortical dysfunction resulting from the original neurological insult, which causes visual loss unexplained by ocular examination. This is a visual "processing" disorder and is referred to as *cortical visual impairment* (Groenveld, Jan & Leader, 1990).

In children with spasticity and low vision, the picture is further complicated by the fact that not only do the diagnoses of ocular problems and/or cortical visual impairment interfere with the efficient use of vision, but so do the neuromotor problems inherent in spasticity, i.e., the high postural tone. The more severe the spasticity, the greater the interference with the use of the eyes (Blackwell, 1982; Duckman, 1987; Erhardt, 1987; Geniale, 1991).

This chapter will discuss the management of the child with cerebral palsy and low vision whose spasticity is sufficiently severe to affect the efficient use of vision.

The specific objectives are to

- briefly review treatment frameworks relevant to management of a population with cerebral palsy and low vision;
- outline features of spasticity and how these features compromise visual functioning;
- identify several key patterns of abnormal movement that are characteristic of the child with cerebral palsy and spasticity, which interfere with the effective use of vision; and
- describe in detail, management options that give the child the best possibility for optimum use of vision.

The management options that will be presented are designed for interdisciplinary teams involved in planning individual programs for the child with low vision and spasticity. The scope does not include teaching specific treatment techniques, but rather offers ways to apply relevant treatment frameworks. The management guidelines are not appropriate for other types of cerebral palsy (e.g., ataxic, athetoid). Only "possibilities for management" are outlined, and not all options will be relevant to every child.

Treatment Frameworks Relevant to the Management of the Child with Spasticity and Low Vision

By definition the child with low vision can "increase visual functioning through the use of non-optical aids, environmental modifications, and/ or training techniques" (Corn, 1980). Therefore, effective treatment of the child whose low vision is partly attributable to his spasticity must not only contain strategies to address the ocular disorder and/or cortical visual impairment (as discussed in sections of this book), but also techniques to simultaneously manage the problems caused by his spasticity.

Because of the complexity of the problems associated with the combination of low vision and spasticity, techniques of management require the application of knowledge derived from several treatment frameworks, including sensory integration, neurodevelopmental therapy, a systems approach, and motor control theory.

Management of Sensory Processing Components

The frameworks of sensory integration and systems theory acknowledge the importance of appropriate sensory input to organize and create a motor response that is adaptive to environmental demands (DeGangi & Dunn, 1993; Fisher, Murray, & Bundy, 1991), thus providing the feedback to reinforce learning (Case-Smith, 1996; Chapparo & Ranka, 1996). Given that the population under discussion has a sensory impairment affecting motor control and learning, it is valuable to incorporate treatment frameworks that are concerned with optimizing sensory processing.

Those familiar with the child with cerebral palsy and low vision observe that he may typically experience a variety of arousal and sensory modulation problems. (DeGangi & Dunn, 1993, DeGangi, 1994). In some children the original cortical damage, and/or medication, causes levels of alertness to fluctuate and sleep/wake cycles to be affected. The child may be easily overloaded by the stimuli from an environment over which he has little physical control. Limited experiences and immobility can lead to poor motivation and feelings of "learned helplessness." Including philosophies from a sensory integrative approach to therapy ensures that:

• Intervention procedures address the assessed underlying dysfunction (e.g., techniques to reduce arousal problems or difficulties with sensory modulation).

• The environment is "engineered" so that the child is motivated by his own choice of activity, that the child directs his responses (i.e., he is *active*), and that an adaptive response is demanded.

• The therapist is constantly monitoring the child's ability to process the sensory input as indicated by the child's adaptive responses to the environment. This is of particular relevance for the child who has cortical visual impairment, due to his difficulty with modulation of visual input, and suffers the likelihood of "sensory overload."

• The activity offers a challenge and that it is the child's participation and success in effortful, meaningful activities that helps increase self-esteem.

• There are diverse experiences and opportunities for increasing the variety of adaptive responses, in order to promote the likelihood of generalization and transfer of learning and so reduce the child's dependency and "learned helplessness."

Management of Neuromotor Components

Traditionally neurodevelopmental therapy (Bobath, 1984; Campbell, 1987; Geniale, 1991) and more recently in Australia, motor control literature (Shepherd, 1995) have been associated with the management of movement disorders. When considering the needs of the child whose movement disorder (i.e., spasticity) is affecting his efficient use of vision, such treatment frameworks can combine with the sensory integrative approach discussed above to provide comprehensive strategies directed toward minimizing the deleterious effects of spasticity on movement.

Specific strategies are expanded in a later section; however, the fundamental concepts require review.

Current Neurodevelopmental Therapy (NDT) treatment ensures that, since there is no time to waste on the child's learning to achieve tasks meaningless to life roles, only those missing motor patterns essential for completion of functional tasks are developed. *The therapy does not follow* a *"developmental sequence"* (Mayston, 1994). For example, in normal development a child would gain head and eye control in prone before sitting or standing. In practice, though, a child with vision compromised by spasticity may find it far more difficult to dissociate his eyes to "look ahead" in prone than when he is in a partially supported upright position. The consequent emphasis in programming, then, would not be in developing prone activity, but rather the upright positioning responses that are much more meaningful to the child's life role functions.

Specific functional, normal, or *preferred movement patterns* are developed through NDT as a substitute for movements which may exacerbate existing abnormal movement patterns. Preferred movement patterns are incorporated throughout the child's daily routine in order to provide opportunities for practice, and thus learning.

The child has the best neuromotor and biomechanical possibility to use a preferred movement pattern when systematic "handling" techniques are used as a "preparation" for the initial stages of learning desired movements. Preparation involves elongation of shortened musculature and mobilization of joints and is achieved during gentle vestibular and tactile input.

From our knowledge of sensory integrative theory, then, this preparation is also a valuable means of modulating the child's arousal level to promote the attending skills critical to learning.

NDT also ensures that the child is *independent and active* so that motor learning can take place. The therapist therefore takes away contact and handling as the child practices the preferred movement through unassisted repetitions.

Environmental adaptations (including choice and placement of equipment and strategies for when and where carers must take away support) are made i.e., placement and type of equipment, and strategies for when and where carers must take away support (Boehme, 1990) and are used to promote movements in a desired pattern. This information from NDT on environmental adaptations offers extensive management options in program planning for children with cerebral palsy and spasticity.

Low Vision Habilitation

Ocular disorders. It is recommended that disorders such as errors of refraction, amblyopia, and field defects are managed along conventional lines (Black,1982), for example, the provision of optical aids. In the case of a pure ocular disorder, it is the visual signals that are impaired and not the "processing" components of sight. These are cases that may benefit from visual enrichment and training (Groenveld et al., 1990). This would typically involve systematic presentation of visual stimuli of abnormal intensity to increase awareness and use of vision.

Like the therapeutic strategies for neuromotor problems discussed above, it is important to consider the value of including "visual training" in *visually dependent functional tasks* that are meaningful to the individual child (Goetz & Gee, 1987; Hall, 1989; Warren, 1995).

Instructional strategies in visually dependent task training introduce the concept of the *critical visual moment*.

The *critical visual moment* refers to those steps in a task when vision is a crucial element in success. Identifying the critical visual moments in tasks has proven very valuable in the management of the child with low vision and spasticity, as the child has significant difficulty with the neuromotor components of sustained visual attention while moving.

It is important to note that many children with an ocular disorder (e.g., nystagmus and field loss) may adopt an *abnormal head posture.* An abnormal head posture may be the child's own management strategy for improving visual efficiency. The vision specialist, the occupational therapist, and the physiotherapist must together determine the interrelationship between an abnormal head posture used to compensate for an ocular disorder, and one adopted due to the use of abnormal movement patterns.

Cortical Visual Impairment (CVI)

Despite the reported value of visual stimulation techniques with children with ocular disorders, it is necessary to stress that such strategies may be inappropriate for those diagnosed with cortical visual impairment (Morse, 1990). If a program of visual stimulation is instituted for a child with cortical visual impairment, the amount of visual input is increased, but the child still has a deficiency in his ability to process the input. The possibility of sensory overload is thus very real. Signs of sensory overload can include the child shutting his eyes, distress, overactivity, or depressed arousal.

Though not documented in low vision habilitation literature elsewhere, it is important here to reiterate the value of a sensory integrative framework to habilitation of cortical visual impairment. Strategies from a sensory integrative framework enable the therapist to engineer appropriate levels of sensory input that the child can modulate.

The child with cortical visual impairment may be unpredictable and inconsistent from day to day in responses to his visual environment. The sensory integrative therapist is alert to such responses and can vary the demands as directed by the child's immediate needs. The child, too, may modulate certain attributes of visual input selectively. Typically the colors red, yellow, or orange and/or object movement help the child orient and then attend to the environment. Using additional knowledge from a systems approach, the sensory integrative therapist can emphasise *visually dependent tasks* in the child's daily routine. Objects are kept the same (e.g., red cup, yellow plate) so that the visual attributes that can be processed become familiar in a environment providing clear feedback to the child through task completion. *Given a visually dependent task, an adaptive response to meet environmental demands is the key indicator of successful visual processing.*

The Effects of Spasticity on the Use of Vision

A child with cerebral palsy with spasticity is identified by a combination of clinical signs, including abnormal muscle patterns elicited by changes in head position ("tonic reflexes"), hyperactive reflexes, abnormally high resistance to passive stretch (high tone), and changes in the actual muscle tissue structure.

In order to address the management of the child with spasticity and low vision it is essential to understand how the features of spasticity affect the use of the eye musculature.

Spasticity occurs in patterns. Spasticity affects the musculature in fairly predictable patterns. It does not affect one group of muscles in isolation. When the child has sufficiently severe spasticity, the resultant restriction of body movements will limit dissociation of the extraocular eye muscles from the predominant patterns of spasticity. The child then may also lack the selective control of eye musculature. Lack of eye musculature dissociation and selectivity of eye movements, plus limited body movement, deprives the child of learning from the visual exploration of his environment.

Spasticity is changeable. Even though the child may present with no stiffness at rest, he may demonstrate the exaggerated stiffness that is recognized as an increase in spasticity when he moves. Fortunately the changeability in stiffness is fairly predictable: the more effort the child uses, the more emotional he is (e.g., excited, angry), the more his movements are in abnormal patterns, the stiffer and more restricted the movement patterns become. It is common that a child who has "straight eyes" at rest, cannot visually fixate to maintain eye contact when he is moving in a stereotypical abnormal pattern.

There is the potential for contractures and deformities. The potential for contractures and deformities is considerable, as the child with spasticity moves in stereotypical abnormal patterns and is subsequently restricted in the variety and range of movements. Certain muscle groups remain, and are used, in a shortened position and contract. The antagonist muscles are overstretched.

In the extraocular muscles, prolonged and persistent deviation of the eyes to one side, or into elevation (due to a predominant abnormal pattern of movement) will cause the shortening of the agonist group and overstretching of the muscles opposing the predominant pattern. *The physiological changes in the shortened or contracted muscle tissue itself, rather than the original cortical insult in cerebral palsy, are now acknowledged to be the cause of many of the deleterious features of spasticity.* Features resulting from these physiological changes include lack of movement, delayed initiation of movement, and poor movement quality.

Lack of movement. As movements are stiff and labored, much effort is required to move, which in turn increases spasticity. The spastic musculature held immobile in shortened positions becomes stiffer still. The overstretched antagonists cannot generate tension, and as the child matures movement becomes more and more limited by the further degenerative changes in the spastic muscle tissue (McCluskey & Schurr, 1994; Shepherd, 1995).

For an easy lifestyle, the child gradually moves less and less. The child becomes unwilling to use his or her eyes, particularly a child with cortical visual impairment. Unless the reluctance to move is addressed, therapy attempts for vision habilitation can be defeated.

Delayed initiation of movement. The inaccurate timing of muscle contractions in the child with spasticity delays the initiation of movement. Motor responses are labored and slow, and the child may often miss the "critical visual moment."

Poor movement quality. With the inaccurate timing and exaggerated force generation caused by the changes in spastic muscle tissue, movements seem uncoordinated. The paucity of balanced antagonist activity due to overstretching causes inappropriate grading of muscle action. Excessive cocontraction causes a spread of unnecessary muscle activation in the spastic muscle tissue. These associated reactions impair movement quality further. For example, when a child is reaching there may be unwanted activation in the eye musculature, causing strabismus.

Suggestions to Modify the Negative Effects of Spasticity

A number of practical strategies for the general management of cerebral palsy with spasticity can be successfully adapted to reduce the degree to which spasticity compromises the use of vision.

Reducing the Use of Abnormal Movement Patterns

Training the use of *preferred movement patterns* will reduce the need for the child to be reliant on those one or two stereotypical movements which prevent the development of dissociated eye movements.

Preparation strategies may be required and demand such hands-on techniques as elongation of shortened musculature and positioning to obtain correct body alignment. Preparation techniques are integrated into an individual service plan by relevant therapists.

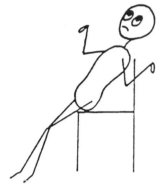

Figure 13.1

However, preparation alone does not directly lead to a preferred movement. Often once the force generated by spasticity is removed by positioning and elongation techniques, the child can be left without effective substitute movements. For example, a child is sitting in a chair extending strongly, mainly at head and hips (Figure 13.1).

After correct positioning the predominant pattern of extension has disappeared. The child no longer sits up, however, but drops forward with his head toward his knees (Figure 13.2).

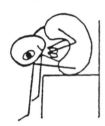

Figure 13.2

The child now must now *learn a new way* (a preferred movement pattern) to move against gravity without the use of unwanted spastic muscle actions.

Preferred movement patterns are designed to make dissociation of body parts possible. For example, visual pursuit movements are made possible by increasing head control using the active extension facilitated by the standing position. Preferred movement patterns need to be learned in order to give the child the possibility of both the dissociation and selectivity of eye movements. A detailed study of those patterns follows.

In order to minimize the use of unwanted patterns to move 1) the team identifies the predominant patterns of spasticity, and 2) those tasks demanding constant repetition of movements in the spastic pattern are avoided, and substitute forms of task completion are programmed. For example, if the stereotypical pattern was identified as involving head turn to the right with eye deviation to the right, the environment would be organized so that this pattern is nonfunctional. People approach the child from the left, and favored objects are presented from the left.

Controlling Factors That Increase Spasticity

The changeable nature of spasticity in all but the most severe cases of cerebral palsy is a key element in the success of adapting the environment to promote more normal use of musculature. When there is severe spasticity, unchanged by any adaptations of learning conditions, other compensatory management options should be investigated (Campbell, 1989). In a daily routine it is unrealistic to expect all the factors which increase spasticity to be controlled. The following instructional strategies and programming considerations help ensure that changeability of postural tone has a positive effect on performance, and not the negative effect of an increase in spasticity.

Reducing effort. Effort during task performance is greater when the task is new to the child. When each interval of the daily program commences with a *familiar* task, the child is able to adjust to confounding environmental conditions such as positioning, lighting, and noise prior to a new challenge. This is particularly important for the child with cortical visual impairment who, as we have seen, has significant sensory modulation problems.

Effort is reduced when the task is made less difficult. Cognitive, visual, and motor demands must be considered as a whole. A cognitive task is easier when visual-motor demands are lessened and vice versa. For example, a child is learning to differentiate visually between the value of coins. Initial learning conditions provide supportive positioning, good lighting, and contrasting backgrounds. The child is required only to point to a carefully positioned coin using a preferred movement pattern. He or she is not required to reach, grasp, and release the coins into appropriate sorting trays.

Note that many tasks in the daily routine do not require the child to "look" throughout their completion. During task analysis, the "critical visual moments" must be identified. This reduces visual-motor demands, as prolonged visual fixation during body movement is very difficult for the child with spasticity. Often the command "keep looking" is unnecessary for efficient task completion. Sometimes it increases task difficulty and consequently spasticity.

Reducing Stress. Anxiety related to a learning environment is controlled in part by choosing appropriate instructional techniques. Physical guidance can be preferable to verbal instructions for the child in the initial stages. Verbal instructions are kept to a minimum, and the adapted conditions of the environment and physical guidance prompt the child. Remember that verbal commands introduce yet another sensory modality to the visual, tactile, and movement stimuli demanded by the task. For the child with cortical visual impairment, verbal commands can cause a sensory overload. It is not uncommon for the child to shut his or her eyes firmly as soon as the command to "look" is given!

During physical guidance, tactile stimulation is best controlled by using gentle but firm holding or pressing techniques initially, then slowing fading pressure. Tapping or sudden changes in grip position and pressure are avoided as this may generate a protective or stress reaction from the somatosensory system. When verbal commands are used, a soft tone of voice reduces the likelihood of a "startle" reaction, which causes a sudden increase in spasticity. The use of soft, calm auditory input assists with reducing the excitatory nature of stimulation.

The child with spasticity is less stressed and therefore performs best when movement control is "subconscious" and his or her attention is directed to the task (not the muscle) action being demanded. Asking the child to "look" is asking him to use his eye musculature. It is far more appropriate to encourage the use of vision by prompting his or her responses with a visually dependent task.

Encouraging Emotional Responses That Do Not Restrict Motor Control

It is important that the child is allowed to experience a normal range of emotional states, so that he can learn to use appropriate motor responses during the expression of emotion. For example, a young child who is angry or excited may respond only with a strong, predominant pattern of extension to express feelings. In such cases a primary objective of the program is that the child learns to use a substitute form of communicating these feelings—either an augmentative or verbal system.

Idiosyncratic manual signs that facilitate preferred movement patterns are an excellent option for communication. With speech pathology involvement to plan priorities and combine communicative and motor needs, the child can experience and learn to express a wide range of emotions without compromising motor function.

The emotional reaction of fear due to poor balance, in the child with spasticity, requires alternative management. Provision of adequate postural support is important when learning a new task, to reduce insecurity and the resultant increase in muscle tension. However, like the fading of physical guidance, it is critical to aim for the reduction of postural support required for task completion, if better balance is ever to develop.

The child's attention is drawn to the task and the task is selected so that it intrinsically challenges balance. For example, a child with predominant flexion, who is wheelchair dependent, is positioned with a door to his side beyond his reach. The situational cue is to "push the door open" by looking, shifting his weight sideways, and stretching out to reach the door. The child's awareness, and thus fear of, the balance demands are reduced because he or she is not being specifically told to "keep balance."

Reducing the Likelihood of Contractures and Deformities

The likelihood of contractures and deformities can be reduced by (1) preventing length-associated changes in soft tissue, through the use of positioning and prolonged stretch (Shepherd, 1995) and (2) maintenance of muscle tissue extensibility by active lengthening of shortened musculature as the child uses preferred movement patterns. For the extraocular eye muscle, the first option is not really a possibility (eyes cannot be splinted or held in positions of stretch). The second option, however, reiterates the importance of practicing preferred movements. During growth spurts, e.g., early childhood and adolescence, physical management regimes to counteract contractures and deformities need extra emphasis as these are periods of high risk for the deleterious changes in soft tissue extensibility.

Increasing Opportunities for Movement

To overcome the lack of movement seen in the child with low vision and spasticity, program objectives train wide ranges and varieties of movement. For example, every time an objective demands a "reach" response, the task demands that the child visually locates an item placed at the extent of his or her reach range to promote a preferred movement pattern.

Programming a *variety of position changes* into the daily routine provides opportunities for the child to experience a greater repertoire of movements, e.g., standing during assembly or at the sink, "sidelying" for playtime. In this way the child is offered a variety of new viewpoints for the visual understanding of the environment and also a gentle enrichment of the low vision.

Increasing the Initiation and Speed of the Motor Response

Only movements that do not reinforce the stereotyped patterns of spasticity should be trained to be completed at higher speeds and higher levels of efficiency. Preferred movement patterns prevent the soft tissue changes responsible for inactivation of the correct muscle force required by intentional movements.

It is essential that team members learn to wait for the child's response. In the first stages of learning the child must be given the time and the opportunity to *start his own movement*. The only way a child can practice initiating movements is to be left to try, over and over again. The skill of waiting for the child is one of the most valuable we can learn.

The child needs many opportunities to practice a preferred motor response if the speed of movement initiation is to be increased. The preferred movement pattern is programmed into as many functional tasks as possible—usually through careful environmental adaptation, and the speed of task completion is included as a criterion for acceptable performance. Often it is slow motor performance that renders a skill nonfunctional, e.g., a child is able to point to a symbol or picture communication board, but is so slow to point that the listener moves away.

Improving Movement Quality

If the balance between agonist and antagonist activity can be improved by reducing the problems associated with muscle length-associated changes, there is a possibility of improving movement quality. The mechanical disadvantage of overstretched eye musculature and its inability, say, to control smooth tracking will be overcome only by *using* the weakened musculature.

The central tenet of management for the population with cerebral palsy with spasticity sufficiently severe to compromise visual functioning is clear: the child must be actively involved in the practice of preferred movement patterns that simultaneously address visual and motor needs, throughout the daily routine.

Management Options for Patterns of Spasticity Compromising the Efficient Use of Vision

This section will describe the predominant patterns of abnormal movement typically used by the child with spasticity and provide management considerations that incorporate those positioning options, preferred movement patterns, and environmental modifications most likely to give the child the best possibility to use his or her vision.

The unwanted stereotypical patterns of movement described do not occur in isolation from each other, and the presence and interaction of patterns is different in every child. The possibilities for management, therefore, must be carefully evaluated by the interdisciplinary team in each child's case. Positioning, movement patterns, and environmental modifications should be modified to address individual needs.

The four abnormal, key patterns of spasticity described are

- predominant pattern of extension
- predominant pattern of flexion
- patterns of asymmetry
- associated reactions.

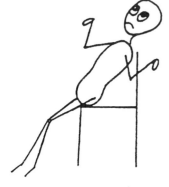

Figure 13.3 Predominant pattern of extension in sitting. Note eyes in elevation.

Predominant Pattern of Extension

A predominant pattern of extension is commonly seen in the younger child (under 7 years of age) with spasticity. Often this child is described as having quadriplegic cerebral palsy. The typical presentation is shown in Figures 13.3 and 13.4.

With the predominant pattern of extension, head hyperextension is accompanied by the eyes moving into elevation.

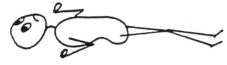

Figure 13.4 Predominant pattern of extension in supine. Note eyes in elevation.

Management options for a predominant pattern of extension

Supine. The supine positions encourage extension throughout the body. If, in the supine position, the extensor spasticity is sufficient to hyperextend the neck, the child is unable to achieve head alignment and the elevation of the eyes is marked. To depress the eyes the child has to overcome the predominant pattern of extension (Figure 13.4).

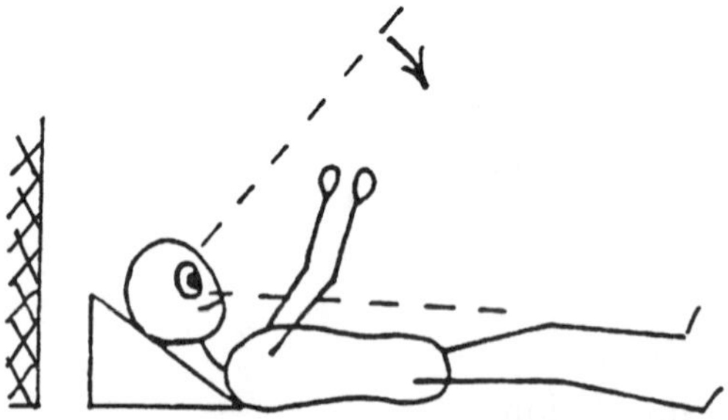

If, in the infant, supine play is considered an appropriate option, the environment can be modified to promote elongation of the neck musculature. The child is placed supine but with the head on a wedge, to promote movements in "chin tuck." The legs can be positioned to encourage external rotation and abduction at the hips (Figure 13.5).

Figure 13.5 Preferred range for visual motor activity in supine.

In the figures, the preferred ranges for optimum use of vision are denoted by dotted lines. These preferred ranges ensure that active eye movements will stretch the eye musculature shortened by persistent use within the identified abnormal patterns of movement.

Considerations in supine

1. The presentation of visual input, e.g., carer's face, encourages the eyes to move into depression.
2. Visual stimuli behind the child's head are minimized to inhibit elevation of the eyes. For example, place child with a blank wall behind his or her head.
3. Ensure that overhead lighting does not compromise the use of vision in the preferred movement range of eye depression.
4. Reach, grasp, and manipulation, e.g., of suspended toys, is encouraged at arm's length above the chest. Bringing the arms well forward to play allows the child to practice moving in a range that will lengthen shortened shoulder girdle and arm musculature as well as promoting visual regard in a range to lengthen contracted eye muscles.
5. Carers approach the child from directions that encourage the child to use a chin tuck action and to use his or her eyes in depression for location or tracking.
6. The child participates actively in an assisted position change, by making eye contact with his eyes in depression, and reaching forward to the carer using chin tuck, shoulder protraction, and elbow extension.

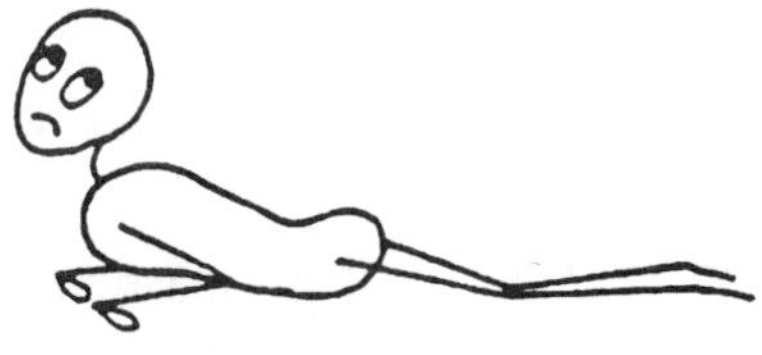

Figure 13.6 Predominant pattern of extension in prone. Note the eyes in elevation.

Prone. Traditionally, activities in the prone position have been used to practice active extension against gravity, since this reflects the normal developmental sequence. However when trying to optimize the use of vision for the child with low vision and a predominant pattern of extension, the prone position creates problems. In prone, though the predominant pattern is one of extension, the upper body is usually pulled tightly into flexion, with upper spine rounded and arms tucked under the body (Figure 13.6). The child then has to use head hyperextension to lift his or her head, as he or she has insufficient upper trunk extension to do so. To look around, therefore, the child reinforces the elevation of his or her eyes.

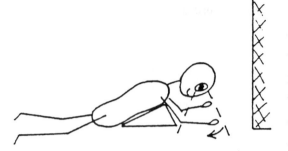

Figure 13.7 Preferred range for visual motor activity in prone. Note the eyes working in midposition and not in elevation.

Current neurodevelopmental therapy practice actually discourages the inclusion of any position that may promote unwanted movement patterns, despite the fact that the position may be a part of normal development. It is clear that *prone activities must be introduced with caution.* There are many more suitable options to develop active extension and antigravity head alignment.

Considerations in prone

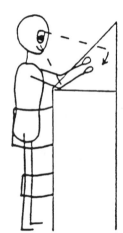

Figure 13.8 Preferred range for visual motor patterns in standing, for the child with predominant pattern of extension.

1. If prone activities are introduced, visual interest is maintained in ranges that promote depression of the eyes, when the head is in correct alignment (Figure 13.7).
2. The child is placed on a wedge, which encourages a stretch into upper spine extension and the possibility for the arms to work away from the body.
3. Forearm propping with elbows below shoulders is encouraged, with the child shifting the weight from side to side as he or she plays with toys placed out to the side of the shoulders.

Standing. It is not uncommon that when extensor spasticity is inhibited (e.g., by sitting with excessive hip, knee flexion and leg abduction) the child collapses forward and finds maintaining an upright position very difficult: he lacks active extension, despite displaying a pattern of extensor spasticity. Active extension is best learned by preferred movements in sit-to-stand activities or assisted, well-aligned standing positions (e.g., prone stander, flexi-stand, or standing frame) (Mayston, 1994).

The pelvis is more easily held vertical due to lower limb extension, thus giving the spine the possibility of good alignment. (Often in sitting, the pelvic tilt makes alignment of head and spine more difficult.) The recommended standing position is shown in Figure 13.8.

Considerations in standing

1. The child takes several minutes to adjust to an antigravity position if he has been reclined or resting.

2. Active extension of the spine is promoted when the child is using arm movements (e.g., reach and grasp) out to the side at shoulder height. (If the child hyperextends the head during reach, the task has been placed too high.) Working with arms out to the side (e.g., something so that wide movement range is demanded).

3. Initially activities only requiring vision for location are provided (e.g., striking a large target). The visual location of the target must not encourage head hyperextension at any point in the movement. To do so will reinforce unwanted muscle contraction.

4. As active extension improves, fixation during reach is introduced (e.g., selection of a toy). The increase in more normal muscle control is reflected in the ability of the eyes to maintain fixation with movement dissociated from predominant extension.

5. Visually directed grasp and release is practiced while the child has the best possibility to maintain active trunk extension (i.e., wide ranges to the side). This gives the child the opportunity to practice visual motor skills in patterns other than those dictated by his predominant extension. The child has the opportunity to learn a variety of movements, as visual motor range is gradually increased.

6. Learning visual-motor skills in wide and varied ranges gives the child the possibility of working in positions to his visual advantage. A child with an ocular disorder such as sensory nystagmus must be able to use his or her hands in the range in which he or she can best see (the null point). If restricted to the ranges of his pattern of spasticity, this may not be possible.

7. Practicing visual-motor movements out to the side also enables the child with cortical visual impairment to use the typically well-developed peripheral vision.

8. Standing is also a valid position for working at an easel, or upright surface: the eyes are looking ahead or in slight depression (Figure 13.8). The child rests one or both forearms on the easel so that weight bearing helps maintain active upper trunk extension and head alignment.

9. The child is not fully supported or static in standing but is in a

position where he or she is active against gravity. Standing stimulates sufficient postural tone to give the child the best possibility to free the eyes from using the predominant pattern of spasticity (Umphred, 1987) and practice using more appropriate muscle movement.

Sitting. Despite the undeniable value of activities in standing, the child's day involves many sessions of sitting (e.g., in wheelchair or posture chair) to participate in functional tasks.

Although much research and development has been directed toward providing comfortable, "inhibitory" and supportive seating for the spastic child, static positioning should be balanced with opportunities to develop active postural control. This is especially true for the child with low proximal tone and spasticity of the extremities (the "atonic spastic" type).

Considerations in sitting

1. In order for the child to develop active control of movements in sitting, he or she is provided with a variety of seating options. All options a) discourage head hyperextension, i.e., with no head rest or back support against which to use extensor thrust and b) ensure good pelvic alignment.
2. In a well designed and supportive seat which includes a head rest and a way to correctly position trunk, pelvis, and limbs, the child may be able to dissociate eyes from head and head from trunk and upper limbs. For orthoptic/ophthalmological/optometric assessment, specific visual training, and some fine motor and cognitive skills, this special seating is essential.
3. The use of the eyes when the child's head is maintained in alignment is obtained by presentation of tasks below or at eye level, either to side or front.
4. Less supportive positions are also included in the daily program so that active extension in sitting is developed.
5. The extensor thrust is minimized if there is no back or head rest against which to obtain leverage from extensor thrust. For example,

the child could be assisted in "high sitting" on the carer's knee, or placed in a forward-leaning seat or on a bench (Figure 13.9).

6. There is a continual adjustment of task components to ensure the pelvis is aligned with the spine and that movements of the upper body are mainly in front of the center of gravity. In this way, active extension is the natural postural response.

7. Activities involving arm movements to the side at shoulder level again facilitate active trunk extension. *Active extension* gives the child the best possibility to "free" his or her eyes and look at what he or she is doing (e.g., shaking hands with a friend while maintaining eye contact).

8. If the child can maintain alignment, then movements toward the front of the body are introduced, such as operating a battery toy with a switch. If shoulders begin to hunch, or head hyperextends, more active extension is practiced by reintroducing activities to the side.

9. The presentation of the visual stimulus at or below eye level (e.g., at an easel) ensures a controlled chin-tuck is practiced, and in this way the child can learn eye movements other than in eyes in elevation.

10. The combination of activity in front of the body, with active extension, helps develop the balance between flexion and extension (co-contraction) necessary for head and trunk control. With the reduction of head hyperextension due to improved head and trunk control, the eyes are freed from the extensor pattern of spasticity in the sitting position.

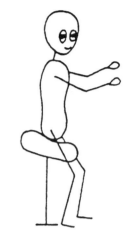

Figure 13.9 High sitting to obtain a biomechanical advantage for active trunk extension

Additional management considerations for the child with a predominant pattern of extension but low proximal tone

1. If the child has low proximal tone, many more opportunities to practice movements that encourage active control against gravity are needed.

2. Standing provides maximum stimulation for trunk activity.

3. The child is given extra time to adjust to a new position. Wait for several minutes before training a specific task.

4. The preferred movement pattern of "reach" out to the side, to facilitate trunk activity, must be programmed frequently throughout tasks.

5. Increased force can be generated in trunk muscles as an overflow from using the hands in a gripping or pushing action, such as gripping a squeeze switch while watching a computer program.

6. Toys are fixed to the work surface (e.g., with a C-clamp or Velcro®) and are designed for holding or pushing.

7. A grab handle is attached to the work surface so that grip and weight bearing with the nondominant hand promotes stability. It is reiterated that the nondominant hand is used in preferred patterns that provide active elongation of shortened musculature.

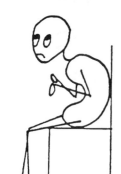

Figure 13.10 Typical compensatory pattern in the child with predominant extension. Note the eyes in elevation, associated with neck hyperextension.

Compensatory patterns associated with a predominant pattern of extension

In order to compensate for the posterior pelvic tilt caused by shortening of muscle tissue, the child when in sitting habitually pulls his upper body forward in order to maintain balance. This causes shoulder hunching and a kyphotic upper spine.

To look "ahead" in sitting, the elevation pattern of the eyes is reinforced. The elevation is also seen as "overuse" of optical righting. For example, the child is using his or her eyes to initiate righting his head to the face vertical position. Due to the flexion of the upper trunk, the "face vertical position" is achieved by neck hyperextension. Neck hyperextension tends to further reinforce elevation of the eyes (Figure 13.10).

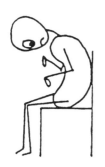

Figure 13.11 With the predominant pattern of flexion the eyes tend to move into depression.

Predominant Pattern of Flexion

The effect of the pattern of flexor spasticity on vision tends to become more apparent as the child is placed for longer periods in the sitting position, or as he progresses to four-point crawling for mobility. The child may be quadriplegic or diplegic. In sitting the child does not "collapse" forward but *pulls* forward with head and trunk flexion, shoulder protraction and upper limb flexion (Figure 13.11).

Most of the children who are sufficiently disabled by spasticity for it to interfere with use of vision are not ambulant and spend their time sitting. The fact that sitting, plus the issue that the use of flexion is so common for the completion of functional tasks, means that the strength of flexor spasticity, and the development of flexion contractures, are extremely difficult to counteract.

The long-term effects of an increase in flexion must be highlighted. The child will become limited in ability to participate in standing transfers, to sit up straight, look ahead, and reach out in any direction. Even tasks demanding vision within flexion become impossible. The chin tuck is so strong that when the eyes are in depression the child can only look toward his or her chest.

The child's program, therefore, concentrates on careful modifications so that the way tasks are learned maximally reduces the component of flexion. By reducing the components of flexion, the child is given the best possibility to use his or her vision during task completion.

Management Options for a Predominant Pattern of Flexion

Supine. As supine tends to promote extension throughout the body, it is a useful position for preparing a flexed child for work.

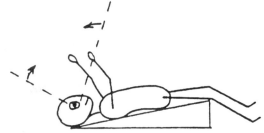

Figure 13.12 Encouraging preferred movement patterns in the child with predominant flexion.

Considerations in supine

1. Slight inversion (e.g., head down) on a wedge assists elongation and alignment. The younger child plays with toys suspended in a wide range at or above eye level (Figure 13.12).
2. Gravity assists the preferred movement of arm out of the shortened protraction pattern.
3. Classroom activities are organized so that the child is encouraged to look to the side and straight ahead. Often eye musculature is so

shortened that eye elevation is not possible until after extended practice.

4. The older child is encouraged to sleep supine or to lie supine to complete gym activities such as pulleys or punch bag, with the equipment placed above him or her and at his or her eye level. This helps to work the arms away from the body and develop upper trunk dissociation from the arms. In turn this decreases flexor pull.

Prone. Because prone and crawling activities exacerbate the pull of the flexor pattern, they are restricted and rarely programmed for visual-motor skill practice. The pull into flexion is often most difficult to inhibit in prone, and thus the prone position does not give the child the best possibility to use his or her eyes.

Standing. It is obvious why the child with predominant flexor spasticity benefits from the standing position. The extension at the knees and hips counteracts flexion contractures, and the pelvis' vertical position gives a biomechanical advantage for aligned trunk extension. In the same way that voluntary movements for extension against gravity must be developed in the child with a predominant pattern of extension, so active extension must be developed in the child with a predominant pattern of flexion. Neither child is able to work with dissociated movements in an upright position.

Often too, the flexor patterns have actually developed to compensate for an earlier predominance of extension (e.g., the child has learned to pull forward strongly so that he can adjust his center of gravity further forward). Developing a balance between active antigravity flexion and extension is again the goal of management. However, because of the predominance of flexor spasticity, *the eye movements are encouraged away from depression.*

Considerations in standing

1. Visual stimuli or visually dependent tasks are designed to get the child to "look ahead."
2. Work is presented to the front of the body, and at an easel (at least a 45° angle) to eliminate the strong chin tuck. For the child with

low vision who must be close to his work, use of an easel is particularly important.

3. If an easel is impractical for the task (e.g., eating, sorting coins), the task is stabilized at least 15 cm away from the body to reduce eye movements into depression.

4. If the work surface is flat, table height is raised to upper chest level to bring the arms away from the body and decrease upper trunk flexion.

5. Active trunk extension is again made easier in initial stages of learning, by movements of the arm out to the side at shoulder level. This movement pattern develops sufficient postural control to then present work lower down or to the front of the body. The object to be sorted is collected from the side and placed to the front, or vice versa.

Sitting. In sitting, the restriction of eye movement caused by flexor spasticity is very marked. However, to meet most functional tasks the child needs to be able to work in sitting. Much effort then is directed to programming movement patterns in sitting, which counteract the effects of a predominant pattern of flexion and thus optimize visual functioning. In individual therapy, considerable time is devoted to both developing motor skills requisite for "good" sitting (e.g., improved pelvic mobility during weight shift) and to developing appropriate seating equipment.

Considerations in sitting

1. In preparation for activity in sitting, good postural alignment is first obtained. The lower back is straightened; the child's weight is on the buttocks, not the sacrum. This reduces the child's need to flex the upper body to maintain the center of gravity. Such preparation is achieved by handling or positioning equipment such as a pelvic strap.

2. Movements of the arms out to the side of the body in ranges up to shoulder height work against the upper body flexor shortening and at the same time stimulate the desired active extension (e.g., pointing to a tilted communication board placed to the side of

the wheelchair tray). Side reach can easily be interspersed through-out daily tasks (Figure 13.13).

3. Due to the biomechanics of reaching with shortened musculature, arm movements *above* shoulder height to the front of the body may increase flexor pull (e.g., the use of a computer touch screen above eye level, or pointing to a high object). The flexor pull means the child cannot look and point ahead simultaneously, so such sequences are omitted from visually dependent tasks.

4. In the wheelchair or posture chair, a cut-out tray or desk is pre-ferred. The cut-out gives a surface so that arms are brought forward, away from the body, and elbows rest on the tray surface. A Dycem® non-slip mat stabilizes elbows. This arm positioning decreases shoulder hunching and excessive chin tuck.

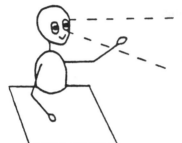

Figure 13.13 Reach patterns to the side to promote active trunk control, and the possibility of eye dissociation from a predominant pattern of flexion.

5. Whenever possible, a tilted work surface (e.g., 45°) reduces the need to use head flexion to see. (Care is taken, though, not to encourage reach above shoulder level to the work surface.)

6. On a flat work surface table activities are secured at least 15 cm away from the body to minimize the need to use the hands close to the chest, as this increases the use of flexion. Where the child needs objects closer to the eyes due to limited distance vision, tray height is raised, but objects are still 15 cm away.

7. Alternatively the child is taught to lean forward from the hips with back straight, rather than hunching his upper body (Figures 13.14 and 13.15).

8. Actions involving upper limb weight bearing or pushing, actively stretch the shortened musculature (e.g., pushing a pressure switch to control an electric wheelchair).

9. A task involving visually directed grasp and release, such as sorting, is presented so that grasp (the flexion component) is completed in the position of partial extension out to the side. Release (the extension component) is completed to the front of the body in the position of greater body flexion.

10. Release is made easier by introducing more extension, for example, as the child presses the object to be released against the work surface (i.e., an assisted release).

11. Floor play in sitting is designed to reduce the elements of flexion in movement patterns. Cross-leg sitting is made easier when the child sits on a wedge (Figure 13.16).

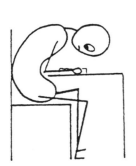 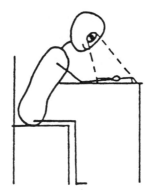 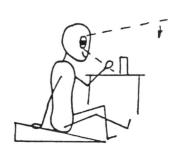

Figure 13.14 The child with strong flexor patterns has difficulty looking at objects close to his body on a waist height tray.

Figure 13.15 Preferred visual motor range for desk work. Note that desk work is placed away from the body and the body is leaning forward from the hips.

Figure 13.16 Cross-leg sitting on a wedge, with toys placed on a low table to optimize visually directed play.

12. In side sitting, cross-leg or long sitting, the need for upper body flexion is reduced by placing activities on a chest height table, or providing activities which do not involve leaning down to the floor (e.g., basketball, or ring toss). However, cross-leg, side or long sitting remain extremely difficult positions for this child, as the degree of hip flexion makes active trunk extension difficult.

Comment on cortical visual impairment

Throughout the preceding sections on predominant flexion and extension patterns the emphasis is on using movement patterns and positioning which promote neuromotor activity. Although giving the child full postural support remains a useful technique when obtaining visual responses for a child with CVI, clinical experience has indicated that many children with CVI use their vision more efficiently *after* a higher level of arousal through postural activity has been achieved. Once the child has adjusted to an antigravity position in which the minimal amount of support is required for good body alignment, the task is introduced. Working in the recommended standing or high sitting positions (see Figures 13.8 and 13.9) appear very successful.

For CVI then, it seems inappropriate to solely use visual enrichment. Rather, first involve the child in work against gravity to increase arousal and give the possibility to dissociate the eyes, then introduce task components reliant on visual responses. Careful design of task sequences may thus obtain the appropriate level of arousal and motor activity, which is a prerequisite to optimizing visual interest and visual motor control in these children.

Patterns of Asymmetry

The motor disorder of cerebral palsy always affects each side of the body differently. The asymmetry of the spasticity is seen both in the presence of abnormal head postures and the delay in the development of midline orientation of the eyes.

Asymmetry with Predominant Extension

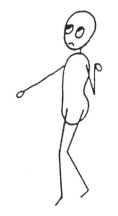

Figure 13.17 An asymmetrical tonic neck reflex pattern.

The NDT approach no longer advocates specific testing of primitive reflexes. In the population of children with severe spasticity, however, there are a significant number whose visual action system is significantly affected by a persistent *asymmetrical tonic neck reflex* (ATNR). The distribution of the spasticity in these children is typically quadriplegic. The ATNR is observed as a head turn to one side, usually the more affected side, accompanied by an extension pattern of the face side of the body, and a flexion pattern on the occiput side (Figure 13.17).

The ATNR is closely associated with a predominant pattern of extension. During the ATNR activity, the eyes move into dextroelevation or laevoelevation (i.e., right or left toward the face side) with elevation due to the increased extensor tone on that side.

Management Options for Patterns of Extension and Asymmetry

In most children the ATNR is a way for the child to achieve trunk and head extension and is used as a point of stability from which the less affected side can work. The pattern is best reduced by developing adequate force generation for symmetrical, active trunk control, as this directly minimizes the use of asymmetrical activity, freeing the eyes from elevation and deviation to right or left. Implementation of the options listed for "predominant pattern of extension" are also relevant.

Supine

Considerations in supine

1. When the child is in supine it is essential to encourage movements in a chin-tuck position to oppose the shortening pattern at the back of the neck caused by the ATNR.
2. Head turn with chin-tuck is encouraged, initially toward the less affected side (e.g., during unilateral play) to oppose the predominant ATNR pattern.
3. With the ATNR arm, visuo-motor activity is obtained as the child reaches out to the extreme of the forward reach range (e.g., sight and hit a target). This brings the shoulder forward off the ground so the child does not push back into an ATNR.
4. Bilateral movements are introduced directly above the chest, with both elbows semiflexed (e.g., tilting a bubble tracking rod or glitter wand).
5. Head turn and eye movements with chin-tuck to the ATNR side are practiced for active lengthening of the extraocular eye muscles in a pattern dissociating the eyes from the head.

Side Lying

Considerations in side lying

1. Side lying is used to optimize visual functioning, only when the stability which the child has historically achieved through using ATNR patterns has been reduced (i.e., chin tuck is maintained by a head pillow and trunk is aligned with appropriate equipment).
2. The child lies on his or her ATNR side, spine parallel to the ground. (Degree of hip/knee flexion will vary with therapeutic decisions and is programmed accordingly.) In this position the pressure of the

child's weight assists myofascial release and elongation of shortened musculature.

The ATNR shoulder is brought forward, and the arm up and away from the body (Figure 13.18).

3. Activities are presented between face and waist level so the eyes move in ranges other than dextroelevation or laevoelevation, and chin-tuck is maintained.

4. The activities are raised 10 cm off the floor (e.g., battery toy on low platform) to encourage midline orientation of the eyes.

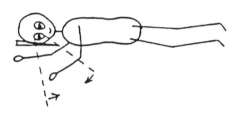

Figure 13.18 Ranges for preferred movement patterns in side lying.

Upright Positions

Considerations in sitting and standing

1. The development of active trunk control counteracts ATNR activity. This is again more easily learned in standing than sitting.
2. Presentation of visually dependent tasks ensures that visual fixation promotes chin-tuck and head turn.
3. Initially head turn is elicited to the less affected side, and the midline.
4. Visually directed arm movements to either side are between shoulder and waist level to promote chin tuck rather than head extension.
5. To promote head alignment, the child is positioned so that upper body weight is forward. Forearm propping (preferably on a tilted work surface) of the ATNR arm is taught. This is necessary for unilateral activities of the less affected arm. The use of a grab handle or nonslip mat under the elbow, assists with the provision of positional stability which will reduce the child's need to rely on the stability achieved through ATNR patterns.

Asymmetry with Lateral Flexion

When this pattern is sufficiently severe to affect vision, it is most commonly seen in the child with extremely limited mobility of the pelvis. As the pelvis cannot move during weight shift, the child compensates using strong lateral (side) flexion and chin-tuck to stop himself or herself from falling to the side. The child obtains even more stability by tucking his or her arm into his or her side (Figure 13.19).

This pattern, with its excessive components of flexion, tends to be accompanied by the eyes moving into depression, sometimes with a slight deviation to the laterally flexed side. Implementation of options listed for predominant pattern of flexion are relevant here.

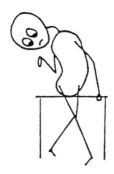

Figure 13.19 Pattern of asymmetry with lateral flexion. Note the eyes in depression.

Supine

Considerations in supine

1. Reclining (inverting) the child down a wedge (Figure 13.12) allows gravity to elongate the shortened side and obtain symmetry.
2. The child practices looking and using arm movements above the head to the shortened side to learn movements involved in elongation, e.g., knocking down bowling pins, using pulleys in the gym.

Side Lying

Considerations in side lying

1. The child lies on the shortened side, the floor arm is up and away from the body, and the lower limb is extended at the hip to stretch the contracted musculature.
2. Activities are placed well away from the body at eye level or above eye level to reduce the pull into flexion.
3. Elongating the shortened side is also possible when the child lies on the less affected side. In this position, arm movements are out to the front.
4. Later the child should complete movements above eye level or up overhead to the side of the body, to encourage dissociation of arm/trunk.

Lengthening the shortened side using reach breaks up the flexor pattern and assists the dissociation of body parts, including the eyes and head.

Upright Positions

Considerations in sitting and standing

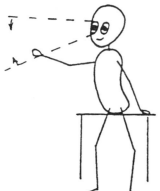

Figure 13.20 Elongation of the weight-bearing side optimizes visually directed reach.

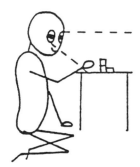

Figure 13.21 Side sitting, with reach across midline to toys on a low table, optimizes visually directed play.

1. Each time visually directed reach and grasp to the affected side is demanded, the environment is arranged so that arm movements elongate the weight bearing side of the body. This opposes the pull into side flexion and teaches the child the preferred pattern of movement during weight shift (Figure 13.20).

2. For example, equipment to prepare morning tea is placed on surfaces at or above midchest height. The child approaches in his wheelchair so that he or she is side-on, and therefore collects items from his or her side. The child must reach to the extent of his or her range and shift weight to the side with which he or she is reaching.

3. Gradually the child is introduced to forward reaching. Objects must be placed at a sufficient distance and height that lateral flexion of the trunk is not substituted to provide the range required to collect the object.

4. During school work, the more affected elbow rests on the desktop, or preferably the easel, in front and away to the side of the body at an angle of about 45° to the axilla. This prevents lateral flexion.

5. The less affected arm has the best possibility for visually directed activity to the affected side when midline cross reach is demanded at a level higher than the shoulder.

6. Side sitting on the floor to the affected side is a preferred position only when activities are placed on a chest-height table on the affected side (Figure 13.21). If tasks are placed on the floor the child uses lateral flexion to reach down to them.

7. Activities can also be placed in a table to the front.

8. If side sitting to the unaffected side, the principles of introducing preferred patterns are the same—keep activities up at chest level or above, to prevent lateral flexion with reach. This time though, activities are best presented at the unaffected side, not the front.

Associated Reactions

Associated reactions are increases in patterns of spasticity in the affected parts of the body during the use of less affected body parts, and as a response to effort, stress, and emotion. Associated reactions are observed in children with less severe spasticity, for example, because these children are more able to "move." Associated reactions are most marked in the distal parts of the body, e.g., hands, feet, and eyes. These reactions interfere with the use of vision as they cause an increase in eye signs, most commonly in strabismus or squint.

Management Options for Associated Reactions Tasks

Involve the body parts affected by the associated reaction. Associated reactions are most effectively reduced by involvement of the affected body part in the task. It is useful to present a task that demands the use of the child's visual fixation during preferred patterns of movement. The more motivated the child is to use vision, the more quickly dissociated eye movements develop. These dissociated eye movements reduce associated reactions. From clinical experience, children with ocular disorders have a greater motivation to use their vision than children with cortical visual impairment. Programming preferred movement patterns for children with cortical visual impairment requires a detailed understanding of their interests and choices.

Training involves the child initially using his or her eyes for "location," with the object to be located placed to encourage "looking" in a direction opposing the associated reactions in his or her eyes. The program provides frequent opportunities for the child to practice visual location—the child visually searching for desired objects rather than the objects being placed on the desk where he or she expects them to be. Repeated use of the eyes for visual location gradually reduces effort. The child is using less effort as the looking response becomes more automatic. From the earlier part of the section that discussed the features of spasticity, it is clear that the less effort that is used, the less the spasticity, and hence the less the associated reactions.

Visual fixation can then be practiced. Initially the provision of activities where the hands are well stabilized helps provide a steady base from which selective fixation can be achieved. The upper limbs can be used for stabilization in a pattern opposing the tendency for muscle shortening, such as weight bearing on an open hand while pressing the keys of an electronic communication system with the less affected hand. Any management options that optimize the use of vision while reducing movement in patterns dictated by spasticity will decrease associated reactions as they give the child the best possibility for maximal use of the affected body part—the eyes.

Decrease the effort required to complete the task. Associated reactions are reduced when the task is redesigned to decrease effort.

For example, motor components of the visually dependent task are made less demanding. The child points with arm resting on a surface rather than pointing with arm in midair. The child uses an electric rather than manual wheelchair for early orientation and mobility skills.

To decrease effort, visual components of the task are reduced. *Critical visual moments* are identified to minimize expectations using vision. Visual cues are enhanced by lack of background clutter, increased contrast, and optimum lighting. Cognitive components are simplified, sequences are limited, and visual discriminations are made less complex.

There is then a systematic introduction of graded motor, cognitive, and visual components of functional tasks in the program. This system monitors the degree of overall effort demanded and counteracts the child's tendency to exhibit associated reactions under stressful learning conditions.

Train preferred movement patterns. Associated reactions are only reflections that the child is using patterns of spasticity. They are least marked when the most "normal" or preferred patterns of movement are being used. This reiterates the central tenet of an NDT treatment framework.

The reduction of effort in motor performance must not be equated with the child being inactive, but rather with the child being active in certain preferred ways. If the child lacks the ability to generate force after his reliance on patterns of spasticity has been reduced by the conditions of task performance, then any activity will be effortful and associated reactions will increase. Preferred movement patterns must therefore be introduced and *practiced*, if reduction in associated reactions is to occur.

Summary and Conclusion

This section of the chapter has examined one aspect of the complex management required by the child with cerebral palsy and low vision. The management strategies presented were related specifically to the child with cerebral palsy whose spasticity is sufficiently severe to interfere with his use of vision.

The child with low vision can increase visual functioning through the use of nonoptical aids, environmental modifications, and specialized management techniques. Effective management of the child whose low vision is partly attributable to spasticity therefore should not only contain strategies to address ocular disorder and/or cortical visual impairment, but also aids and techniques to manage those patterns of spasticity further interfering with efficient use of vision.

The nature of spasticity is such that it affects the body musculature in fairly predictable patterns. It does not just affect, arm, leg, or extraocular muscles in isolation. As a result, the management of spasticity that interferes with the use of already impaired vision necessitates the use of treatment perspectives that address the problems associated with abnormal patterns of movement, and with abnormal sensory processing. A combination of sensory integrative, neurodevelopmental therapy, and a systems approach to learning has proved valuable.

There are features of spasticity directly relevant to visual functioning that should be understood by all members of the interdisciplinary team in order to plan the most effective individual program. Features such as the likelihood of contractures and the consequent physiological changes in muscle tissue, the difficulty with the initiation of movement, and the presence of associated reactions, may significantly impair a child's performance unless appropriate management strategies are instituted.

The implementation of management strategies is simplified by the identification of several stereotypical patterns of spasticity. In the population of children studied, there appear to be key patterns of spasticity or abnormal movement that interfere in predictable ways with the efficient use of vision. These patterns can be described as predominant patterns of extension, of flexion, of asymmetry, and associated reactions. In each child these patterns rarely appear in isolation, and the dominant pattern may vary according to the child's positioning or his stage of development. The presence of these key patterns and their interaction is different in every child.

For the key patterns of abnormal movements identified, management options suggest

- the way to position the child
- the directions of movement or preferred movement patterns
- the ranges in which he should look
- the relevant environmental modification.

All management options give the child the best possibility to use his or her vision.

Familiarity with both the characteristics of the key patterns identified, and with the specific management options described, seems essential if the interdisciplinary team is to ensure accurate assessment and appropriate individual program development.

The child who has cerebral palsy with spasticity and low vision has complex programming needs. Traditionally programs for this population of children have tended to delineate visual habilitation from motor management. Hopefully, this chapter has provided a practical introduction to strategies that simultaneously address the interrelated visual and motor programming needs of the child with cerebral palsy and low vision.

REFERENCES

Black, P. (1982). Visual disorders associated with cerebral palsy. *British Journal of Ophthalmology, 66,* 46–52.

Bobath, B., & Bobath, K. (1984). The neurodevelopmental treatment. In D. Scrutton (Ed.), *Management of the motor disorders of cerebral palsy.* London: Heinemann.

Boehme, R. (1990). *An approach to treatment of the baby.* Tucson, AZ: Therapy Skill Builders.

Campbell, P. (1987). Integrated programming for students with multiple handicaps. In L. Goetz, D. Guess, & K. Stremel-Campbell (Eds.), *Innovative program design for individuals with dual sensory impairments.* Baltimore, MD: Paul H. Brookes.

Campbell, P. (1989). Dysfunction in posture and movement in individuals with profound disabilities. In F. Brown, & D.H. Lehr (Eds.), *Persons with profound disabilities.* Baltimore, MD: Paul H. Brookes.

Case-Smith, J. (1996). *Fine motor development and assessment seminar.* Unpublished course notes, Brisbane, Australia.

Chapparo, C., & Ranka, J. (1996). *The perceive, recall, plan and perform system.* Unpublished course notes, Sydney, Australia.

Corn, A.L. (1983). Visual function: a theoretical model for individuals with low vision. *Journal of Visual Impairment and Blindness.* 373–376.

DeGangi, G. (1994). *Documenting sensory motor progress.* Tucson, AZ: NDTA Therapy Skill Builders.

DeGangi, G., & Dunn, W. (1993). Sensory integration and neurodevelopmental therapy for educational programming. *Classroom applicatons for school based practice.* Royeen, C. (Ed). Bethesda, MD: American Occupational Therapy Association.

Duckman, R.H. (1987). Visual problems. In E.T. McDonald (Ed.), *Treating cerebral palsy: For clinicians by clinicians.* Austin, TX: Pro-Ed.

Erhardt, R.P. (1987). Sequential levels in the visual motor development of a child with cerebral palsy. *American Journal of Occupational Therapy, 41,* 43–48.

Fisher, A.G., Murray, E.A., & Bundy, A.C. (1991). *Sensory integration: Theory and practice.* Philadelphia: F.A. Davis.

Geniale, T. (1991). *The management of the child with cerebral palsy and low vision.* North Rocks, Australia: North Rocks Press.

Goetz, L. & Gee, K. (1987). Functional vision programming. In L. Goetz, D. Guess, & K. Stremel-Campbell (Eds.). *Innovative program designs for individuals with dual sensory impairments.* Baltimore: Paul H. Brookes.

Goetz, L. & Gee, K. (1987). Teaching visual attention in functional contexts: acquisition generalization of complex visual motor skills. *Journal of Visual Impairment and Blindness,* 115–117.

Groenveld, M., Jan, J.E., & Leader, P. (1990). Observations in the habilitation of children with cortical visual impairment. *Journal of Visual Impairment and Blindness,* 11–15.

Hall, A., Bailey, I.L. (1989). A model for training vision functioning. *Journal of Visual Impairment and Blindness,* 390–396.

McDonald, E.T. (1987). *Treating cerebral palsy: For clinicians by clinicians.* Austin,TX: Pro-Ed.

Mayston, M. (1994). *Bobath certificate course: Student notes.* Unpublished course notes, Melbourne, Australia.

Morse, M.T. (1990). Cortical visual impairment in young children with multiple disabilities. *Journal of Visual Impairment and Blindness,* 200–202.

Shepherd, R.B. (1995). *Physiotherapy in paediatrics, 3rd edition.* Oxford, Great Britain: Butterworth Heinemann.

Umphred, D.A. (1987) Neurophysiologic bases of modern treatment procedures. In E.T. McDonald (Ed.), *Treating cerebral palsy: For clinicians by clinicians.* Austin, TX: Pro-Ed.

Warren, M.L. (1995). *Evaluation and treatment of visual dysfunction.* Sydney, Australia. Unpublished course notes.

14 Functional Aspects of the Eye Diagnosis

Eleanor E. Faye, MD, FACS

When working with older adults who may have a variety of deficits, the most difficult to evaluate is sight. A person can report visual problems without identifying the cause; self-reported problems could range from a need for new glasses, to normal aging changes, to pathological changes in the eye or the brain.

The obvious solution is universal periodic eye examinations both as a preventive and as a means of early detection of the disorders that traditionally accompany aging: cataracts, macular degeneration, glaucoma, and retinopathy of diabetes mellitus.

No eye complaint is innocuous until proven so. The difficulty in evaluating any older person is that normal aging results in changes in eye tissues that are probably normal but may signal the onset of serious vision impairment. Whether it is eyeglasses, medications, or surgery, everyone needs eye care.

Symptoms and their functional implications must be evaluated by professionals such as ophthalmologists or optometrists who either refer patients for vision rehabilitation or are actively involved in the treatment program. The functional evaluation should answer the following questions: What does a symptom mean in terms of providing the best environment for the person? How must tasks be modified to be accessible to the person with visual impairment? What optical devices and visual aids are useful and how do they fit into an individualized program?

This section first discusses normal aging changes and describes typical symptoms. Second, it reviews characteristic low vision devices. And third, it discusses various eye disorders, their typical symptoms, and prescription devices.

Visual Changes Associated with Normal Aging

Is there such an entity as normal aging of the eye, that is, decreased visual function, unrelated to ocular disease? The answer is not clear-cut because many changes in the eye may not initially affect visual activity; only if the changes reach a significant level do they cause visual malfunction (Marmor, 1995). In addition, aging does not affect all persons or all systems uniformly or equally. Therefore, it is useful to differentiate between a normal aging process and an anticipated loss of function from outright pathology.

Results from the Framingham Study (Leibowitz et al., 1980) dispel the myth that all aging persons can eventually expect to have an eye disease. Of the most common conditions—cataract, macular degeneration, glaucoma, and diabetic retinopathy—only 19% of adults between 65 and 74 years of age have at least one disease. After age 75, the number rises to 50%. With increasing age comes increased prevalence of cataract and macular degeneration (in other words, these conditions are age-related), although many older adults remain free of functional deficits well into their 80s.

Lens, Cornea, and Vitreous

Optical media changes associated with normal aging occur in the lens, cornea, and vitreous. As these clear structures age, they develop microscopic changes in the protein molecules (Boettner & Wolter, 1980). These particles absorb light and scatter shortwave-length light rays (blue or ultraviolet light) (Wolf, 1960). This microscopic change reduces the quality of light reaching the retina, but, more significantly, it causes glare from light sources such as lamps, headlights, and windows. When working with older adults, it is important to note the level of illumination and type of lamp that provides the most comfort and best contrast. For example, a person may need more light for reading but complain of glare if the intensity is above the comfort level or if the light is at an angle that reflects from the surface of the page. Fluorescent and halogen light sources, which have a high proportion of blue light, may cause fatigue and discomfort for an older person who has no specific eye disorder (Hemenger, 1984).

Another normal structural change in the aging person may be a reduction in the size of the pupil due to sphincter atrophy. When the pupil can no longer dilate significantly in low-light conditions, a delay in light and dark adaptation results. This delay becomes an important consideration with hallway lighting, with orientation when entering an unfamiliar building or room, or with traveling on a cloudy day or at night.

Presbyopia

The condition of middle-aged sight (*presbyopia*) is well-known to anyone in their mid- to late-40s. The lens of the eye in youth responds promptly to a near object by contraction of the muscle of accommodation in the eye, which allows the lens to become more convex (i.e., stronger) to accommodate for near range. Most near work involves print, computer images, diagrams, and drawings. As the lens becomes more rigid with age, it loses its elasticity and can no longer adapt to near range. This deficiency can be simply remedied by the introduction of reading glasses (single lenses, half-eye frames, bifocals, trifocals, and progressive lenses) to compensate for this normal aging phenomenon (Hofstetter, 1965).

Visual Acuity

Visual acuity changes that occur with aging are corrected with the prescription of conventional eyeglasses for distance, intermediate (arm's length), and near range. The average eye tends to become more far-sighted with age (*hyperopia*), resulting in the inability to focus a clear image for either distance or near. A *myopic* (near-sighted) person tends to become less myopic with age, that is, a decrease in the power of the myopic correction may be needed. Therefore, refraction for glasses should be done every 2 years to be sure the older person is wearing the optimal correction and not blaming poor vision on age or eye disease (Owsley & Sloan, 1980).

Before working with an older person in any area of rehabilitation, it is important that the person knows which glasses to use for a given activity, that the prescription is up-to-date, that the glasses are clean and scratch-free, and that the frame fits properly. An older person with corrected vision may not score 20/20 acuity because of normal corneal and lens changes, yet be unaware of any functional disability. It is important in evaluating an individual's symptoms to realize that the standard visual acuity test bears so little resemblance to the real world that a person's self-reported history of visual performance is more significant than a measured visual acuity. Performance may be better than the acuity would suggest or, in some instances, worse. The essential point is to insist on a complete eye examination to reveal the source of the vision complaints and not allow an older person to blame age for poor performance.

Contrast

Aging reduces the adult's ability to discern contrast of objects against a background. Several factors are involved in discerning contrast, such as structural changes in the cornea and lens as well as a diminished sensitivity of retinal receptors that reduces sensitivity to light and color. Contrast is further reduced significantly in the presence of cataracts, corneal disease, and retinal pathology (Owsley, Sekuler, & Siemsen, 1983).

When working with older adults, whether it is sewing, arranging a place setting, doing art work or hobbies, reading, watching television, or using a computer, contrast must always be a consideration. Colors should be selected for optimal contrast, for example, dark colors against a light background or the converse. Black and white offers the best contrast.

Color Vision

Color vision does change with age. The aging lens usually becomes pale yellow or amber (without being affected by a cataract). This change would affect colors in the blue-yellow range. Light blue may be seen as aqua; yellow may be called white; navy blue may appear black. An older person may want to label items of clothing that could be easily confused. Another potentially serious problem is identifying pills and medications by color rather than by shape, size, or a clearly marked label. A yellow pill may appear to be white or beige. A blue pill may appear to be light green and a red pill, brown.

Visual Field

With age comes a gradual reduction of the field of view (peripheral field) as sensitivity decreases in the peripheral receptors. While a visual field test may be normal, in real-life situations the person does not recognize movement or objects in the far edge of the field because of this age-related loss of sensitivity. The implications of the insensitive peripheral field require being especially alert to hazards and moving objects while walking and driving. Reaction time is often insufficient to protect one from an accident (Ball, Owsley, & Beard, 1989).

At some point in an older person's life, the aging process may progress to actual pathology. Symptoms cease being simply a nuisance and begin interfering with activities that are customarily simple. If an examination reveals pathology that cannot be corrected either medically or surgically or with conventional eyeglass correction, the resulting decrease in visual function is called *low vision*.

The Evaluation Process

Many types of low vision and many approaches to treatment exist. The ideal approach to vision rehabilitation takes data from measurements of functional deficits in visual acuity, refraction, contrast, and visual fields and applies the data to a performance evaluation. Each person is different, not only in the degree of damage to the system but in motivation and response, so no such thing as a routine low vision evaluation is possible. Tests can be done routinely, but the *interpretation* is always matched to the person being evaluated.

A comprehensive evaluation starts with refraction and evaluation of the level of visual acuity (Rosenthal & Cole, 1996). Vision for distance and near is tested with high-contrast Snellen vision charts. Although the data from these charts are not as important as contrast data, the data serve to verify the refraction and to provide some idea of distance acuity as well as near acuity. It is useful to follow patients over time to document changes from the baseline vision.

After best corrected acuity is verified, the central visual field may be tested using an Amsler grid (see Figure 14.1). The presence of distortion, scotomas, and low-contrast areas in the central (macular) vision is as important as acuity because defects in the central field may affect reading or seeing detail more than the actual reduction of acuity.

Defects in the peripheral field may affect mobility. When peripheral vision is affected by an eye disorder, such as glaucoma, retinitis pigmentosa, stroke, or neurological brain damage, the visual field provides essential information suggesting the need for mobility skills training. In addition, knowledge of visual field defects allows the instructor to anticipate possible difficulties for the patient in coping with the demands of traveling.

Tests of retinal sensitivity are called contrast sensitivity tests (contrast sensitivity function or CSF). A number of tests are available, but the principle of all the tests is the same, to measure the eye's ability to determine borders and backgrounds (Bodis-Wollner & Camisa, 1980) (see Figure 14.2A). Although the entire retina is sensitive to gradations

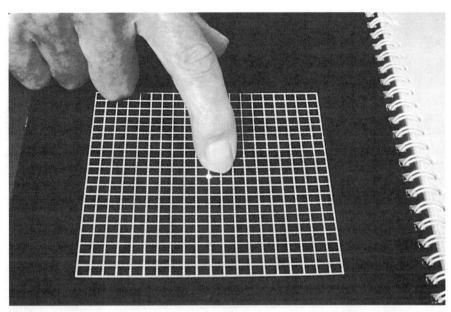

Figure 14.1 The Amsler Grid held at 33 cm (13 in.) measures distortion and scotomas over the 20-degree area of the macula. The patient is asked to describe the appearance of the grid first binocularly, followed by each eye separately. The patient may also draw a picture on the recording sheet. Photography courtesy of The Lighthouse, Inc. Reprinted with permission.

of contrast, the most sensitive area is the fovea and surrounding macula. The sensitivity of retinal cells decreases toward the periphery.

CSF has been used to great advantage in low vision since 1984, when a study of patients with low vision showed that a correlation between response to magnification and contrast sensitivity existed (Ginsburg, Rosenthal, & Cohen, 1987). The need for more magnification and greater contrast in print as well as the need for lighting can be predicted quite accurately by the CSF results (see Figure 14.2B). Responses that fall below the age-related normal area indicate reduced sensitivity to magnification. If at least three targets are seen, the person will probably respond to optical magnification. If two targets or fewer are identified (subthreshold), the patient will need more magnification than is available in optical devices. We now know that many diseases decrease the CSF to such a degree that, by analyzing the curve, we can predict that CSF will be insufficient for a person to read print or see distant objects clearly even with maximum magnification. The diseases that most often affect the CSF are cataracts, corneal dystrophy, macular degeneration, glaucoma, and diabetic retinopathy.

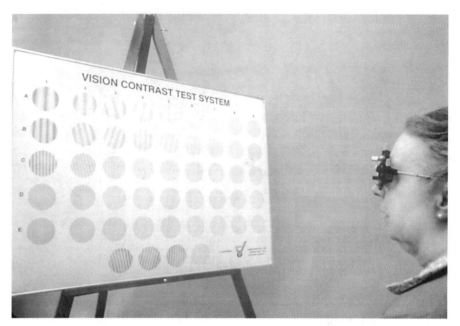

Figure 14.2A Contrast sensitivity in low vision is best tested with grid targets covering five frequencies from low to high and a range of targets of diminishing contrast. The test is administered at 1 m if visual acuity is 20/60 or less. Both eyes are measured, followed by a binocular measurement. Photography courtesy of The Lighthouse, Inc. Reprinted with permission.

The need for special mobility training can also be predicted objectively. When the curve is subthreshold on any test, the examiner can assume quite accurately that the person will not be able to respond to clues in the environment or to benefit from optical magnification.

Once the diagnosis has been confirmed and the function tests completed, the visual rehabilitation process can begin. However, before discussing the diseases and their effect on treatment, we must look at the tools that are used: low vision adaptive devices.

Low Vision Adaptive Devices: Functional Considerations

In the course of the low vision evaluation before introducing devices to the patient, the examiner has considered the pathology and its effects on the patient's ability to perform. All the function tests have been analyzed, the power of the device calculated, and devices are now evaluated in relation to functional capacity and task.

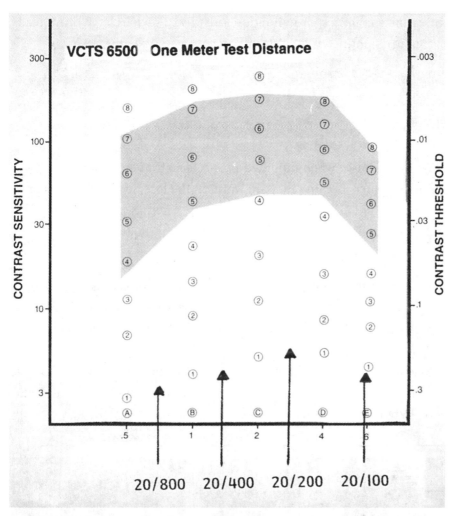

Figure 14.2B The contrast test is recorded on a special form calibrated for low acuities. The shaded area represents the age-related norm from the highest response seen in young people to the lower responses seen with increasing age. Any responses under the shaded area are abnormal. If a person sees two targets or less (subthreshold), optical magnification probably will not be effective. Photography courtesy of The Lighthouse, Inc. Reprinted with permission.

The purpose of applying the low vision evaluation data is to understand what the deficits are and to channel the patient's ability to use residual vision. Each patient has interests, motivation, intelligence, coping history, and complex intangibles that must be considered. Once the devices are selected, the patient must learn adaptation skills, whether reading with magnifiers or using, or simple adaptive equipment around the house.

Basic devices for low vision are either optical, such as magnifying lenses and sunglasses, or nonoptical (adaptive), such as large print, reading stands, lighting, and electronic travel aids (Williams, 1996).

Spectacles

Magnifying lenses when mounted in spectacle frames must be used in a specific manner. Because they are worn on the face, the working distance is close to the lenses, that is, 13 in. or less, often as close as 2 or 3 in., and both hands are involved in holding reading material.

Because of these optical limitations, patients who read using both eyes must be aided by base-in prisms in the glasses (see Figure 14.3). The prisms support the effort the eyes must make to converge at such a close distance. The monocular patient who uses the better eye alone also must hold material close to the eye at the focal distance of the lens. (Focal distance in millimeters is related to dioptric strength using the formula f = 100/D.) The illumination should be positioned so light falls directly

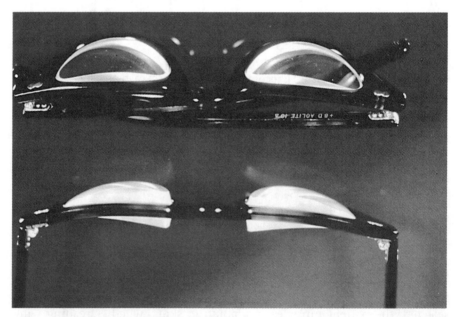

Figure 14.3 Prism half-glasses are available in powers of 4 to 12 diopters to allow binocular use of vision for near work. Base-in prism, shown from the front and from above, allows both eyes to converge at the close reading distances required (less than 10 in.). Photography courtesy of The Lighthouse, Inc. Reprinted with permission.

on the page without creating glare. The person has to learn to read slowly at first, usually one word at a time, and to move the paper slowly past the eye or to scan with a lateral head movement. The difficulty in adjusting to this way of reading is offset by the large reading field and greater reading speed compared with using handheld devices such as a hand magnifier. Patients with macular degeneration usually prefer a spectacle aid unless the disease is far advanced or an extraordinary amount of light is needed; such a person might prefer an illuminated stand or hand magnifier. If the disease involves a peripheral field loss with a small central field, a spectacle may not be appropriate, because an image close to the eye is larger than the available central field.

Hand Magnifiers

Most patients, regardless of their eye condition, will use a hand magnifier for a variety of short-term tasks. A hand-held lens is held away from the eye, increasing the work space between the eye and lens (see Figure 14.4). For many patients, the increased viewing distance is more comfortable

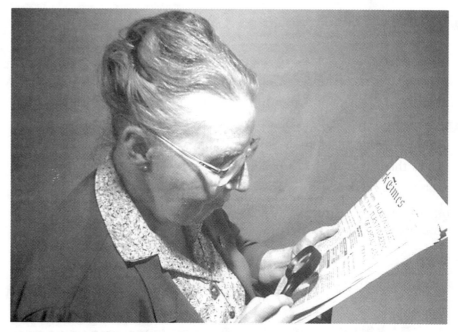

Figure 14.4 The hand magnifier is held at its focal distance and is useful for short-term tasks. It may be used either with or without glasses. Patients with tremors or arthritis may have difficulty holding a magnifier. Photography courtesy of The Lighthouse, Inc. Reprinted with permission.

than a comparable spectacle. The first step for a patient is to practice doing practical tasks, such as reading a stove dial or a thermostat. Although patients traditionally use magnifiers for shopping and reading mail, labels, recipes, and menus, many learn to read efficiently enough to enjoy reading but scan at a slower pace than with spectacles.

Patients may use a hand magnifier with distance glasses, with their reading glasses, or without glasses. With distance glasses, the magnifier must be held as far from the print as possible; with reading glasses the magnifier must be held closer to the print; and without glasses the patient must hold the lens at whatever distance the image appears sharpest. Patients with constricted fields often prefer to use magnifiers instead of spectacles closer to the eye because the visual field with a magnifier farther from the eye covers a greater area. Patients who have lost central field (macular degeneration) are efficient users of magnifiers, which can be nonilluminated or illuminated. If patients have tremors or orthopedic or neurological deficits, hand magnifiers are probably *not* the device of choice.

Stand Magnifiers

A stand magnifier can be thought of as a hand magnifier mounted on a base that rests on a page. The base holds the lens at or close to its focal distance so the patient does not have to maintain that distance manually. The premounted lens is stable and easy to maneuver for patients with a tremor or arthritic hands. Many stands have built-in illumination, which makes them the lens of choice for a person who needs a uniform light source (see Figure 14.5). Many patients with macular degeneration and glaucoma benefit from a stand magnifier and will use their own conventional reading glasses in conjunction with the stand to view the image clearly.

Telescopes

The telescope tends to be overemphasized as a low vision device although to many experts it is synonymous with low vision rehabilitation. Tele-

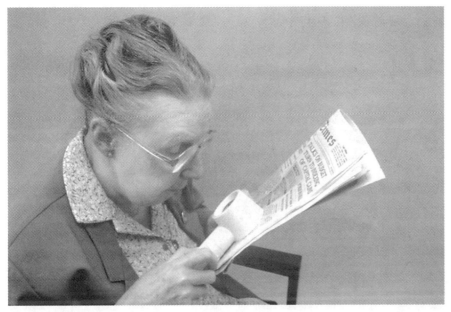

Figure 14.5 A stand magnifier rests directly on the surface of the page, maintaining its focal distance without effort on the part of the patient. The stand illustrated has self-contained battery illumination. Photography courtesy of The Lighthouse, Inc. Reprinted with permission.

scopes have charisma. They not only look as if they were a low vision aid, but they have a special optical characteristic that no other device has—the capacity to focus at any distance from infinitely far to very near. Of particular importance is the intermediate or arm's length work distance, which is beyond the visual range of the average low vision patient. Typical examples of focusing at this distance are looking at shelves in a supermarket or library, reading music, looking at display cases in stores and museums, looking at computer screens, and doing home repairs.

Telescopes are most often prescribed as monoculars, but they can also be mounted in a spectacle frame to free both hands (see Figure 14.6). They can have a set focus, be focused by hand, or, most recently, be designed with an auto-focus feature. Because of their light weight, spectacle-mounted telescopes may be preferable to binoculars for sporting events, movies, lectures, and art exhibits. Before computer programs were available in enlarged type, telescopes were useful at the range for reading a computer screen, although the field limitation always required special visual skill training.

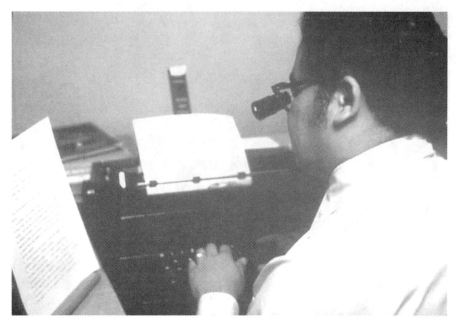

Figure 14.6 The spectacle telescope is used for tasks that require intermediate (arm's length) work distances. Most telescopes are focusable from distance to near range. For simple distance viewing a handheld monocular is practical. Photography courtesy of The Lighthouse, Inc. Reprinted with permission.

Aside from cost, telescopic devices have two optical disadvantages— a restricted field and little leeway in the working distance. Telescopes mounted in a frame also block out the surrounding field when the patient is looking through them, which could present a hazard in mobility unless special instruction is included in the rehabilitation.

Closed Circuit Television

Using a television monitor to reproduce reading material is another alternative to the telescope. A number of options are available with closed circuit television reading machines (CCTV). It is possible to sit at a normal distance from the screen either by moving the reading material by hand on an x-y table or by using a small handheld camera to scan the material. Some newer sets have features, such as a calculator, calendar, clock, and note pad that allows selective areas of text to be magnified. Most patients prefer white or yellow letters on a dark background for best contrast. Current sets have many other options such as a color monitor and a variety of colors for the text. CCTV provides the greatest range of magnification (up to 60×) and best contrast of any low vision aid.

Techniques in Rehabilitation

Low vision magnifying lenses are prescribed for the many activities that require the use of magnification. Daily living, however, encompasses many mundane tasks for which magnification with optical devices is impractical. Part of the rehabilitation will emphasize moving closer to an object to visualize it more clearly (such as sitting closer to television), or using objects that are designed with enlarged letters or numbers (such as clock faces, timers, large print books, and computer programs) (*Consumer Products Catalog*, 1994–95; Williams, 1996).

Tasks such as shopping, cooking, and personal care can be more frustrating than the inability to read because they are time-consuming, and the patient's performance is not like it used to be. Tasks that help the patient adapt more efficiently are marking objects, arranging items in an orderly fashion in the kitchen, bathroom, and closet, and emphasizing nonvisual skills and auditory signals. Patients should also be encouraged to explore options for themselves and to think about listing priorities as they work with the instructor to evolve new approaches to old skills.

Common Eye Diseases and Visual Function

Prescribing low vision devices requires assessing the effect of the eye pathology. The presence of eye pathology influences what the doctor can prescribe and, in some cases, even limits the type of device that can be used. The patient's response can be only as good as the level of visual function, regardless of motivation and enthusiasm. Each of the common eye diseases has characteristics that should be considered by the clinician and instructor.

Three major categories exist, and each category has specific characteristics that affect the approach to designing a remedial plan (Faye, 1995; Faye, 1996). The three groups cover all the structures of the eye, visual pathways, and visual cortex of the brain.

Group 1: *Cloudy optical media,* includes corneal diseases, pupillary abnormalities, cataracts, and opacities of the vitreous humor. Group 2:

Central visual field defects, includes macular degeneration of all types, macular edema, macular hole, cysts, and neurological scotomas from the optic nerve to the macula (cecocentral scotomas). Group 3: *Peripheral visual field defects,* includes advanced glaucoma, advanced retinitis pigmentosa, diabetic retinopathy with retinopathy in the peripheral retina or laser treatment in that area, postsurgical detached retina, stroke, and any other brain damage in the optic pathways or brain.

Cloudy Media

Although cataracts alone are not low vision conditions, the presence of a cataract may complicate the management of a primary eye disease such as glaucoma or macular degeneration. In addition to the scotoma caused by the primary condition, added haze, blur, and reduced contrast is present. Because many levels of disability are experienced with cataracts, not all patients require surgery until the physician feels visual improvement would be significant. Before surgery is needed, the therapist must be aware of a potential difficulty with lighting in the home for a specific task or out of doors. Direct lighting on a task may have to be angled or modified until maximum comfort and illumination level are achieved. Patients usually prefer the yellow spectrum of incandescent light to the blue spectrum of halogen or fluorescent light sources. If vision becomes faded or blurred, the light level may be too high, particularly with light in the blue spectrum. Patients may also use a combination of fluorescent ceiling lights with an incandescent lamp at the work surface to reduce glare or discomfort.

Patients may find simple devices helpful. A black plastic reading slit (typoscope) can reduce the glare of reflected light from the page. Bold pens and black ink can make written materials stand out. Telephone numbers can be written in large print; visors can reduce overhead glare; and neutral gray wraparound sunglasses can reduce glare and perhaps provide better contrast.

Central Visual Field Defects

The macula is responsible for detail vision, color vision, and daylight vision. Although it occupies at most only 20 degrees of a total field diameter of more than 180 degrees, it is solely responsible for keen sight. Eyeglass lenses focus principal rays on the macula for best corrected vision. If macular cones are damaged by atrophy, hemorrhage, laser treatment, or scar tissue, the sight is blocked centrally to a degree commensurate with cell damage. The loss of vision (distortion or scotoma) calls for an adjustment, usually a spontaneous head or eye turn that shifts the vision away from the macula to the edge of the lesion (paramacular area). Since the visual resolution of this area is less precise than the center of the macula, magnified images are needed to interpret the image. During the period of adaptation the person with a macular defect learns to look off center (up, down, sideways) and to use whatever magnifying lenses or devices best suited to the task. Patients need nonoptical techniques that they can apply to activities around the house. Because peripheral vision is unaffected (as a rule), individuals are able to travel around by themselves, perhaps using a monocular telescope for signs, or simply asking for directions when needed. However, these same persons may need to arrange for alternative types of transportation when they can no longer drive. They do not usually need special mobility aids such as a cane unless they want a cane for support or security.

Peripheral Visual Field Defects

Although glaucoma is the most prevalent condition in this category, it must be emphasized that only in the late stages of decompensation of the optic nerve does the patient with glaucoma become a patient with low vision. The advanced stage of glaucoma is unusual in a patient who takes medication faithfully, although a few susceptible individuals have progressive disease in spite of maximum medication or surgery, especially with the so-called *low tension* or *normal tension* glaucoma.

The visual field is obliterated first in the periphery and only gradually advances toward the macula. Not until dropout of macular cells is present is contrast sensitivity reduced to the point that reading becomes difficult or impossible. Traditional magnification is not effective if no healthy peripheral retina registers the image. At the late stage of glaucoma, spectacles are not as effective as CCTV and low-power hand magnifiers. Eventually, no type of magnification works and the person must learn nonvisual techniques. Patients with glaucoma in this latter category need mobility instruction and other rehabilitation services from agencies that specialize in rehabilitation of the visually impaired and blind. Patients have a number of options: human guide technique, cane travel, or electronic sensors. Most patients with glaucoma prefer human guides; the older person may not have the physical strength to manage and care for a guide dog.

Other conditions that fall into this category are retinitis pigmentosa, extensive retinal detachment after surgery, advanced diabetic retinopathy, and neurological conditions that cause peripheral scotomas (stroke or trauma).

The remaining central vision in a patient with retinitis pigmentosa is generally more useful than the same area in a patient with glaucoma because the contrast sensitivity is at or near normal. The best devices for these individuals are computers with a flexible menu of large print programs, CCTV, and sunglasses that block UV light and enhance contrast (Ginsburg et al., 1987).

When patients have diabetes with retinopathy, other medical problems must be considered. Patients may not be able to tolerate much stress; even reading with magnification can be stressful. They may be depressed, taking multiple medications for other systemic problems, and lack energy, which may be interpreted by a therapist as lack of motivation. The same considerations should apply to patients who have had brain trauma, particularly stroke; many seemingly well-functioning persons have difficulty concentrating or retaining what they read. If the patient has a hemianopia (either right or left), he or she needs special prism glasses and retraining in tracking printed material.

The response of *any* person with peripheral field defects depends on the level of contrast perception, which may vary for each individual. Therefore, attention should be given to the use of materials that provide maximum contrast, such as black print on a white background, marking pens, enlarged print, and CCTV with white letters on a dark background (Ginsburg et al., 1987; Williams, 1996).

Instruction in orientation and mobility techniques is needed if independent mobility becomes an issue.

Summary

Concerns about an aging population are escalating as longevity becomes the rule rather than the exception. Any professional involved with geriatric caregiving is faced with recognition of pathology versus normal aging changes: decision making and program planning are often based on a patients functional status. Eye care has traditionally been refraction or surgery and medicine. Only a small segment of the visually impaired population is recommended for comprehensive vision rehabilitation. The increasing demand for low vision care may change the attitude of inertia within the eye care professions and create greater awareness within the various professions involved in general rehabilitation. Visually challenged people of the upcoming generation are not going to be satisfied with the statement that nothing can be done because it is obvious that a judicious combination of low vision adaptive devices and a thorough training in their application, combined with other rehabilitation techniques, will maintain optimum quality of visual function for patients with low vision.

REFERENCES

Ball, K., Owsley, C., & Beard, B. (1989). Clinical visual perimetry underestimates peripheral field problems in older adults. *Clin. Vis. Sci., 4,* 229–249.
Bodis-Wollner, I., & Camisa, J. M. (1980). Contrast sensitivity measurement in clinical diagnosis. In G. Lassell & J. T. W. Van Dalen (Eds.), *Neurophthalmology* (Vol. 1, pp. 373–401). Princeton, NJ: Excerpta Medica.
Boettner, E. A., & Wolter, J. R. (1980). Transmission of the ocular media. *Invest. Ophthmol. Vis. Sci., 1,* 776–783.
Consumer Products Catalog. (1994–95). New York: The Lighthouse.
Faye, E. E. (1995). Low vision. In D. Vaughan, T. Asbury, & P. Riordan-Eva (Eds.), *General ophthalmology* (pp. 388–395). Norwalk, CT: Appleton & Lange.
Faye, E. E. (1996). Pathology and visual function. In B. P. Rosenthal, R. G. Cole, & R. London (Eds.), *Functional assessment of low vision* (pp. 63–75). St. Louis, MO: Mosby.
Ginsburg, A. P., Rosenthal, B., & Cohen, J. (1987). The evaluation of reading capability of low vision patients using the Vision Contrast Test System

(VCTS). In G. C. Woo (Ed.), *Low vision: Principles and applications* (pp. 17–18). New York: Springer-Verlag.

Hemenger, R. P. (1984). Intraocular light scatter in normal vision loss with age. *Appl. Optics., 23,* 1972–1974.

Hofstetter, H. W. (1965). A longitudinal study of amplitude changes in presbyopia. *American Journal of Optometry, 42,* 3–8.

Leibowitz, H. M., Krueger, D. E., Maunder, L. R., et al. (1980). The Framingham eye study monograph. *Surv. Ophthalmol., 24*(Suppl.), 335–610.

Marmor, M. F. (1995). Normal age-related vision changes and their effects on vision. In E. E. Faye & C. C. Stuen (Eds.), *The aging eye and low vision (A study guide)* (Chap. 2, pp. 6–10). New York: The Lighthouse.

Owsley, C., Sekuler, R., & Siemsen, D. (1983). Contrast sensitivity throughout adulthood. *Vis. Res., 23,* 689–699.

Owsley, C., & Sloan, M. E. (1980). Contrast sensitivity, acuity and the perception of real world targets. *B. J. Ophthalmol. Vis. Sci., 19,* 401–406.

Rosenthal, B. P., & Cole, R. G. (Eds.). (1996). *Functional assessment of low vision.* St. Louis, MO: Mosby.

Williams, D. R. (1996). Functional adaptive devices. In B. P. Rosenthal & R. G. Cole (Eds.), *Remediation and management of low vision* (pp. 71–121). St. Louis, MO: Mosby.

Wolf, E. (1960). Glare and age. *Arch. Ophthalmol., 64,* 502–514.

15 Gerontic Occupational Therapy Practice

A Focus on Vision

Beverly P. Horowitz, PhD, OTR/L

Rehabilitation and the Older Adult

In addition to being a diverse population of people of differing backgrounds, cultures, and values, our older patients challenge our knowledge and skills given their high incidence of multiple diagnoses including complex medical and social histories. Statistically, older individuals have a high incidence of visual disturbances. Vision impairment ranks third among chronic conditions for those 70 years and older, after arthritis and heart disease (Colenbrander & Fletcher, 1995; Stuen, 1991). Among nursing home residents, rates of vision impairment are estimated to be more than four times as high as those for community-residing older persons (Branch, Horowitz, & Carr, 1989), and incidence of many types of ocular pathology increases with age. Cataracts, glaucoma, and retinal disorders are much more common among persons over 65 years. Aging commonly alters color perception (Ellis, 1991), visual reaction time, accommodative capabilities of the lens (Kline, Sekuler, & Dismukes,

1982) and has been seen to affect spatial vision (Sekuler & Owsley, 1982). Among persons 65 and older, visual impairments are twice as likely to be associated with other impairments, physical or sensory, and sometimes with cognitive impairments (Kline et al., 1982).

Benefits of Comprehensive Evaluations

Traditional occupational therapy evaluations examine performance areas (activities of daily living [ADL], work, and leisure), performance components (sensorimotor, cognitive, psychosocial, and psychological), and performance contexts, including home, community, and workplace. Performance components related to sensation include sensory awareness, sensory processing (tactile, proprioceptive, vestibular, visual, auditory, gustatory, and olfactory capabilities), and perceptual processing (Commission on Practice of American Occupational Therapy Association, 1994; Trombly, 1995). Evaluations may use medical histories and reports, clinical observation and assessment, questionnaires, nonstandardized instruments, checklists, or standardized assessment instruments (Bachelder, 1994; Law, 1995).

Occupational therapists have traditionally assessed perceptual processing skills as part of comprehensive evaluations, especially for individuals with head injury or central nervous system injury or disease or for individuals with developmental disabilities. Basic textbooks addressing adult physical dysfunction and occupational therapy practice advocate screening of visual foundation skills, including acuity, visual fields, and oculomotor function to assess the integrity of the visual system (Warren, 1996). Baseline information about visual skills is important to obtain for appropriate referral and treatment planning. This baseline information is particularly important in geographic regions and settings where optometrists, ophthalmologists, or vision specialists are not available to perform comprehensive evaluation (Pedretti & Zoltan, 1990, 1996; Ryan, 1993; Warren, 1995b, 1996). In addition to using vision functional checklists for screening, many prominent occupational therapy clinicians and researchers stress the importance of including testing of primary visual skills as part of comprehensive evaluations, because primary visual capabilities form a basis for normal visual perception with an impact on motor planning and praxis (Toglia, 1989; Warren, 1993a, 1993b). These primary visual skills include visual acuity, both near and far; visual fields; and oculomotor function, including alignment, range of motion, convergence, saccades, and pursuits (Quintana, 1995). The role of occupational therapy in either vision screening or assessment of primary visual deficits is not to diagnose the deficit, but to describe its functional effect and formulate the critical questions for the ophthalmologist or optometrist (Warren, 1993b, p. 58). The additional importance of such information for occupational therapy is to aid clinical observation of functional capabilities, to identify visual deficits that can potentially interfere with functional performance and progress in rehabilitation programs, and to prevent faulty clinical assumptions about individual perceptual-cognitive performance and related capabilities, which may be limited because of impaired primary visual skills.

Many individuals can compensate for visual impairments if aware of them; however, individuals who have not had a recent vision evaluation may not be aware of how their visual capabilities affect their daily activities. People with undiagnosed and untreated visual deficits may lose interest in activities because of increased visual stress without recognizing that their loss of interest is because of visual difficulties that may reduce concentration and visual endurance (Warren, 1996). For example, individuals who have decreased acuity or convergence may have difficulty reading normal printed material, thereby making it difficult to perform some ADL tasks independently, including cooking from written recipes, taking medications as directed, reading mail, managing finances and paying bills, or using cleaning products safely (Branch et al., 1989; The Lighthouse, 1991; Warren, 1996). Individuals with impaired oculomotor range of motion may lose visual information in restricted visual fields. Restricted visual fields commonly reduce awareness of movement in the environment in one's peripheral field of vision, thereby compromising safe mobility, especially safe driving. Depending on the severity, restricted visual fields may pose safety concerns for individuals participating in community activities, using public transportation, or marketing, and may impair reading and writing capabilities (Egan, 1992; Horowitz, Reinhardt, & Cantor, 1995; Treml, 1996; Warren, 1996). When mobility within one's community is limited, visual disabilities additionally affect socialization and participation in community activities (Horowitz, Teresi, & Cassels, 1991). Appreciation of the functional ramifications of visual impairments thus aids in identifying reasons for limited functional capabilities and assists in developing strategies to maximize independence and quality of life at home and in the community, while reducing potential for accidents (Branch et al.).

Thus, it is understandable that in addition to hindering ADL independence, visual impairment, especially significant visual losses, is reported to affect social and psychological well-being. Such losses are associated with reduced feelings of self-worth and clinical depression, including psychomotor retardation and agitation, fatigue and loss of energy, and impaired thinking or concentration, especially for individuals with severe visual loss (Branch et al., 1989; Kline et al., 1982; Rosenthal, 1995). Many of these symptoms are seen in older persons who have primary diagnoses of cerebral vascular accident (CVA), head trauma, Alzheimer's disease, non-Alzheimer's dementia, or Parkinson's disease (Mace & Rabins, 1991; Satin, 1994; Scott & Dow, 1996). Historic associations between blindness and total personal and economic dependence, including biblical associations of blindness with infirmity, poverty, and total dependence may be related to these emotional responses (Branch et al.).

Vision Screening

Regardless of age, the visual system provides basic sensory input to support visual perception, purposeful movement, and functional capabilities. The importance of vision screening within occupational therapy has historically been from the perspective of evaluation and treatment of individuals with neurological impairments, especially from head injuries, and those post-CVA (Lampert & Lapolice, 1995; Warren, 1993a). In regard to neurological conditions, rehabilitation departments commonly treat older persons with primary diagnoses of CVA, and others with primary diagnoses related to other central nervous system diseases or insults, including Parkinson's disease, anoxia, and brain tumor (Hooks, 1996; Miller & Kirchman, 1991; Schlageter & Zoltan, 1996; Woodson, 1995). These older persons are at particularly high risk for vision impairments because of advanced age and neurologic disease or insult.

The increasing appreciation of the importance of visual screens and assessments as part of generic occupational therapy evaluation relates to gerontic practice from multiple perspectives. Older individuals recovering from disease or insult to the brain with potential perceptual-cognitive dysfunction need particularly careful screening of primary visual skills to identify deficits that can affect functional capabilities and for referral for further evaluation, especially because of the prevalence of ocular pathology with increasing age (Ellis, 1991; Kline et al., 1982). For those with irreversible vision impairment with resulting functional limitations, vision rehabilitation with a focus on multidisciplinary rehabilitation interventions can improve functional capabilities for appropriate rehabilitation candidates. Interventions may include the use of compensatory strategies and assistive devices, including optical aids to enhance vision (Beaver & Mann, 1995; D'Allura, McInerney & Horowitz, 1993; Lampert & Lapolice, 1995; Warren, 1995b). Additionally, these impairments can then be differentiated from higher order perceptual-cognitive dysfunction to support appropriate treatment planning that can help individuals to use compensatory strategies to maximize their existing vision or to use other strategies to compensate for total vision loss (Quintana, 1995; Warren, 1996).

As with any clinical screen, occupational therapy visual screens are but a gross measure of visual capabilities. They are best performed after a careful review of all pertinent medical information, including patient and family interviews regarding the vision history and including the individual's subjective perceptions about his or her visual capabilities. Additionally, therapists need to observe whether the individual has head or postural deviations; has difficulty making eye contact or maintaining gaze; complains about eye discomfort, redness, tearing, and so forth; has difficulty negotiating narrow hallways; or undershoots or overshoots when reaching for objects (Chamoff, 1996; Pedretti & Zoltan, 1990). Occupational therapy visual screens for older persons are most beneficial when they include ADL assessments that address capabilities in basic self-care; work and productive activities including, home management, care of others, educational and vocational activities; and leisure (Warren, 1995a, 1996).

Comprehensive visual screens require assessment of both near (16 in.

or less) and far (20 ft or more) acuity using usual letter or symbol charts to test each eye and both eyes together, both with and without corrective lenses (Quintana, 1996). However, visual acuity is more than the ability to correctly identify letters on a Snellen chart; it is a highly complex process. Contrast sensitivity is now increasingly appreciated as very important in regard to acuity, particularly for older persons (Quintana, 1996; Pelli, 1987). Sine wave grating charts of varying contrasts and orientations are available to assess visual acuity related to contrast sensitivity.

Visual fields are most accurately tested through computerized automated perimetry; but when this is not possible, they have traditionally been grossly assessed clinically through confrontation testing (Warren, 1996). During confrontation assessment, the examiner sits in front of the patient and asks the patient to fixate on the examiner's nose and report when he or she perceives a stimulus in the periphery. Visual fields extend approximately 65° upward, 75° downward, 60° inward, and 95° outward when the eyes are focused straight ahead. Therapists can grossly rate capabilities as intact, impaired (perception past 45° but not to full extent), or severely impaired (perception between midline and 45° only) (Chamoff, 1996).

Visual screens may assess ocular alignment by observing for the corneal light reflex. The therapist sits in front of the patient with a penlight held about 12 in. in front of the patient's eyes. The patient needs to fixate on the light with the head held straight ahead. The reflection should be the same in both eyes when alignment is normal. Alignment can be grossly rated as intact or displaced, noting if one or both eyes deviate and the severity of deviation.

During ocular range of motion, the examiner typically assesses the extraocular muscles of each eye by having the patient follow a slowly moving target that makes a large H. Eyes are tested individually and together for complete assessments. Again, the therapist can grossly rate performance as intact with full range of motion, impaired (incomplete), or severely impaired or absent, if there is paralysis or compensatory head or neck movement.

Convergence, or the nearest point for binocular visual fixation, can be clinically assessed by having the individual follow a target, commonly a dowel, held in midline at 18 in. from the eyes and slowly moving toward the nose. The examiner measures the nearest point of binocular fixation before one eye breaks off from fixation. Convergence near points under 6 in. will usually not interfere with near vision. Fatigue and concentration difficulties may complicate accurate visual screening.

Saccades, rapid changes in fixation from one point in the visual field to another, are assessed using two dowels with different colored tips held 12 in. in front of the patient, 8–10 in. apart from each other. The examiner again sits in front of the patient and asks the patient to alternate fixation from one dowel to the other. Abilities need to be assessed in all visual field quadrants. Three-point rating scales can be used here as well to indicate if abilities are generally intact, if impairment is noted in under-shooting or overshooting with the particular quadrant noted, or if the patient cannot alternate fixation from target to target with the quadrant noted.

Visual pursuits, often called *visual tracking*, assess the quality of eye movement for fixation on moving targets. The therapist observes the ability of the patient to visually follow a moving target in all directions for a distance of at least 12 in. A penlight or dowel is commonly used for the moving target and is held 12–16 in. from the patient. Eye movements should be smooth with very limited associated head or body motion. Again, ratings can be made on a three-point scale: generally intact; impaired, when uneven eye movement is present, head or body moves, or cuing is needed; or absent, when the individual cannot follow the target even with cues. This part of the visual screen requires concentration and may be influenced by fatigue.

Implications for Practice in Varied Settings

Occupational therapists commonly work with older adults in skilled nursing facilities (SNFs), adult day-care programs, home-care programs, and assisted living settings (Benzing, 1992; Cutler Lewis, 1989; Hunt, 1994; May, 1993; Miller & Kirchman, 1991; Osorio, 1991; Paulson, 1991;

Walker & Howland, 1992). Vision impairments increase statistically with age and are particularly prevalent among nursing home residents (Balistreri, Stuen, & Fangmeier, 1995). Thus, occupational therapists in gerontic practice commonly work with persons with visual impairment, many of whom have not been identified as visually impaired (Bachelder & Harkins, 1995; Ellis, 1991; Horowitz, Balistreri, Stuen, & Fangmeier, 1995). Vision impairment for individuals with concomitant motor and cognitive deficits or both possess added stresses for individuals who cannot fully use other systems to compensate for visual impairment. This inability to compensate may be especially relevant regarding mobility and ambulation for individuals who already have impaired balance, given the important role of vision in postural adjustment (Carr & Shepherd, 1987).

Within SNFs, individuals who do not receive intensive restorative rehabilitation are often seen for consultation to support overall plans for rehabilitation care with attention to safety, maximizing capabilities, and quality of life as part of the federal Omnibus Budget Reconciliation Act of 1987 mandates (Epstein, 1991; Moon-Sperling & Crispen Pinson, 1991). Often these residents have cognitive and motor deficits that affect ADL capabilities, deficits particularly noted in persons with Alzheimer's disease (Szekais, 1991). However, because of the idiosyncratic rate of functional decline and simultaneous age-related visual changes, many of these individuals may benefit from a hierarchical evaluation system, including attention to primary visual skills, adapted to their cognitive abilities, given the relationships among vision, postural skills, related motor control, and ADL independence (Branch et al., 1989; Carr & Shepherd, 1987; Horowitz et al., 1991). Appropriate recommendations can then be made regarding the kinds of strategies that can maximize safety and independence.

Shortened hospital stays and Medicare and Medicaid reimbursement regulations, combined with greater knowledge of the benefits of rehabilitation for appropriate candidates, has dramatically increased the number of occupational therapists providing home-care treatment (May, 1993). Older persons receiving home care have been found to have statistically higher rates of vision-related problems than well older persons (Horowitz & Cassels, 1985). Comprehensive evaluation of aged individuals by occupational therapists, with increased attention to visual skills, can identify visual deficits for appropriate referral and treatment and would also identify individuals who could benefit from environmental modifications or compensatory strategies to increase safety and functional capabilities (Bachelder & Harkins, 1995; Lampert & Lapolice, 1995; Warren, 1995a).

Depending on setting, treatment teams often include the physician; patient; family members where possible; and occupational therapy, physical therapy, speech therapy, nursing, social work, recreation, and dietary staff. In some cases the team includes an audiologist, a dentist, a psychologist, and a member of the clergy, and in certain cases a consulting ophthalmologist or optometrist (Gallo et al., 1988; May, 1993; Miller & Kirchman, 1991). The frequent lack of ophthalmologists, optometrists, or other vision specialists among team members reflects the fact that nursing home residents commonly do not receive regular vision assessments, with resulting underestimation of the prevalence of visual impairments among the nursing home population (Horowitz, Baliestreri, Stuen, & Fangmeier, 1995). Increasing awareness of the importance of regular vision assessment to prevent disability and to support compensatory strategies for maximum functional abilities, in conjunction with greater dialog between the aging network and vision and other rehabilitation professionals, may help ameliorate this problem. Recognizing this problem and its effect on functional independence may increase vision rehabilitation referrals and encourage rehabilitation departments to include regular vision assessments with appropriate referral or in-house treatment for visual disabilities as part of comprehensive rehabilitation services (Branch et al., 1989; McGinty, Bachelder, & Harkins, 1995; Warren, 1995a, 1995b).

Compensations for Visual Deficits, Low Vision and Blindness Within the SNF Environment

Compensatory strategies to support increased independence for older persons with visual impairments within SNFs may incorporate aspects of universal design for all or be specific to individual need. For example, within nursing homes large-print, high-contrast written and pictorial information and guides can support independent mobility and orientation to location, including one's own room, the dining room, the recreation room, and bathrooms, and help inform residents about scheduled recreation events. Visual guides may be part of individual treatment programs or may result from ongoing consultation with professional staff. In regard to maximizing independence in eating, mealtime has both self-care and social components. Thus, functional dining rooms optimally require well-lit environments (with minimal glare) for individuals to interact and dine with other residents in a pleasant social atmosphere. Occupational therapy programs focusing on increasing eating skills for individuals with significant acuity deficits may recommend visual contrasts between table surface (place mat or tablecloth) and utensils, plate and food, and napkin to enable individuals to optimally locate and visualize their meal. Place settings designed with monochrome aesthetics and without visual contrasts make it difficult for individuals with visual impairment to differentiate objects (Beaver & Mann, 1995; Cutler Lewis, 1989).

Low Vision and Blindness

Visual loss is a neutral term that describes the entire continuum from visual disorders to visual handicaps, but *blindness* by definition means total loss of vision (Colenbrander & Fletcher, 1995). Historically, *legal blindness* was defined in the mid-20th century for Social Security purposes as visual acuity of 20/200 or less in the better eye with the best correction, or a visual field limited to 20 degrees or less (Bennett, 1991; Colenbrander & Fletcher, 1995; Fonda, 1981). In actuality, legal blindness is a term often used erroneously to refer to severe vision loss, not total loss of vision. The dichotomy in terminology between normal vision versus blindness was eliminated in 1975 by the World Health Organization (WHO) when it recognized the need to redefine terminology and added the term *low vision* for the large grey area that forms a continuum between normal vision and blindness.

Low vision encompasses a wide range of visual capabilities including moderate low vision, severe low vision, and profound low vision. The low vision population is increasingly common and increasingly aged, and is approximately 10 times more prevalent than total blindness (Colenbrander & Fletcher, 1995). Low vision seriously affects self-care and independent living, including mobility and reading capabilities, and has other functional implications (Pelli, 1987; Warren, 1995a). Within this low vision continuum, moderate low vision refers to a range from 20/80 to 20/160 that requires people to bring print closer than 25 cm (10 in.), which is uncomfortable for prolonged reading without prisms within eyeglasses. Those with reduced acuity have severe low vision covering a range from 20/200 to 20/400. Binocularity cannot be maintained at this distance other than with the use of a video magnifier or closed circuit television (CCTV). While people with this level of low vision can read, reading is slow. Radio, audiotapes, cassette players, and compact discs are often used to obtain information and for recreation to reduce reliance on vision. Individuals with more severe impairment have profound low vision, with a vision range from 20/500 to 20/1000. At this level individuals cannot read recreationally and CCTV becomes necessary for reading. Those with greater vision loss are called near-blind if they have less than 20/1000. While these people have some vision, it is often unreliable, and assistive devices and technological aids are needed to compensate for visual loss. The term *blindness* should be reserved for individuals with no vision at all (Colenbrander & Fletcher, 1995).

Individuals with vision loss have traditionally received services through specialized community-based vision rehabilitation programs, including state vocational services, and Veterans Administration programs within community-based programs, outside of the medical system and apart from most medical rehabilitation centers (Bachelder & Harkins, 1995; Warren, 1995a). While occupational therapists have historically been involved in vision rehabilitation, few occupational therapists have extensive experience working in vision rehabilitation (Warren, 1995a). Presently, low vision services are available through traditional vision rehabilitation programs and the medical health care system; however, community awareness of resources and services has been a problem. One possible reason is that traditional vision rehabilitation programs have historically existed outside of medical centers and physical medicine programs (Horowitz et al., 1995; Stuen, 1991). Only recently has the health care system expanded beyond treatment of ocular disorders to more broad-based rehabilitation services for the low vision population.

Increased ability to provide low vision services within medical rehabilitation centers has been supported by Medicare's recent expansion of coverage for occupational therapy services for individuals with primary vision loss. In 1990 the Health Care Financing Administration expanded the definition of physical disability to include visual impairment, thereby enabling persons with low vision to obtain Medicare reimbursement for vision rehabilitation. This was due in large part to the efforts of Dr. Donald Fletcher, an ophthalmologist and low vision specialist who was frustrated by unsuccessful efforts to secure occupational therapy services for his patients because of Medicare's differentiation of visual impairment and disability from other disabling conditions warranting rehabilitation services. This 1990 redefinition included low vision as a disability similar to other disabilities that merited rehabilitation, thereby expanding access to vision rehabilitation (Lampert & Lapolice, 1995; Warren, 1995a). As with other disabilities and diagnoses that benefit from rehabilitation, reimbursement under Medicare Part B requires that a medical necessity for occupational therapy treatment exists, that the condition results in disability or a functional reduction in one or more ADL tasks or unsafe performance of one or more tasks, and that a reasonable likelihood exists for significant functional improvement in a reasonable time frame (May, 1993; Warren, 1995b).

Occupational Therapy Services and the Older Adult with Low Vision

While individuals with low vision have unique and special needs, older persons with low vision often have different needs than the visually impaired of prior generations, who were generally younger and did not commonly have multiple health problems. Today's older adults with low vision are typically retired and often do not have family responsibilities. Although the majority of older persons are independent and relatively healthy (Warren, 1995a), increasing age is correlated with increased prevalence of illness and more complex medical histories with greater risk for impairments and disability separate from visual disability. Traditional consumer-oriented rehabilitation services and programs for the blind and visually impaired have focused on the exclusive needs of the blind and visually impaired, including their psychosocial, mobility, vocational, and ADL needs (Bachelder & Harkins, 1995; Crews, 1991). They have operated as separate agencies, generally removed from medical health care delivery systems and rehabilitation medicine departments. Funding sources commonly include a combination of charitable organizations, private donations, and decreasing government funds, in contrast to medical rehabilitation services that are reimbursed by Medicare and other third-party payers for prescribed restorative rehabilitation treatment. Historically agencies for the blind and visually impaired developed primarily in urban areas. Despite the outreach efforts of many agencies, access is often difficult for the very aged and multiply impaired individuals, especially for those residing in nonurban areas (Bachelder & Harkins, 1995; Lampert & Lapolice, 1995).

Our growing aging population at greater risk for vision impairments and disability presents challenges to traditional vision rehabilitation agencies. Growing numbers of older adults will increase the demand for vision rehabilitation services in both urban and nonurban areas (Bachelder & Harkins, 1995) and additionally present these agencies and their staffs with the need to understand a wide range of medical problems with resulting medical and functional implications to fully address the vision rehabilitation needs of older adults. For example, diabetes is the leading cause of blindness among adults 25–74 years. Older diabetic adults with secondary vision loss often need comprehensive rehabilitation programs to maximize ADL independence and safety. It is important that diabetics with low vision learn the importance of regular skin inspection to prevent skin ulcers, a common problem for diabetics. Their high incidence of cardiac complications, neuropathy, and lower extremity amputation underscores the need for accessible rehabilitation programs that provide services for their multiple, complex needs including the integration of low vision rehabilitation with other rehabilitation regimes (Cate, Sikes Baker, & Gilbert, 1995). Thus, a unified approach to rehabilitation, including low vision rehabilitation, that utilizes collaborative approaches among health care professionals is particularly important for aged persons with multiple medical problems. Currently this comprehensive approach is available only in very limited numbers of rehabilitation centers (Bachelder & Harkins, 1995; Warren, 1995a, 1995b). Changes in Medicare's definition of disability in 1990 to include low vision as a condition that can benefit from rehabilitation have encouraged an expansion of low vision rehabilitation centers throughout the country supporting occupational therapy's role in providing rehabilitation services to low vision clients (M. Warren, personal communication, September 18, 1995; Warren, 1995a).

Low vision evaluations are goal oriented in that they seek to determine an individual's capabilities in order to help individuals achieve their specific functional goals. The evaluations focus on obtaining specific information to promote vision enhancement or compensation, not to alter the impairment. Because adaptations, optical aids, and technological solutions are often task specific, it is most important to understand specifically what the client wants to achieve from vision rehabilitation so that services address client goals, thereby motivating the client to work to learn a new way to obtain visual information (Beaver & Mann, 1995; Couturier & Gresset, 1987). As in other rehabilitation programs, low vision rehabilitation succeeds because of knowledgeable rehabilitation teams using appropriate enhancement, compensatory, and technological aids to their best advantage. However, success also requires the consistent work and effort of the client to use his or her existing vision coupled with support from family and friends for vision rehabilitation goals. Successful rehabilitation outcomes, thus, generally result from learning new ways to perform activities, planning daily routines to maximize success, and using new tools and technological aids, which takes patience, concentration, energy, and motivation (M. Ellis, personal communication, September 28, 1995; Flax, Golembiewski, & McCaulley, 1993; Rosenthal, 1995).

Occupational therapists who work in the newly expanding field of low vision rehabilitation may receive referrals as part of a comprehensive team approach to evaluation and treatment or may have a more limited role in the evaluation process, primarily focusing on intervention strategies to promote maximum performance (Flax et al., 1993; E. Reymann, personal communication, September 29, 1995; P. Salchow, personal communication, October 10, 1995; Warren, 1995b). Differences in roles among low vision centers may depend on the availability of specialized low vision professionals; the availability of occupational therapists in the particular locale; and the organizational philosophy, education, and expertise of the occupational therapist (C. Griffith, personal communication, October 13, 1995; Warren, 1995a, 1995b). While our generic professional education provides us with the requisite knowledge for routine visual screens, work with the older population requires specialized knowledge for both vision evaluations and assessment of the functional implications of specific diagnoses with resulting low vision (Lampert & Lapolice, 1995; Warren, 1995b). Therapists who want to use low vision acuity charts or standardized tests for that population, including the Pepper Visual Skills for Reading Test (VSRT) or the Minnesota Low Vision Reading Test (MN Read), need training and practice in the administration of these tests and their interpretation, as with any specialized tool or standardized test (Warren, 1995b; see Figure 15.1).

In addition to specialized visual assessments, occupational therapy functional assessments typically include checklists or other types of ADL assessments to determine capabilities regarding the ability to shop, prepare meals, manage one's home and money, and participate in community activities (Cate et al., 1995; E. Reymann, personal communication, September 29, 1995; Warren, 1995b). Evaluation of the environment (performance context) is particularly important for this population because the physical environment, including housing design, as well as social and cultural context in which ADL are performed, can affect success, energy expenditures, safety, and self-esteem (Dodd, 1993; Lampert & Lapolice, 1995; Long, 1995). While these functional assessments are geared to the specific needs of this population, ADL assessments in general are basic aspects of occupational therapy practice with all populations (Commission on Practice of American Occupational Therapy Association, 1994).

Occupational therapists working with patients with low vision need an appreciation of the functional ramifications of low vision (contrast sensitivity, field, sensitivity to light, need for magnification), which is often influenced by the type and requirements of the task and environmental considerations. Such considerations include the availability of adequate light and the kind of visual stimuli in the environment (contrast, glare factor, movement, visual clutter) and social expectations regarding performance of task (Cutler Lewis, 1989; Lampert & Lapolice, 1995). Other considerations may include noise level, the presence and influence of others, and the ability to be optimally positioned for tasks.

MNREAD™ ACUITY CHART 1

M size		Snellen logMAR for 40cm (16 inches)	
	My father asked me		
4.0	to help the two men	20/200	1.0
	carry the box inside		
	Three of my friends		
3.2	had never been to a	20/160	0.9
	circus before today		
	My grandfather has		
2.5	a large garden with	20/125	0.8
	fruit and vegetables		
	He told a long story		
2.0	about ducks before	20/100	0.7
	his son went to bed		
	My mother loves to		
1.6	hear the young girls	20/80	0.6
	sing in the morning		
	The young boy held		
1.3	his hand high to ask	20/63	0.5
	questions in school		
	My brother wanted		
1.0	a glass of milk with	20/50	0.4
	his cake after lunch		
0.8	I do not understand why we must leave so early for the play	20/40	0.3
0.6	I to mean than four hundred miles from my home to the city	20/32	0.2
0.5	Use what wants to to wash the chicken before we go back	20/25	0.1
0.4	They would love to see the thing you said have given	20/20	0.0
0.32		20/16	−0.1
0.25		20/13	−0.2
0.20		20/10	−0.3
0.16		20/8	−0.4
0.13		20/6	−0.5

Figure 15.1 This test appears on a two-sided 14″ × 11″ card. It has been reduced by 70% to be shown here.

Although some programs, including Visions in New York City, have included occupational therapy in their rehabilitation programs for some time, occupational therapy generally has not played an extensive role in vision rehabilitation (Warren, 1995a). Most occupational therapists working in vision rehabilitation seem to be either members of new programs or have recently joined existing programs. Given this recent increased involvement in the field, occupational therapy approaches to vision therapy programs vary in different programs, often adapting to the program's target population needs and the availability of vision rehabilitation professionals.

Some low vision programs provide outpatient low vision rehabilitation within the context of integrated comprehensive medical rehabilitation services. Other programs offer rehabilitation services in community-based rehabilitation programs such as Lighthouses for the Blind, the American Foundation for the Blind, and the Association for Education and Rehabilitation of the Blind and Visually Impaired (Cate et al., 1995; M. Ellis, personal communication, September 29, 1995; Ruben, 1990; Vicci, 1995; Warren, 1995a, 1995b). These programs often serve somewhat healthier, more independent community-living individuals who seek vision rehabilitation to enable them to perform specific tasks more easily and improve the quality of their lives (Couturier & Gresset, 1987; Warren, 1995b). However, even among this community-living group a majority often have secondary medical problems with additional physical impairments that require both adaptation of low vision aids and devices as well as multifocused treatment programs that address all of the factors (physical as well as psychosocial) that prevent maximum independence and safety (Warren, 1995b). Older persons seeking such low vision rehabilitation services often do so despite societal myths about the inevitable consequences of vision loss and disability in old age, including a limited understanding about low vision rehabilitation among physicians and within the medical community in general (Horowitz & Cassels, 1985; Silver, 1987).

Specific treatment often focuses on strategies to effectively use

1. existing vision through the use of enhancement techniques, which often include vision scanning exercises for individuals with a diagno-

sis of macular scotoma so they can maximally use eccentric vision to view objects (Schuchard, 1995; Warren, 1995b)

2. optical devices (magnifiers, reading telescopes, video magnifiers) for reading; specific ADL needs including preparing meals, housekeeping, and taking medication; recreation; and writing for basic information. High-technology solutions to specific problems are available, including CCTV, screen enlargement systems that display information onto a computer screen at a variety of magnification levels, and computer applications for written communication (Beaver & Mann, 1995; Maley, Ray, & Greene, 1991)

3. low-tech writing aids and communication or high-technology aids for home and financial management and overall written communication

4. retraining in methods of performing self-care tasks, including care of clothing and fall prevention

5. retraining in methods of caring for one's home and environment safely

6. training in ways to access community programs and leisure activities (Flax et al., 1993; Lampert & Lapolice, 1995; Maley et al., 1991; E. Reymann, personal communication, September 29, 1995; Warren, 1995b).

Treatment may address lighting needs, environmental modifications (especially for fall prevention and home safety), and work and task simplification to reduce stresses that may occur when full concentration is needed for lengthy daily tasks (Lampert & Lapolice, 1995; Maley et al., 1991; Rosenthal, 1995). Often simple adaptations can be made to increase safe mobility including use of contrasting colors. For example, dark colors against light-colored backgrounds make objects easier to see. Window treatments can be used in combination with lighting changes (including type of lighting, placement of light, appropriate wattage for task) to provide appropriate illumination while minimizing the effect of glare (Beaver & Mann, 1995; Cate et al., 1995; Lampert & Lapolice, 1995). Individuals can be advised to remove or tack down scatter rugs where possible and to minimize lengthy electrical cords and clutter to provide passageways for safe ambulation. Simple adaptations and low-technology assistive devices can be used to enhance visual capabilities. These adaptations may include the use of nonoptical devices such as audiocassette recorders, high-contrast markers, writing guides, talking watches, and notebooks or optical devices prescribed for the individual needs of the client to maximize vision for activities requiring reading and writing. High-technology aids include the use of computer technology to provide large print or speech output; CCTVs for video magnification of printed, handwritten, and graphic information; or television low vision enhancement systems (LVES) (Beaver & Mann, 1995; Herzberg, 1990; Warren, 1995b).

Counseling programs and support groups address the psychosocial ramifications of vision loss and disability and are integral components of vision rehabilitation. Inclusion of family members and significant others is beneficial as a means of providing both information and support for families to help their loved ones become more independent. Rehabilitation teachers and social workers with the assistance of trained volunteers often run these programs (Flax et al., 1993; Horowitz & Cassels, 1985). Trained volunteers are used for patient education and to facilitate support groups to maximally use scarce resources (Stuen, Consorte, & Bosley, 1995). Occupational therapy education and clinical training provide us with the prerequisite training to be partners in these educational and mental health programs. Our expertise in supporting ADL independence is a tremendous asset because we commonly work with persons coping with both the physical and emotional aspects of disability and reduced independence (Burack-Weiss, 1992; D'Allura et al., 1993; Warren, 1995b).

Aged persons with low vision often require attention to the multiple impairments that together hinder function. Such multiple impairments may make outpatient rehabilitation unrealistic for homebound persons. These individuals may be able to visit a vision rehabilitation center for evaluation purposes but may need vision rehabilitation home-care services. Vision rehabilitation is often provided by community-based agencies for the blind and visually impaired, such as the Lighthouses. However, these agencies are often unable to provide home-care services outside their geographic areas. Home-care occupational therapy rehabilitation services for patients with low vision are now reimbursable by Medicare, provided a physician has ordered such treatment and the individual qualifies for such home-care services by being homebound and requiring the services of a skilled professional to achieve a significant improvement in functional performance (May, 1993). However, home-care occupational therapy vision rehabilitation is not commonly found because of a limited number of occupational therapists trained in vision rehabilitation. Occupational therapists have the generic education and training to facilitate ADL independence and improve the quality of life for older persons with low vision. However, vision rehabilitation is an area of practice that requires additional education and training, including knowledge of traditional community vision rehabilitation centers.

The ability of occupational therapy to integrate low vision rehabilitation with traditional gerontic occupational therapy practice enables occupational therapists to provide integrated treatment and services that can address the needs of persons with low vision with multiple rehabilitation needs, particularly necessary in the home-care environment, thus differentiating occupational therapy from traditional vision rehabilitation professionals whose background is primarily with the visually impaired population. As discussed earlier, diabetics with diabetic retinopathy and resultant low vision often have neuropathies and other medical complications that particularly support a holistic medical rehabilitation program, including low vision rehabilitation (Cate et al., 1995). The multiple needs and growing numbers of aged individuals with low vision often require the services of many types of programs and professionals. A collaborative relationship between newer medically oriented low vision rehabilitation programs and traditional community-based programs is optimal for individuals to maximally benefit from community resources. Agencies for persons who are blind or with low vision often have programs that include *orientation and mobility* (O&M) *training,* self-help support and family groups, and counseling programs. Traditionally vision rehabilitation teachers or O&M instructors teach O&M. O&M instructors, who have specific certification credentials, are affiliated with community-based vision rehabilitation agencies (Parthasarathy, 1995). These teachers and O&M instructors provide instruction in community travel and use of public transportation systems and often provide training in the use of technological aids, some of which send out light beams or ultrasound waves to alert the user to obstacles (Beaver & Mann, 1995; Flax et al., 1993).

Specialized programs for the blind and those with profound low vision, with resulting mobility problems, may include guide dog programs that evaluate persons to determine their suitability for using guide dogs, and then teach individuals how to care and work with their guide dog for independent travel in the community. These programs are typically not part of general vision rehabilitation programs but function as independent programs (Flax et al., 1993). Occupational therapists are generally not involved in guide dog programs and do not usually instruct individuals in white cane use or sighted guide techniques.

Summary

Recent research documents high rates of low vision among nursing home residents (Dugan & McGrann, 1993; Horowitz, Balistreri, Stuen, & Fangmeier, 1995). Some vision rehabilitation programs within SNFs focus on the low vision needs of their nursing home residents but will provide rehabilitation services to community-living outpatients, including comprehensive evaluation by ophthalmology, occupational therapy, and low vision rehabilitation professionals (J. Festa, personal communication, October 30, 1995; E. Reymann, personal communication, September 29, 1995). Treatment plans and services may include the same modalities as those provided in other outpatient vision rehabilitation programs or may be tailored to the needs of nursing home residents, who are generally older and less physically able with higher rates of dementia than community-living older persons (Guralnik & Simonsick, 1993). As with other rehabilitation programs, treatment plans need to be based on the results of a full evaluation, medical and social history, and individual goals and needs, considerations particularly relevant for those nursing home residents with plans to return to their homes with limited social supports.

For long-term care nursing home residents, high rates of cognitive impairments may complicate their ability to qualify and benefit from admission to vision rehabilitation programs established for individuals with intact memory and cognitive capabilities. Medicare reimbursement for rehabilitation, regardless of diagnosis, requires a reasonable expectation of significant functional improvement, which may be compromised if cognitive deficits limit the learning of new strategies to maximize safety and ADL independence (M. Ellis, personal communication, September

27, 1995; Horowitz, Balistreri, Stuen, & Fangmeier, 1995; Paulson, 1991). Low vision programs may benefit from using the individual's strengths, structuring tasks and environmental supports to maximize functional capabilities and safety, and using compensatory low vision techniques, optical aids, and technology. Emphasis on teamwork and structure of the environment is needed for optimal rehabilitation interventions for this population because dementia and cognitive impairments both reduce the ability to learn new tasks (Cutler Lewis, 1989; Epstein, 1991; Szekais, 1991).

Broadly based programs, with attention to the psychosocial ramifications of low vision, including depression, social isolation, and low self-esteem, may serve best the needs of nursing home residents with low vision and multiple medical problems and impairments. These programs need to include individual treatment for appropriate candidates, while focusing on fall prevention and safety during performance of ADL, on environmental adaptation, and on family and staff inservice training (Burack-Weiss, 1992; Dugan & McGrann, 1993; Flax et al., 1993; Stuen, Fragmeier, & Horowitz, 1991; Tideiksaar, 1992; Watzke & Kemp, 1992). This approach is similar to other kinds of nursing home occupational therapy programs using a systems approach to maximize independence, safety, and quality of life for nursing home residents. These ongoing rehabilitation programs are supported by the Omnibus Budget Rehabilitation Act of 1987 with its focus and mandate on the rehabilitation and quality-of-life needs of all long-term care residents (Epstein, 1991; Moon-Sperling & Crispen Pinson, 1991).

Traditional occupational therapy education coupled with specialized education and training in low vision rehabilitation can provide occupational therapists with the basic knowledge and capabilities for analyzing those tasks that have become difficult or impossible for persons with low vision. Our traditional focus on activity analysis and appreciation of the requisite environmental attributes to develop strategies that promote task success are particularly beneficial, especially given the impact of visual stimuli (lighting, contrast movement, and visual clutter) on the functional performance of this population (Lampert & Lapolice, 1995). This activity analysis coupled with evaluation of individual performance components (Commission on Practice of American Occupational Therapy Association, 1994) would then lead to a treatment program that addresses ways to capitalize on individual strengths, the benefits of assistive devices and vision aids, and methods of adapting or coping with environmental variables to support safe and successful participation in desired tasks (Barnes, 1991; Beaver & Mann, 1995; Dugan & McGrann, 1993; Mann, 1994; Smith, 1991; Warren, 1995b).

Despite skill in task analysis, broad-based education and knowledge, and expertise as rehabilitation professionals, one occupational therapy leader in vision rehabilitation (Warren, 1995b) challenges us to develop our own frame of reference for occupational therapy practice in low vision rehabilitation. Warren (1995b) calls on occupational therapists to develop a comprehensive theoretical framework and treatment methodology for occupational therapy practice that can "encompass the biopsychosocial needs" of the low vision population and guide our perspectives so we may make distinct, unique contributions to the field of low vision rehabilitation (p. 859).

Although occupational therapy does not have a particular frame of reference to guide practice in vision rehabilitation, the values and belief in the need for human engagement in meaningful self-directed tasks and support for individuals to maximize competencies for successful life tasks and life roles provide us with a clear identity and overall perspective on rehabilitation treatment in general (Cynkin & Robinson, 1990; Trombly, 1995). Regardless of frame of reference, philosophy, or type of low vision program, however, collaborative efforts by multiple disciplines are most beneficial to serve the complex needs of older persons with low vision (Lampert & Lapolice, 1995). This view is in keeping with recommendations of gerontologists and geriatricians who see multidisciplinary treatment approaches as optimal for rehabilitation of older persons (Gallo et al., 1988; Miller & Kirchman, 1991). Given occupational therapists' generally recent entry into low vision rehabilitation, it is important for occupational therapists to network with vision professionals and become knowledgeable about community resources and traditional vision rehabilitation agencies and programs, including the Lighthouses for the Blind, the American Foundation for the Blind, and the Association for the Education and Rehabilitation of Persons with Visual Impairment and Blindness, and with Veterans Administration programs for collaborative work and appropriate referral (Bachelder & Harkins, 1995; Warren, 1995b). One in four adults 75 years or older reports functional vision impairment (Horowitz et al., 1995). Given the high rate of low vision among aged persons, the paucity of vision rehabilitation programs and professionals, and frequent multiple impairments of aged individuals with low vision, health care professionals can best provide services by using the expertise of all available vision rehabilitation specialists. The changing health care environment creates stresses as we all cope with new terminologies, new reimbursement practices, and bureaucratic changes; however, it need not prevent like-minded professionals from working together to provide needed rehabilitation treatment and services to growing numbers of visually disabled older adults.

Resources

Minnesota Low Vision Reading Test (MN Read), Minnesota Laboratory for Low Vision Research, Department of Psychology, University of Minnesota, Minneapolis, MN 55455, (612) 625-4516.

Pepper Visual Skills for Reading Test (VSRT), Pennsylvania College of Optometry, 1200 West Godfrey Avenue, Philadelphia, PA 19141, (215) 276-6291.

National Consumer Advocacy Organizations and Health Organizations

American Council of the Blind (ACB), 1155 15th Street, NW, Suite 720, Washington, DC 20005, (202) 467-5081, (800) 424-8666 (Legislative News Number).

American Diabetes Association, 1660 Duke Street, Alexandria, VA 22314, (703) 549-1500, (800) 232-3472.

American Foundation for the Blind, 15 West 16th Street, New York, NY 10011, (212) 620-2000, (212) 620-2155, (800) 232-5463.

Association for Education and Rehabilitation of the Blind and Visually Impaired (AERBVI), 206 North Washington Street, Suite 230, Alexandria, VA 22314, (703) 548-1884.

Association for Macular Diseases, Inc., 210 East 64th Street, New York, NY 10021, (212) 605-3719.

Council of Citizens with Low Vision, Riley Tower 2, Suite 3200, 600 North Alabama Street, Indianapolis, IN 46204-1415, (317) 638-8822, (800) 733-2258.

Foundation for Glaucoma Research, 490 Post Street, Suite 830, San Francisco, CA 94102-1409, (414) 986-3162.

Helen Keller National Center, 111 Middle Neck Road, Sands Point, NY 11050-1299, (516) 944-8900.

The Lighthouse National Center for Vision and Aging, 800 Second Avenue, New York, NY 10017, (212) 808-0077, (800) 334-5497.

Lions Clubs International, 300 22nd Street, Oak Brook, IL 60570, (312) 571-5466.

National Association for the Visually Handicapped (NAVH)–East Coast, 22 West 21st Street, New York, NY 10010, (212) 889-3141.

National Association for the Visually Handicapped (NAVH)–West Coast, 3201 Balboa Street, San Francisco, CA 94121, (415) 221-3201.

National Eye Care Project, PO Box 9688, San Francisco, CA 94101-9688, (800) 222-EYES (222-3927).

National Federation of the Blind (NFB), 1800 Johnson Street, Baltimore, MD 21230, (301) 659-9314.

National Society to Prevent Blindness, 500 East Remington Road, Schaumburg, IL 60173, (312) 843-2020.

Neuro-Optometric Rehabilitation Association (NORA), William E. Leadingham, OD (secretary), 1330 Carter Avenue, Ashland, KY 41105-1069.

Rehabilitation Research and Training Center on Blindness and Low Vision, Mississippi State University, PO Drawer 6189, Mississippi State, MS 39762, (602) 325-2001.

Retinitis Pigmentosa Foundation, Fighting Blindness, 1401 Mount Royal Avenue, 4th Floor, Baltimore, MD 21217, (410) 255-9400, (410) 225-9409 TDD, (800) 683-5555.

Veterans Administration Programs are located at regional centers. For further information contact:

Director, Blind Rehabilitation Service/124, VA Central Office, 810 Vermont Avenue, NW, Washington, DC 20420, (202) 273-8483.

Visions/Services for the Blind, 817 Broadway, New York, NY 10003, (212) 477-3800.

Dog Guides

Guide Dog Foundation for the Blind, 371 East Jericho Turnpike, Smithtown, NY 11787, (800) 548-4337.

Guide Dogs for the Blind, PO Box 151200, San Rafael, CA 94915-1200, (415) 499-4000.

Guiding Eyes for the Blind, 611 Granite Springs Road, Yorktown Heights, NY 10598, (914) 245-4024.

Leader Dogs for the Blind, 1039 Rochester Road, Rochester, MI 48307, (313) 651-9011.

The Seeing Eye, Inc., PO Box 375, Morristown, NJ 07960, (201) 539-4425.

Consumer Products and Assistive Technology

Aids Unlimited, 1101 North Calvert Street, Baltimore, MD 21202, (410) 659-0232.

America Online, 8619 Westwood Center Drive, Vienna, VA 22182-2285, (800) 827-6364.

American Foundation for the Blind, Consumer Products, 15 West 16th Street, New York, NY 10011, (212) 862-8838.

American Foundation for the Blind, National Technology Center, 15 West 16th Street, New York, NY 10011, (212) 620-2080.

American Printing House for the Blind, 1839 Frankfort Avenue, Louisville, KY 40206, (512) 895-2405, (800) 223-1839.

Ann Morris Enterprises, Inc., 36 Horseshoe Lane, Levittown, NY 11756, (516) 292-9232.

Assistive Devices for Reading, National Library Service, Reference Circular No. 93-01, Library of Congress, Washington, DC 20005.

Bossert Specialties, Inc., PO Box 15441, Phoenix, AZ 89060, (800) 776-5885.

Brytech (Sensory 6), E. L. Bryenton & Associates, Inc., Suite 102, 28 Concourse Gate, Nepean, ON, Canada K2E 7T7.

CompuServe, 5000 Arlington Center Boulevard, Columbus, OH 43220, (800) 848-8990.

Dazor Manufacturing Corporation, 4483 Duncan Avenue, St. Louis, MO 63110, (314) 652-2400.

Descriptive Video Service, WGBH-TV, 125 Western Avenue, Boston, MA 01134, (617) 492-2777.

Don Johnson, Inc., 1000 North Rand Building-115, PO Box 639, Wallconda, IL 60084-0639, (800) 999-4660.

Diabetes Supplies, 8181 North Stadium Drive, Houston, TX 77054-1826, (713) 622-5587, (800) 622-5587.

Eschenback Optic of America, Inc., 904 Ethan Allen Highway, Ridgefield, CT 06877, (203) 438-7471.

Hoolean, 260 Justin Drive, Cottonwood, AZ 86326, (800) 937-1337.

Independent Living Aids, Inc., 27 East Mall, Plainview, NY 11803, (800) 537-2118.

Innovative Rehabilitation Technology (wide angle mobility light), 1411 West El Camino Real, Mountain View, CA 94940, (800) 322-4784.

Job Accommodation Network, West Virginia University, 809 Allen Hall, PO Box 6123, Morgantown, WV 26506-6123, (800) 526-7234.

The Lighthouse, Low Vision Products, 36-02 Northern Boulevard, Long Island City, NY 11101, (718) 937-9338, (800) 829-0500.

Lions Vision Center (Low Vision Enhancement System-LVES), Johns Hopkins Wilmer Eye Institute, 550 North Broadway, 6th Floor, Baltimore, MD 11101, (800) 829-0500.

L. S. & S. Group, Inc., PO Box 673, Northbrook, IL 60065, (708) 498-9777 (in Illinois), (800) 468-4789.

Maxi Aids, 42 Executive Boulevard, PO Box 3209, Farmingdale, NY 11735, (800) 522-6294.

National Library Service for the Blind and Physically Handicapped (NLS), 1291 Taylor Street, NW, Washington, DC 20542, (202) 707-5100, (800) 424-8567.

Nurion Industries (Laser Cane & Polaron), Station Square, Building #3, Paoli, PA 19302, (610) 640-2345.

Prodigy Services Company, PO Box 791, White Plains, NY 10601, (800) 284-5933.

Recording for the Blind (RFB), 20 Roszel Road, Princeton, NJ 08540, (800) 452-0606.

Resources for Rehabilitation, 33 Bedford Street, Suite 19A, Lexington, MA 02173, (617) 862-6455.

Rochester Visual Horizons (Panasonic Panaboard), 180 Metro Park, Rochester, NY 14623, (716) 424-5300.

Science Products for the Blind, PO Box 888, Southeastern, PA 19399, (800) 888-7400.

Smith Kettlewell Eye Research Institute, Rehabilitation Engineering Research Center, 2232 Webster Street, San Francisco, CA 94115, (415) 561-1619.

Streamlight, Inc., 1030 West Germantown Pike, Norristown, PA 19493, (215) 631-0600.

Telesensory, 455 North Bernardo Avenue, Mountain View, CA 94043, (415) 960-0920, (800) 227-8418.

Vis Aids, 10209 Jamaica Avenue, Richmond Hill, NY 11418, (718) 847-4734, (800) 346-9579.

REFERENCES

Bachelder, J. M., & Harkins, D. (1995). Do occupational therapists have a primary role in low vision rehabilitation? *American Journal of Occupational Therapy, 49,* 927–929.

Barnes, K. (1991). Modification of the physical environment. In C. Christiansen & C. Baum (Eds.), *Overcoming human performance deficits* (pp. 702–745). Thorofare, NJ: Slack.

Beaver, K., & Mann, W. (1995). Overview of technology for low vision. *American Journal of Occupational Therapy, 49,* 913–921.

Benzing, P. (1992, September). A day-care respite program for persons with dementia as a level 1 fieldwork experience. *Gerontology Special Interest Section Newsletter, 15,* 1–3.

Branch, L., Horowitz, A., & Carr, C. (1989). The implications for everyday life of incident self-reported visual decline among people over age 65 in the community. *The Gerontologist, 29*(3), 359–365.

Burack-Weiss, A. (1992). Psychosocial aspects of aging and vision loss. In E. Faye & C. Stuen (Eds.), *The aging eye and low vision* (pp. 29–34). New York: The Lighthouse.

Carr, J., & Shepherd, R. (1987). *Movement science foundations for physical therapy in rehabilitation.* Rockville, MD: Aspen.

Cate, Y., Sikes Baker, S., & Gilbert, M. (1995). Occupational therapy and the person with diabetes and vision impairment. *American Journal of Occupational Therapy, 49,* 905–911.

Chamoff, C. (1996, February). *The role of the occupational therapist in the identification and treatment of visual dysfunction.* Presented at Touro Colleges School of Health Sciences, Dix Hills, NY.

Colenbrander, A., & Fletcher, D. (1995). Basic concepts and terms for low vision rehabilitation. *American Journal of Occupational Therapy, 49,* 865–869.

Commission on Practice of American Occupational Therapy Association (1994). *Uniform terminology for occupational therapy* (3rd ed.). Bethesda, MD: American Occupational Therapy Association.

Couturier, J. A., & Gresset, J. (1987). Visual enhancement and disability: Enhancement and substitution. In G. Woo (Ed.), *Low vision—Principles and applications* (pp. 134–146). New York: Springer-Verlag.

Crews, J. (1991). Measuring rehabilitation outcomes and the public policies on aging and blindness. In N. Weber (Ed.), *Vision and aging: Issues in social work practice* (pp. 137–151). New York: Haworth Press.

Cutler Lewis, S. (1989). *Elder care in occupational therapy.* Thorofare, NJ: Slack.

Cynkin, S., & Robinson, A. (1990). *Occupational therapy and activities health.* Boston: Little, Brown.

D'Allura, T., McInerney, R., & Horowitz, A. (1993). *Lighthouse low vision services: Are they effective?* New York: The Lighthouse Research Institute.

Dodd, A. (1993). *Rehabilitating blind and visually impaired people.* New York: Chapman & Hall.

Dugan, M. C., & McGrann, P. (1993). Testing vision rehab—Long-term care. *OT Week, 6*(3), 14–16.

Egan, M. (1992). Keeping older people driving—Safely. *OT Week, 6*(48), 14–15.

Ellis, N. (1991). Aging, functional change, and adaptation. In J. Kiernat (Ed.), *Occupational therapy and the older adult* (pp. 76-94). Gaithersburg, MD: Aspen.

Epstein, C. (1991). Specialized restorative programs. In J. Kiernat (Ed.), *Occupational therapy and the older adult* (pp. 285–300). Gaithersburg, MD: Aspen.

Flax, M., Golembiewski, D., & McCaulley, B. (1993). *Coping with low vision.* San Diego, CA: Singular Publishing Group.

Guralnik, J., & Simonsick, E. (1993). Physical disability in older Americans. *Journals of Gerontology, 48,* 3–10.

Hooks, M. (1996). Parkinson's disease. In L. Pedretti & B. Zoltan (Eds.), *Occupational therapy: Practice skills for physical dysfunction* (4th ed., pp. 845–851). New York: Mosby.

Horowitz, Baliestreri, Stuen, & Fangmeier. (1995). Visual impairment & rehabilitation needs of nursing home residents. *Journal of Visual Impairment & Blindness,* 7–15.

Horowitz, A., & Cassels, L. (1985). *Vision education and outreach: Identifying and serving the visually impaired elderly.* New York: The Lighthouse Research Institute.

Horowitz, A., Reinhardt, J., & Cantor, M. (1995). *The Lighthouse National Survey on Vision Loss.* New York: The Lighthouse.

Horowitz, A., Teresi, J., & Cassels, L. (1991). Development of a vision screening questionnaire for older people. *Journal of Gerontological Social Work, 17*(3/4), 37–56.

Hunt, L. (1994). Home health care. In B. Bonder & H. Wagner (Eds.) *Functional performance in older adults* (pp. 286–295). Philadelphia, PA: FA Davis.

Kline, D., Sekuler, R., & Dismukes, K. (1982). Social issues, human needs, and opportunities for research on the effects of age on vision: An overview. In R. Sekuler, D. Kline, & K. Dismukes (Eds.), *Aging and human visual function* (pp. 3–6), New York: Alan R. Liss.

Lampert, J., & Lapolice, D. (1995). Functional considerations in evaluation and treatment of the client with low vision. *American Journal of Occupational Therapy, 49,* 885–890.

The Lighthouse. (1991, Fall). A few practical tips for: Print legibility and low vision. *Lighthouse News.*

Long, R. G. (1995). Housing design and persons with visual impairment: Report of focus-group discussions. *Journal of Visual Impairment & Blindness,* 59–69.

Maley, K., Ray, J., & Greene, J. (1991). Uniting occupational therapy and optometry. *OT Week, 5*(39), 14–15.

Mann, W. (1994). Technology. In B. Bonder & M. Wagner (Eds.), *Functional performance in older adults* (pp. 323–337). Philadelphia: F. A. Davis.

Mann, W., & Lane, J. (1991). *Assistive technology for persons with disabilities.* Bethesda, MD: American Occupational Therapy Association.

May, B. (1993). *Home health and rehabilitation.* Philadelphia: F. A. Davis.

McGinty, J., Bachelder, J., & Harkins, D. (1995). The issue is—Do occupational therapists have a primary role in low vision rehabilitation? *American Journal of Occupational Therapy, 49,* 927–931.

Miller, M., & Kirchman, M. (1991). Geriatric rehabilitation programs. In J. Kiernat (Ed.), *Occupational therapy and the older adult* (pp. 99–122). Gaithersburg, MD: Aspen.

Moon-Sperling, T., & Crispen Pinsen, C. (1991, September). Implications of OBRA '87: Expansion of services and opportunities. *Gerontology Special Interest Section Newsletter, 14,* 1–3.

Osorio, L. (1991). Adult daycare programs. In J. Kiernat (Ed.), *Occupational therapy and the older adult* (pp. 241–258). Gaithersburg, MD: Aspen.

Parthasarathy, R. (1995). Rehab with a vision: Opening eyes to vision problems in rehab patients. *Advance, 11*(45), 14–15.

Paulson, C. (1991). Home care programs. In J. Kiernat (Ed.), *Occupational therapy and the older adult* (pp. 220–239). Gaithersburg, MD: Aspen.

Pedretti, L., & Zoltan, B. (1990). *Occupational therapy: Practice skills for physical dysfunction.* St. Louis, MO: Mosby.

Pedretti, L., & Zoltan, B. (1996). *Occupational therapy: Practice skills for physical dysfunction.* St. Louis, MO: Mosby.

Pelli, D. (1987). The visual requirements of mobility. In G. Woo (Ed.), *Low vision: Principles and applications* (pp. 134–146). New York: Springer-Verlag.

Rosenthal, B. (1995). Low vision and depression. *Aging and Vision News, 7*(1), 3–4.

Ruben, B. (1990). OT brings insight to the field of visual impairment. *OT Week, 4*(15), 4–5.

Ryan, S. (1993). *Practice issues in occupational therapy.* Thorofare, NJ: Slack.

Schlageter, K., & Zoltan, B. (1996). Traumatic Brain Injury. In L. Pedretti (Ed). *Occupational therapy: Practice skills for physical dysfunction* (pp. 807–836). St. Louis: Mosby.

Schuchard, R. (1995). Adaptation to macular scotomas in persons with low vision. *American Journal of Occupational Therapy, 49*(9), 870–877.

Sekuler, R., & Owsley, C. (1982). The spatial vision of older human. In R. Sekuler, D. Kline, & K. Dismukes (Eds.), *Aging and human visual function* (pp. 186–202). New York: Alan R. Liss.

Silver, J. H. (1987). The city study. In G. Woo (Ed.), *Low vision: Principles and applications* (pp. 450–462). New York: Springer-Verlag.

Smith, R. (1991). Technological approaches to performance enhancement. In C. Christiansen & C. Baum (Eds.), *Overcoming human performance deficits* (pp. 748–786). Thorofare, NJ: Slack.

Stuen, C. (1991). Awareness of resources for visually impaired older adults among the aging network. *Vision and aging: Issues in social work practice,* 165–179.

Stuen, C., Consorte, L., & Bosley, K. (1995, October). *Insights: A peer volunteer vision education training program.* Presentation at the Annual State Society on Aging of New York Conference, Albany, NY.

Stuen, C., Fragmeier, R., & Horowitz, A. (1991, November). *Infusion of vision rehabilitation into the nursing home setting.* Paper presented at the Gerontological Society of America Scientific Meeting, San Francisco, CA.

Szekais, B. (1991). Treatment approaches for patient with dementing illness. In J. Kiernat (Ed.), *Occupational therapy and the older adult* (pp. 192–219). Gaithersburg, MD: Aspen.

Tideiksaar, R. (1992). Avoiding falls. In E. Faye & C. Stuen (Eds.), *The aging eye and low vision* (pp. 55–60). New York: The Lighthouse.

Toglia, J. (1989). Visual perception of objects: An approach to assessment and intervention. *American Journal of Occupational Therapy, 43,* 587–595.

Treml, L. (1996). Accessibility and safety. In C. Emlet, J. Crabtree, V. Condon, & L. Treml (Eds.), *In-home assessment of older adults* (pp. 17–40). Gaithersburg, MD: Aspen.

Trombly, C. (Ed.). (1995). *Occupational therapy for physical dysfunction* (4th ed.). Baltimore: Williams & Wilkins.

Vicci, V. (1995). Vision and rehab—Do you see what I see? *Advance, 11*(45), 14, 46.

Walker, J. E., & Howland, J. (1992, March). Exploring dimensions of the fear of falling: Use of the focus-group interview. *Gerontology Special Interest Section Newsletter 15,* 1–3.

Warren, M. (1993a). A hierarchical model for evaluation and treatment of visual perceptual dysfunction in adult acquired brain injury, part 1. *American Journal of Occupational Therapy, 47,* 42–54.

Warren, M. (1993b). A hierarchical model for evaluation and treatment of visual perceptual dysfunction in adult acquired brain injury, part 2. *American Journal of Occupational Therapy, 47,* 55–66.

Warren, M. (1995a). Including occupational therapy in low vision rehabilitation. *American Journal of Occupational Therapy, 49,* 857–859.

Warren, M. (1995b). Providing low vision rehabilitation services with occupational therapy and ophthalmology: A program description. *American Journal of Occupational Therapy, 49,* 877–889.

Warren, M. (1996). Evaluation and treatment of visual deficits. In L. Pedretti (Ed.), *Occupational therapy practice skills for physical dysfunction* (4th ed., pp. 193–212). St. Louis, MO: Mosby.

Watzke, J., & Kemp, B. (1992). Safety for older adults: The role of technology and the home environment. *Topics in Geriatric Rehabilitation, 7*(4), 9–21.

Woodson, A. (1995). Stroke. In. C. Trombly (Ed.), *Occupational therapy for physical dysfunction* (4th ed., pp. 677–704). Baltimore: Williams & Wilkins.

16 Occupational Therapy and Collaborative Interventions for Adults with Low Vision

Tressa Kern, MS, OTR, and
Nancy Weber Miller, MSW

Introduction

A current challenge for occupational therapists is to use their existing talents and training in working with patients with low vision—whether vision impairment is the patient's primary or secondary disability—while a more comprehensive knowledge base, integrating scientific, medical, practical, and research wisdom, is developed.

In this chapter, the term *low vision* will be used to refer to the full continuum of vision loss from partial sight, to legal blindness, to total blindness. According to *The Lighthouse National Survey on Vision Loss* conducted by Lou Harris Associates in 1994, one in six adults, 45 years of age and older (17% of the U.S. population, or 13.5 million people) reports having a moderate or severe vision impairment. One in four persons (25%) over the age of 75 years reports experiencing moderate to severe vision impairment. Rough estimates indicate that 10% of people with low vision (functional vision loss) are under the age of 21; 30% are between 21 to 64 years of age; and 60% are over the age of 65.

Moderate impairment is the inability to recognize a friend across a room, trouble seeing even when wearing glasses, or reported blindness in one eye. Severe vision impairment is the inability to recognize a friend standing at arms length, inability to read ordinary newsprint while wearing glasses, or reported blindness in both eyes (The Lighthouse, 1995). Practically all individuals with low vision, even persons with legal blindness, can benefit from a low vision examination, prescription of devices, and environmental modifications.

It is of greatest importance that occupational therapists familiarize themselves with and use the existing research and literature in low vision, blindness, and vision rehabilitation. Resources for obtaining up-to-date information should include journals (i.e., *Journal of Visual Impairment and Blindness* (JVIB), *Journal of Vision Rehabilitation, AER Re-View*), and books in the field of vision rehabilitation, adult services, and aging. Some examples are Rosenbloom and Morgan (1986); Weber (1991); and Orr (1992).

The protocols and knowledge base presented in this chapter were developed to provide vision rehabilitation in the home and community settings but can be applied easily in any setting (e.g., hospital, rehabilitation center, nursing home, or adult day-care).

In the United States, the definition of *legal blindness* is central visual acuity of 20/200 or less in the better eye with optimal corrective glasses or a visual field of 20° or less in diameter. This means that a person can identify at 20 ft. what a person with normal vision can identify at 200 ft., or that the field of vision is limited to a small area. Being blind does not mean having no vision. People who are classified as "functionally blind" may have a visual acuity better than 20/200 corrected in the better eye, but because of various conditions cannot read ordinary print or function without adaptations. This group of people with vision loss frequently uses low vision aids. Regardless of degree of blindness, no further damage is done by using any remaining (residual) vision.

The term *legal blindness* has been used since 1935 to determine eligibility for a variety of governmental and private benefits and services for persons with low vision. Recent publications, practice experience, and research emphasize that functional vision assessments, rather than isolated clinical measurements of distance vision, provide more relevant information about an individual's ability to use vision in daily life. In the past decade, the term *low vision* has been used to describe individuals who are neither totally blind nor fully sighted, and who may or may not meet the clinical criteria for legal blindness, but whose residual vision cannot be corrected to normal by regular eye glasses or contact lenses. What represents usable vision depends not only on visual functions that can be clinically measured but also on the person's ability, motivation, and life circumstances. Low vision can be considered any condition in which a person's visual function is not adequate for his or her visual needs.

Persons with *congenital* blindness, that is blindness from birth or shortly thereafter, have no previous visual experience. There is a wide range of learning styles and a variety of differences in personal and experiential backgrounds, and, thus, in levels of concept and language development. For example, congenitally blind persons may use, or appear to comprehend, words and concepts that they may not actually understand because of limited real life experiences (e.g., colors).

Persons with *adventitious* blindness have lost their sight after visual maturation. Having sight memory, adventitiously blind individuals will often draw from their background and life experiences in adapting to vision loss.

Implications of Low Vision

The roots of low vision care for people with partial sight were established at the beginning of this century. The first devices were developed in 1908 when magnifiers were created. Optometrists and ophthalmologists began prescribing magnifiers and telescopes in the 1920s. The first optometric clinic for low vision was opened in 1953 at the Industrial Home for the Blind (now known as Helen Keller Services) in Brooklyn, New York. In the same year, the first ophthalmologic clinic for low vision was founded at The Lighthouse in New York City. In the 1960s, the first use of advanced technology to provide magnification for persons with low vision came with the development of closed circuit television, which projected magnified text onto a screen.

To best serve the low vision patient, the occupational therapist should incorporate medical (neurological and other) research findings on the effects of various diseases on visual ability (the basis of the impairment) while assessing and then ameliorating the disability through rehabilitation. In the ideal situation, after the disease itself has been diagnosed and addressed, the next step should be a low vision evaluation by a qualified optometrist or ophthalmologist. We should recognize that this evaluation is not part of the traditional medical system familiar to occupational therapists. The low vision examination will include, but not be limited to, the following:

- detailed history of the eye and medical history of the present impairment or pathology
- social history including education level, employment history, hobbies, interests inventory, ADL, interpersonal relationships, and socialization choices
- self-reported difficulties with ADL, mobility, and environmental challenges
- hierarchical list of goals
- distance visual acuity, including preferred gaze position and best lighting environment (conditions and contrast for optimal vision function)
- standard evaluation of accommodation (focusing), pupils, muscle efficiency, balance, and color and stereo vision
- keratometry (measure of the curvature of the exterior cornea) and retinoscopy
- manifest refraction (determining the appropriate lens power) and telescopic refraction (use of telescopic devices if appropriate)
- comprehensive eye health evaluation, such as tonometry, biomicroscopy, dilated fundus evaluation, and assessment of visual fields
- near vision evaluation.

The summary of the low vision evaluation must include an optical prescription for distance and near. It may also include prescription for tints and filters, telescopes, prisms, special lighting, stand and hand magnifiers, and other optical and nonoptical devices. Finally, recommendations for follow-up and monitoring for changes in visual status must be included.

Standardized tools for assessing vision function are used by optometrists and ophthalmologists, including those with specialized training in low vision, as part of the low vision examination. Examples of the most commonly used assessment tools (such as the Hirschberg Test, Polaroid® tests, the Worth 4 Dot Test) can be found in Anderson (1982); Duane (1990); and Faye (1984).

Assessment, Planning, and Treatment Considerations

Once the functional vision assessment is made, the occupational therapist will need to include in the treatment plan methods to help the patient adapt to the vision disability through environmental and behavioral techniques. Maximizing the use of residual vision will include consideration of

- lighting (overhead, body level, natural, and artificial)
- contrast
- glare
- preferred field of view (best gaze posture)
- adaptations of reading materials (print size, use of color, fatigue factors, time needed for recognition)
- the use of large print, Braille, or recorded media.

Important for the patient are recommendations for nonprescriptive optical aids such as bold line paper, specialized pens, reading stands, and writing guides.

In addition, a comprehensive treatment plan should take into account the following environmental factors:

- gross object and room dimension recognition (shape, size, doorways, furniture)

- contrast recognition (floor, wall, whether doors are closed or open, carpet or flooring, objects: dark on light, light on dark)
- placement of objects and depth perception (at body level, overhanging, low, in front of, to the side)
- fine object and character recognition (people, name and numbers on doors, writing)
    - use of muscle (motor) memory in navigating familiar environments
    - use of sight memory with the adventitiously blind population
- need for alternative words and descriptors for a congenitally blind individual who may not have developed conceptual understanding for words such as "look," "see," "here," and "there" without changing the intent of the instruction.

Vision Screening Checklist and Task Analysis

Generically trained occupational therapists are not technically skilled and do not have an adequate background or the knowledge to complete a low vision examination and evaluation or to recommend the use and application of prescribed low vision aids (i.e., telescopes, binocular magnifiers) or to prescribe them. However, one tool that the authors have found to be useful in determining an informal assessment of functional vision, applicable in any setting (home, clinic, or day care), is a Functional Vision Screening Checklist and Task Analysis, such as the example that follows.

It is important to the adequate completion of a self-reported functional Vision Screening Checklist to incorporate direct questions to elicit anecdotal information that goes beyond the clinical diagnosis. Suggested questions include:

1. Do you have trouble seeing?
2. How long have you had this trouble?
3. Do you know the cause? Has an eye doctor diagnosed or treated you?
4. Which eye is affected most?
5. What *can* you see?
    (a) headlines of a newspaper: blurry or clear?

(b) newsprint?

(c) details on a television screen?

(d) food on your plate?

(e) clothing or colors?

6. Do you see better straight ahead (central vision) or if you look to one side (peripheral vision)?

7. Can you see the color red (bright color)? What color am I wearing?

8. Does lighting make a difference? Does bright light help? Does glare bother you? Indoors? Outdoors?

9. What were you doing or what did you do for yourself *before* your vision problem (housecleaning, cooking, dressing, shopping, laundry, reading, independent travel)? What about now?

10. Can you read these numbers (have 1-inch numbers written in bold marker, preferably black-on-white, and smaller numbers)?

11. When you are walking on the street, do you depend on others or do you use your own vision? How do you know when to cross?

12. Does your vision change from day to day?

13. Describe any special glasses or devices you use to see better (optical aids).

14. When did you have your last eye exam? Date _____ .

Occupational therapists must begin to develop their own tools for assessing vision function as it applies to the total medical model. Until standardized tools are specifically developed, it would be prudent to apply or use a functional vision screening checklist.

According to Warren (1995a),

If occupational therapy is to make a unique and lasting contribution to this area, we must develop our own frame of reference for addressing the needs of persons with low vision . . . that must be compatible with our other theories regarding adaptation to disease and environment, and must go beyond merely advocating the use of adaptive devices and techniques. Our frame of reference . . . must focus, in part, on how the central nervous system is best able to adapt to a loss in one of its major information gathering systems. (pp. 858–859)

One of the most useful screening, assessment, and curriculum instruments for identifying a patient's need for occupational therapy (and physical therapy) was developed by therapists at the Alabama Institute for Deaf and Blind to be used by nontherapists. The Screening for Physical and Occupational Therapy Referral (SPOTR), developed by the National Independent Living Skills (NILS) grant project 1981–1984, was designed to provide an objective, cost-effective method of referral for therapy, evaluation or services for individuals with sensory impairment 16 years and older. However, the SPOTR is based on a fundamental belief in a multidisciplinary approach to evaluation and training of independent living skills. Because it is designed specifically to be used with a population that is visually impaired, hearing impaired, or both, it is a particularly useful and unique assessment tool for occupational therapists working with low vision patients. Traditionally, most assessment tools have been inappropriate for this population because of the lack of normative data, strict standardization, and test dependence on visual skills (Woosley, Harden, & Murphy, 1985).

Until such time as the complete scientific base is established and communicated to all occupational therapists, the current standard of practice with people with low vision should include collaboration with other disciplines including the physician, ophthalmologist, optometrist, rehabilitation teacher (RT), orientation and mobility (O&M) specialist, low vision instructor, social worker, rehabilitation counselor, and psychologist.

The Traditional System for Serving People with Low Vision

The traditional community-based structure of the system to serve adults with low vision is funded by the federal Rehabilitation Act of 1973 vocational rehabilitation dollars, the Veterans Administration hospitals, and very limited medical and health care system dollars, which generally cover only the eye disease diagnosis, exams and surgeries. Since 1990, coverage by Medicare Part B for occupational therapy services for individuals with primary vision loss can be accessed because of the Health Care Financing Administration's expansion of the definition of physical disabilities to include vision impairment. This expanded definition is due in large part to the efforts of ophthalmologists such as Dr. Donald

Fletcher. No subsequent home- or community-based rehabilitation has generally been funded through medical insurance. Therefore, the private, not-for-profit system for serving people who are blind or visually impaired in their home and community (funded through vocational rehabilitation monies and other sources) has flourished parallel to the health care system.

Other potential funding streams for home-based occupational therapy do exist; they include grants to vision rehabilitation not-for-profit agencies from local city or state legislative and county initiatives, or as a defined service under Medicaid home and community-based waivers, or inclusion in housing grants under the category of home modification and accessibility.

Services for persons with low vision are delivered by numerous private voluntary agencies, state agencies, and consumer groups. Services differ greatly from one state or community to another. One of the simplest ways to access services for a person with low vision is to consult the American Foundation for the Blind *Directory of Services*, 1993, or call 1-800-AFB-LINE (1-800-232-5463) for a list of local organizations.

Curricula exist for training nursing home personnel to identify and serve residents with vision loss (Duffy & Beliveau-Tobey, 1991). Senior centers serve older constituents, including those with low vision (Ludwig & Schneider, 1991). Vision rehabilitation agencies throughout the country provide training and public education to reach the millions of older adults with severe vision loss.

People with Low Vision: An Attractive Service Area

With managed care and reductions in reimbursement rates, the effort of hospitals and clinics is to increase market share, increase their patient base, and compete for patients. A person with a vision impairment is now a desirable patient. Occupational therapists in clinical settings are going to continue to see an increasing number of people with vision problems, related to the demographics of an aging society. Dramatic increases exist in the over-80 age group in which severe vision loss affects

25% of the population. Ethnic minority populations (especially African American and Hispanic) have experienced an increase in vision impairment because of greater risk of diabetes and glaucoma and because of the correlation between low income and disability.

As the population of older people with vision loss is growing because of increased longevity, collaboration at the local, state, and national level between the aging network and the vision rehabilitation system is crucial. In each community, opportunities exist for joint programming, cross-referral, and shared expertise between providers of service to older adults and providers in the field of vision rehabilitation (Orr, 1992).

The occupational therapist's comprehensive knowledge of the physical, cognitive, sensory, and psychosocial aspects of disability enables him or her to implement interventions that will enhance the outcomes for an individual involved in the process of vision rehabilitation.

It is essential that occupational therapists working with low vision patients acquire additional specialized knowledge. This includes ocular pathology causing vision loss, treatment procedures and application of modalities, and the use of prescribed optical devices. Occupational therapists who work directly with optometrists and ophthalmologists specializing in low vision or who work in vision rehabilitation agencies usually receive inservice training, as well as experiential learning. In the absence of direct interaction with low vision rehabilitation professionals, occupational therapists should study low vision rehabilitation journals and textbooks and participate in continuing education courses to gain the skills needed to work with the patient with low vision (Warren, 1995b).

Occupational therapists must also become knowledgeable about the other professionals working in the vision rehabilitation system. These professionals include rehabilitation teachers, O&M specialists, rehabilitation counselors, and low vision instructors.

The History and Role of the Rehabilitation Team Members

Four fields of expertise have been part of rehabilitation training for people with impaired vision: rehabilitation teaching, O&M, rehabilitation counseling, and low vision instruction. Each of these fields has a long history of professional preparation and expertise.

Rehabilitation teaching differs from other physical rehabilitation in its emphasis on the effect of visual impairment on ADL, on the family, and on the patient's life situation. University courses in rehabilitation teaching started in the United States in the 1930s and a full degree program was established in 1963. Rehabilitation teaching programs throughout the country confer a master's degree in rehabilitation teaching or a master's degree in special education or rehabilitation counseling with an emphasis (concentration or certificate) on rehabilitation teaching. Curriculum, practicum, and internship requirements for personnel preparation programs are maintained by the professional organization called the Association for the Education and Rehabilitation of the Blind and Visually Impaired (AERBVI). Rehabilitation teachers work with youth, adults, and older adults to teach many specialized adaptive and alternative skills, such as

- communication skills: use of Braille, sensory development and listening skills, adaptations for reading and writing, abacus, mathematical systems, and computer use
- personal management skills: clothing care and grooming, medication management, child care, eating and social skills
- home management skills: meal preparation, home mechanics, marking systems, labeling, record keeping, and safety procedures
- leisure activities skills: hobbies, games, handcrafts, and accessing community activities
- orientation and movement skills within the home
- training in the use of optical devices: magnifiers, telescopes, closed circuit television (CCTV), image enhancers, and similar prescribed devices
- training in the use of assistive devices specific to low vision or total blindness
- guidance and counseling: adaptation to vision loss and encouraging family support.

Areas are shared by occupational therapists and rehabilitation teachers. Both teach patients to appropriately use all their remaining physical capacity and senses and how to analyze and organize tasks and situations for maximum independence in daily living. Rehabilitation teachers focus only on specialized training and knowledge of alternative approaches for youth and adults with vision loss. Their comprehensive knowledge consists of teaching techniques, technology, and devices designed specifically for people who are totally blind or have low vision.

For people with low vision, a challenge is to gather auditory, tactile, and other sensory data that will keep them oriented in space. The next task is to learn to protect themselves by mastering techniques to guard against hazards, for example, stairs, curbs, vehicles, and edges of subway or train platforms. O&M specialists teach both skills. In the 1950s, the numbers of veterans with vision impairments returning from World War II prompted the development of long cane mobility techniques. Master's level university programs to train professionals in O&M began in 1961. Personnel preparation and certification are offered, such as rehabilitation teachers, through AERBVI.

Orientation techniques enable travelers to use sensory information to establish their position in space in relation to the physical environment and thereby help them determine their position in relation to all significant objects in their environment. Mobility techniques for people with low vision are designed to allow them to travel safely and independently from one place to another. People with low vision generally rely on the use of long canes, sighted guides, electronic travel aids, or dog guides. O&M specialists also teach the interpreting of sounds and other environmental cues to create a mental map while remaining alert to danger signals.

Mobility instruction includes orienting individuals to the layout of their home, immediate environment (e.g., hospital or nursing home room and floor plan), or the community, and general training in basic sighted guide techniques, self-protection, or cane skills for travel needs.

Rehabilitation counselors not only provide counseling specific to occupation and employment goals but administer interest inventories; offer career guidance; teach interviewing and on-the-job skills; introduce workplace technology; help with job placement; develop referral relationships with employers; and assist with planning, interviewing, and adjusting to work and the workplace. In some rehabilitation agencies, the rehabilitation counselor serves as the intake coordinator and case manager, while in other agencies the social worker performs that function.

Low vision instructors work with and are supervised by ophthalmologists and optometrists in low vision clinics and vision rehabilitation agencies. Low vision instruction is a specialization, not a formal discipline, and has no academic degree. Most training is provided through continuing education.

The Joint Commission on Allied Health Personnel and Ophthalmology (JCAHPO) promotes training programs and educational standards, certifies technicians in ophthalmology, and recently created a new certified specialization, called *low vision assisting*. Instructors and technicians cannot prescribe low vision devices. They are trained to describe and demonstrate optical and nonoptical aids and to explain the limitations of them. They teach patients the proper use and maintenance of prescribed devices and optical aids, generally in a clinic setting. Correct techniques of reading, writing, and using telescopes are part of the instructor's role in restoring the patient's functioning. The instructor introduces nonoptical aids such as lighting, reading stands, or large print materials (Faye, 1984) to supplement or augment the effect of optical aids. The availability of a variety of low vision training techniques and complex optical devices requires the provision of assistance to help patients understand how to use them. For example, strong magnifiers require the user to hold the reading material much closer than customary, or in the case of a scotoma (central blind spot), the patient will have to learn to use peripheral vision or eccentric view in order to see clearly. Eccentric viewing techniques capitalize on the remaining healthy retina in diseases that have damaged part of the retina. The role of low vision instruction has become an integral part of low vision care. For example, in macular degeneration the central (straight ahead) vision is unclear. By having patients use their eccentric or peripheral vision, they can reestablish clarity.

The Occupational Therapist's Role in the Multidisciplinary Team

It is important for the occupational therapist to intervene and participate in the rehabilitation process for individuals with low vision when

- an additional functional limitation exists or a physical condition affects the individual with low vision
- a person with low vision ages, with concomitant sensory and physical age-related functional impairments, or both
- a person with multiple impairments ages and exhibits functional vision impairments.

An occupational therapist is unlikely to work with the person with low vision when no other functional impairments or medical conditions exist, unless no rehabilitation teacher is available, or the occupational therapist has received additional specialized training. This training must include knowledge regarding the anatomy, function and dysfunction of the eye, visual deficits, low vision optical aids, and adaptive equipment.

The rehabilitation teacher implements a client-centered functional approach while the occupational therapist uses and applies a clinical, neurologically based treatment approach. Traditionally, occupational therapy is one of the rehabilitation professions complementary to medicine. Occupational therapists along with physical therapists, speech therapists, and various paramedical staff commonly form a rehabilitation team whose aim is to return the patient to his or her greatest level of independence. Occupational therapy's specific goal (VISIONS, 1984) with a patient with low vision is to improve the patient's functional skills by

- evaluating performance capacities and deficits in physical function in the patient's own environment, for example, the occupational therapist evaluates safety in all transfers and bathing activities, eating and dressing skills, communications, and personal management
- establishing a comprehensive rehabilitation plan that takes into account the physical, cognitive, sensorineural, and vision limitations affecting the patient
- establishing with the patient specific goals that may include functional skills in ADL, O&M, and restoration of physical function in which a deficit or impairment is determined
- selecting tasks, activities, or exercises appropriate to achieve defined needs and goals and facilitating learning through a variety of treatment methods in order to achieve desired outcomes or objectives; specific sensorimotor activities and exercises and postural alignment techniques

are used to improve gait and navigational skills in preparation for orientation and mobility training

• devising, designing, selecting, and obtaining special assistive devices or equipment related to ADL activities

• evaluating response and progress

• assessing and measuring change and development in functional independence

• sharing findings and their relevance to other professionals and assistants in the rehabilitation team.

Specific teaching techniques are used by the occupational therapist to meet behavioral objectives and will vary depending on the patient's level of physical ability and sensory loss, in addition to vision loss.

The occupational therapist provides transfer training; eating skills and positioning; splinting; energy conservation and work simplification techniques; environmental modifications; increasing range of motion, strength, and endurance for completion of tasks; and fine motor coordination. The rehabilitation teacher is not qualified to provide this training or these skills.

The importance of the occupational therapist's intervening and participating in the rehabilitation process for individuals with low vision is based on the unique expertise occupational therapy provides in teaching adaptive living skills, using adaptive equipment, and modifying the physical environment. Current rehabilitation practices and blindness-based rehabilitation services for people with low vision sometimes overlook or fail to recognize the valuable expertise occupational therapy brings to the rehabilitation process (Kern, 1996). Occupational therapists themselves may circumvent or avoid working with the individual with low vision because of limited experience, education, or exposure to clients with this disability. Occupational therapists should take advantage of the increasing opportunities for continuing education, for example, workshops and seminars sponsored by the American Occupational Therapy Association. In addition, the AERBVI offers continuing education classes (see the Resources at the end of the chapter).

In any interdisciplinary relationship, each colleague brings to the experience a particular expertise. Specifically, in the rehabilitation of people with low vision, an occupational therapist brings a medically based body of knowledge but lacks the specific hands-on knowledge of blindness or low vision. Similarly, the O&M specialist, rehabilitation teacher, and low vision instructor, whose backgrounds are specific to blindness, have a foundation of medical education but have a more limited ability to comprehensively assess performance capacities and functional limitations unrelated to blindness.

It is important to acknowledge the common philosophical base between these disciplines. In occupational therapy, it is a general assumption that "the goal is to achieve a person-environment fit that enables the older person to function as competently as possible" (Rogers, 1981, p. 664). Like occupational therapy, the vision rehabilitation system operates on the assumption that independence is determined by the patient served and not by the professional. All of the disciplines use life experience as part of the therapeutic process. The shared knowledge base used by all members of the rehabilitation team working with the adult patient with low vision is drawn from the principles of andragogy. *Andragogy* is the study and implementation of conditions relevant to adult learning. The learning is problem-centered. It is a process for problem finding and problem solving in the present. Andragological principles lead to the creation of a self-directed adult learning environment in which there is reciprocity in the teaching-learning relationship—a helping rather than a directive relationship. The outcome sought by all of the professionals involved in service delivery to patients with low vision is the patient's achievement of autonomy in the life skills of their choice (Kern & Shaw, 1985).

As occupational therapists, we are not unfamiliar with adult learning theory or self-help concepts and are historically accustomed to functioning within a multidisciplinary rehabilitation team. However, occupational therapists have a great deal to learn about vision loss and its impact on the patient's independence and rehabilitation outcomes.

Whenever a multidisciplinary approach is used, the following concerns must be addressed: overcoming differences in language usage by various disciplines, developing agreed-upon methods for managing conflicting recommendations, supporting role sharing and role release, minimizing territoriality, addressing competition for the same patients, acknowledging differences in financial reimbursement or insurance coverage, and ensuring methods for developing goals jointly between the professionals and with the patient. These same concerns apply to the overlap in role delineation and expertise between occupational therapists and physical therapists as well as occupational therapists and rehabilitation teachers.

The collaboration between occupational therapists and other professionals in the field of low vision services can take place in work settings, where they are on the staff with rehabilitation teachers, O&M specialists, rehabilitation counselors, and low vision instructors (e.g., in not-for-profit vision rehabilitation agencies). Occupational therapists may also be recruited on a consultant basis by a vision rehabilitation agency or by a state commission for people who are blind or have low vision. Unless occupational therapists have completed specialized training, occupational therapists should make referrals to rehabilitation teachers, O&M specialists, and low vision instructors for their patients with low vision who need these services.

One reason for the greater involvement of occupational therapists in vision-related services is that many of the specialists who provide vision training, such as rehabilitation teachers or O&M specialists, are not available in less populated, rural areas or to serve the isolated elderly population. The more universally prevalent rehabilitation specialists are physical and occupational therapists. Older people report struggling with the everyday instrumental tasks that are necessary to maintain a household in the community when they experience vision loss. Clear evidence of unmet needs exists (Branch, Horowitz, & Carr, 1989). In addition, occupational therapists may be reimbursable, whereas rehabilitation teachers may not.

Unique Techniques Used by the Occupational Therapist with Specialized Training and Experience in the Vision Rehabilitation System

Referral and Evaluation

Low vision rehabilitation as a distinct practice area within occupational therapy has not yet been formalized. However, even without specialized training, the occupational therapist can use traditional problem-solving skills to assist the person with low vision. For example, basic ADL skills training using greater or lesser adaptations for visual functioning is still needed. It must be understood that training will take longer as the person with low vision learns compensatory techniques that are specific to his or her remaining visual functioning.

A comprehensive low vision evaluation requires specific, specialized knowledge of vision and low vision with education and training in optometry, ophthalmology, and the low vision rehabilitation field. Clinical measures of visual skills, however, provide only fundamental information about a patient's vision. The measures are incomplete and do not represent a complete picture of the individual. The functional effect of a vision impairment is likely to be best measured outside the clinic, preferably in the home environment. Some system for doing so needs to be built into every service program (Orr, 1992).

Occupational therapists must consider the functional implications of the eye condition as well as the patient's motivation and the degree to which he or she understands and accepts the impairment. Also important to take into account is the degree to which the vision impairment interferes with the person's goals for functional independence (Lampert & Lapolice, 1995). Once the patient's desires and capabilities are taken into account, the occupational therapist must apply this knowledge to the evaluation process.

Adaptations for visual functioning include attention to color contrast; lighting, including reduced glare; placement of objects; use of cognitive, muscle, and motor memory in lieu of vision; and use of residual vision. The occupational therapist's functional assessment, through interview and observation, can and should always include the observation of visual skills in the performance of self-care and homemaking skills. For example, reading ability, which in many situations might be thought of as leisure activity, does influence a person's ability to maintain independence—reading labels, written instructions, appliance dials, time pieces and watches, thermostats, mail, phone numbers, and phone dials.

In addition to using a vision screening tool and completing a traditional occupational therapy evaluation, the therapist needs to focus on the functional impact of the vision loss on ADL. One way of accomplishing this is through task analysis. An example of a functional task analysis familiar to occupational therapists, which may be useful in both clinical and home-based environments, is the task of telephone dialing as a measure of both physical and visual status (American Foundation for the Blind, 1972). This task will incorporate the use of central vision, sensory integration skills, manual dexterity, eye-hand coordination, and proprioceptive and kinesthetic abilities. The examiner can use a large-print telephone dial overlay (available for both rotary and Touch-Tone phones that are not hand held) for the assessment. Overlays are available free of charge from the local telephone company for people with special needs.

Technique: Place a rotary or Touch-Tone phone on a table in front of the patient. Ask whether he or she can see it and ask him or her to dial his or her own phone number, if possible, or 911, or "zero" for "Operator."

Observe how the patient reaches for the telephone. Does the patient grope or immediately find the receiver?

Ask, "Can you see the numbers?" Ask the patient to find the number "6" (middle of the dial). Can he or she dial? If not, can the patient trail fingers in a circular movement (rotary) or line by line (Touch-Tone phone) to locate numbers?

If the person has difficulty dialing a number or locating a reference number, ask him or her to locate "zero" for "Operator." If placement of fingers on the dial or pad of the phone is difficult because of arthritis, neuropathy, or other condition, this should be noted and distinguished from the visual process.

Integrating skills: Can the patient hold the receiver? Coordinate dialing and holding receiver? Directly return receiver to cradle? Does he or she use vision or is it necessary to use both hands for this task? Do verbal instructions help? Tactual clues? If the patient exhibits difficulty, place a large-print phone dial overlay onto the phone and repeat a portion of the evaluation.

Note the lighting conditions during the administration of the task analysis. Does increasing the illumination (i.e., using higher wattage bulb) or changing the position of the light source (e.g., moving it directly over phone) improve the patient's performance of the task?

In practice, illumination preferences and needs are highly individual. The patient is the best guide for information on helpfulness and comfort with types and levels of lighting.

Skill Areas and Training

All of the specific detailed techniques for training adults with vision impairment in daily living skills are available and accessible to occupational therapists in texts (in print and on cassette) from the VISIONS CIL Publications Series (see Resources).

The following goals and objectives are developed for people with low vision in the same way they would be developed for any other patient. The therapist must take into account that the length of time in accomplishing a specific task will be affected by the vision impairment.

Instructional Guidelines

• Identify yourself as soon as you enter the room. Speak directly to the patient, not with your back to him or her or directing your conversation to another part of the room.
• Your speaking voice need not be louder than normal.
• Let the patient know you are leaving. Do not leave your patient in the position of talking to himself or herself. This points to the vision loss in an unhelpful way and can contribute to frustration and lowered self-esteem.
• Tell the patient what you are going to do *before* you administer any test, assessment, or direct care.

- Do not worry about using words such as "look" or "see." These are often the simplest words to use to get your point across. Chances are the patient will use these words, too.

- Speak directly to the patient with low vision, not through a companion or caregiver.

- If you must leave the patient alone, make sure he or she is oriented to the surroundings or can maintain contact with the environment.

- Use specific words and directions. Avoid expressions such as "over there" or "over here" or "right here" or "straight ahead." These phrases are too vague and should be used sparingly.

- Offer specific directions such as "Your comb is on the left side of the dresser toward the back." Say, "Let me show you," and guide the patient to it; or, "Let me take your hand," and place it on the object. You might say, "To your right," or "Left" or tap the object and say, "It's here" to help the patient to determine the direction from which the sound comes.

- Do not be misinformed. Eyes cannot be weakened or damaged by use of residual vision.

- Allow enough time to learn the task. Do not rush through the lesson.

- Build a clear mental image (word picture) of the object you are working with and the steps involved in the project before you attempt to teach a skill whenever possible.

- Try not to overprotect the patient. A constant question is always present of how much assistance to provide. Let the patient do as much as possible independently. The patient may create techniques suited to individual needs. Do not prevent him or her from using those techniques unless they are unsafe.

- When ordering labels or rewriting phone numbers for better visibility, 14-point type (1 in. in height) is a good choice.

- Provide as much information as possible when serving food. Use a clock reference point describing the food on the plate or items on the table, for example, "Your meat is at 6 o'clock, vegetables at 9 o'clock, and potatoes at 1 o'clock."

- Always specifically state that you are putting food, liquid, or any item in front of the patient before doing so, and let the patient know it is there.

Following are some of the basic activities that people with low vision generally do for themselves and must be addressed by the therapist. It must also be remembered that these are by no means the only skills the patient with low vision should learn. Nor will every patient do all of them. The tasks and the suggested procedures are not the only method for performing each specific function. Personal preferences, other physical or sensory impairments, and the habits of the individual will influence the best techniques for teaching the skills.

Self-care tasks: bathing, nail care, toothpaste application, medication management, makeup application, shaving, cleaning and maintaining eye or limb prostheses, hair care.

Sample procedure for toothpaste application would be

1. The patient removes the cap from the tube of toothpaste and places it in a secure location.
2. The patient grasps the bristles of the toothbrush, which are upward, between the thumb and index finger of one hand, making sure the bristle tops are slightly below the holding fingers. (These fingers will become "guides" in determining where to apply toothpaste.)
3. The patient curls the remaining fingers of that hand around the toothbrush handle.
4. With the toothpaste tube in the other hand, place the tip of the tube between the tips of the fingers (guides), which are holding the toothbrush.
5. Squeeze the bottom of tube gently (this may take practice) until toothpaste covers the top of bristles between the "guides."
6. Remove the tube. Place it in a secure location.
7. After teeth have been brushed or dentures washed, place the cap on the tube of toothpaste and return the tube to a specified, consistent location.

Note: If the patient demonstrates difficulty in locating his or her mouth, that proprioceptive skill must be addressed.

Eating skills and table behavior: seating self at table, use of utensils, setting a table, buffer techniques, using seasoning, pouring liquids, serving, cutting and slicing techniques, carrying containers of food or liquid, table orientation, and food locating.

The procedure for filling and pouring containers of hot and cold liquid are similar. However, hot liquids require more care and training. Sample procedure for pouring liquids would be

1. Using the finger method: Rest the thumb and middle finger gently on opposite edges (inside and outside) of the cup or glass. Use the index finger to locate and guide the spout or container from which you are pouring over the edge of the cup, pouring slowly in spurts, moving the index finger into the cup or glass, and continue pouring until the liquid reaches the tip of the index finger.
2. Using the weight method: As experience is gained in filling and pouring, the desired amount of liquid can often be judged by the weight of the container.

Two very useful adaptive devices are the "Say When" liquid level indicator available from The Lighthouse, Inc., or Maxi-Aids, and the Hot Shot Single Cup Beverage Maker available from Maxi-Aids.

Kitchen skills and meal preparation: labeling and storing foods; identifying and using utensils, pots and pans, and appliances (toaster, broiler oven, microwave, blender, can opener); setting dials; fitting a plug; measuring ingredients; regulating gas and electric burners; using a timer; following recipes and cooking instructions; cutting; chopping; slicing.

The method and amount of labeling of canned and packaged foods will vary with each individual. Some people prefer to have everything labeled; others want very little labeling and depend on memory. Sample procedure for labeling foods would be

1. Use a Dymo-writer to produce labels on plastic strips. This is useful for permanent identification.
2. Use rubber bands placed around cans, for example, one for peaches, two for pineapple, and so on.
3. Paste or tape assorted shapes or small objects, such as paper clips or buttons onto containers, with each having a specific meaning to the person.

4. Use plastic lids that are used for storing open cans of food and come in various sizes. If they are permanently marked, they can be slipped onto the tops of cans at the time of purchase.
5. Similar techniques can be used for packaged food. The size, shape, and location of packaged foods are usually guides to the contents.

Home management and domestic tasks: shopping, preparing to wash dishes, washing dishes, exercising basic cleaning skills (sinks, counter tops, stoves, and windows), loading and operating the dishwasher, doing the laundry (preparing and separating clothes, operating the washing machine and dryer, hand washing clothes, ironing, identifying and organizing clothing, hanging and separating clothes, ironing), needle threading, packing a suitcase, making a bed, sweeping, using a vacuum cleaner.

Keeping dishes clean and sanitary is important and requires special attention when visual scanning for cleanliness is not possible. Sample procedure for washing dishes would be

1. Apply detergent to sponge or pad. To clean glassware and cups, insert a sponge or nonabrasive cleaning pad into the bottom of the cup or glass. Do not force a hand into the glass because pressure can break it. Twist the sponge back and forth to remove dried-on food. Place the sponge or pad in the sink. Rinse the cup or glass thoroughly and place it upside down on the drying rack or in a secure location.
2. Wash both front and back of plates or bowls thoroughly, using a sponge or cleaning pad to remove dried-on foods; using a repeated circular motion is best. Place the plate or bowl in the sink and rinse thoroughly.
3. Keep all sharp knives and pointed kitchen forks or other utensils in one spot in the sink and wash them separately from other utensils. Rinse them with hot water. Wash and place sharp ends down in a dish drainer or utensil drainer.

Communication skills and money management: using a tape recorder, using a reading machine, using a computer or calculator, using a telephone, writing a signature, making out and signing checks, reading mail, identifying coins and bills, making change, telling time, using talking devices (e.g., clocks, watches, timers).

Sample procedure for identifying coins and bills

1. Coins may be identified by size, thickness, and texture (milled or smooth edges). The dime and penny differ in size and the quarter is larger than the nickel. The dime and quarter are milled around the edge; the nickel and penny are smooth.
2. Bills can be folded for identification to different lengths and arranged in a definite pattern in the compartments of the billfold or wallet. A sighted individual must identify or confirm the bill denomination the first time it is used. A "talking" (voice output) bill identifier can be used, but they are very expensive.

    a. Since the dollar bill is most often used, it should be left unfolded and can be placed as is in the front of the billfold.

    b. The five-dollar bill is folded in half so that it is the same height as the dollar bills when placed in the billfold. It goes in the same section as the dollar bills on the right side of the compartment with the folded edge up.

    c. The ten-dollar bill is folded twice and placed, folded edge up, on the left side of the bill compartment.

    d. The twenty is folded the same way as the ten, but placed in the back compartment on the right side.

Selection and Use of Nonoptical Assistive Devices

"A number of studies have documented that the proper use of devices, techniques, and training methods can successfully maximize the use of remaining vision in persons with low vision. Training in the use of magnification, illumination, and contrast, along with environmental modifications, has been found to be effective" (Goodrich & Mehr, 1986, p. 121). To provide the most comprehensive training, occupational therapists must become familiar with low vision and other assistive devices to enhance the use of residual vision or to compensate for lack of vision. A sample list follows, but it does not begin to enumerate all of the available devices.

Self-care devices: talking glucose monitors, insulin injection aids, medication organizers, eye drop guides, talking thermometers, talking scales, magnifiers, high magnification make-up mirrors, shaving systems, dressing aids.

Eating devices: "Say When" liquid level indicator, sectioned dish, food bumpers, adapted dishes, and utensils.

Cooking and food preparation devices: tactile microwave and toaster or broiler oven, temperature control cookware, beverage makers, adapted food processors and blenders, pan and pot holders, oven mitts, cool handles, pan grips, measuring devices, cutting devices, knife guides, tongs, heat diffuser, adapted peelers and slicers.

Domestic tasks: adapted switches, wall plates, tactual thermostat, reachers, needle threaders and other sewing devices, ironing guides.

Communications: adapted television remote; key finding, writing, and signature guides; coin and key holders; low vision, talking, Braille, and large-print watches, clocks, and timers; adapted and variable-speed cassette recorders; location finders; adapted or bold markers and pens; labelers; clothing identifier's; book rests and holders; voiceprint speakers; adapted or large-print telephones and amplifiers.

Environmental Adaptations and Lighting

"Usually the challenge in providing adequate lighting is to provide optimal illumination without producing glare. Methods of increasing light on a task include bringing the light closer to the task, adding more lights, and changing the background of the task so that contrast is increased (for example, with a solid white or light-colored placemat under a dark mug." (Watson & Berg, 1983, p. 343)

When people have difficulty seeing, they will often become frustrated and inefficient in the performance of daily tasks. Improved lighting, both quality and quantity of light, should help. Correct lighting is probably the most important nonoptical visual aid both for people with normal vision and for people with impaired vision. However, increased quantity of light may do little to help a person with vision impairment see an object if there is added glare or insufficient color and shading contrast between the object and the background. Often increasing the wattage of incandescent bulbs additionally increases glare (Carter, 1983). Therefore, just increasing the wattage of the bulb may not be the best solution. Moreover, a person can have the most accommodating lenses and lighting for the purpose of reading, but if the desk or table upon which the book rests has a color value the same as the written page, neither glasses nor magnifiers nor other optical devices nor lighting will help the person see better. However, a desk simply darker in color than the page would be a tremendous help. Any improvements in lighting, color, or contrast must be practical, simple, and economical. One rule to follow is that white lettering on black background is better seen than the reverse.

The Kitchen

The kitchen is notorious for its lack of color contrast. Walls, ceilings, sinks, refrigerators, cupboards, and counters are usually a light color and provide little or no background contrast for light-colored objects, liquids, and foods. Therefore, persons with low vision have great difficulty in measuring quantities, portioning foods into desired amounts, reading gauges, judging cooking time, and addressing physical hazards and safety.

These suggestions can help. To the wall area above a kitchen counter, attach a sheet or dark-colored Contact® paper. If the existing wall is brightly colored, apply a sheet of white Contact® paper to create contrast for pouring dark or light colored liquids or for measuring or cutting foods. In the dining area, recommend light-colored dinnerware on a dark table or tablecloth or the reverse. Avoid patterned place mats, tablecloths, or dinnerware, as they tend to confuse the eye. The simplicity of solid, high-contrast colors is best. Although it is difficult in the kitchen, use incandescent lighting instead of fluorescent whenever possible. Avoid very bright, glaring lights from overhead light sources that can cast heavy shadows. Place the light source below eye level if at all possible.

The Bathroom

Lighting in the bathroom is probably more difficult and complicated than any other area in the house. The most common lighting arrangement found in the bathroom is the wall light fixture located above the mirrored medicine cabinet. This provides the lighted reflected image for grooming. The higher above the eyes the light fixture is located, the worse it is for the person with low vision, because it deepens the shadows of the facial features. An alternate lighting arrangement is the mirrored medicine cabinet with built-in fluorescent light fixtures on either side. This illuminates the face more uniformly and eliminates facial shadows. Placing light fixtures lower will always improve the ability to use residual vision. As in the kitchen, the tendency in the bathroom runs to light-colored walls. Apply Contact® paper for contrast. To reduce glare, whenever possible, use low-gloss finishes, paint, or wall covering.

The Living Area

Use scattered light sources throughout the room rather than overhead lighting of any kind. Use desk and floor lamps with adjustable arms, if possible, in order to specifically direct illumination for reading. If possible, use dimmer switches to reduce glare by increasing or decreasing light levels in relationship to the task. Shield light sources, such as windows, from direct view. A dark, open weave drape or adjustable blind will reduce the sun's glare and add contrast to its surroundings. Modify surfaces to reduce reflection.

Overall Environment

It is important to remember that vision and visual needs may fluctuate dramatically during periods of the day, or from day to day (Sicurella, 1977).

The following suggestions are practical recommendations regarding other changes in the environment. It is important to respect the concerns of an individual with aesthetics and familiarity in the placement of objects and furnishings in the living areas of the home.

- Leave furniture and personal items in the same place and location once they have been positioned safely. This helps orient the person with low vision to the environment and reduces tripping accidents and falls. Advise family members, caregivers, housekeepers, and maintenance persons not to move furniture or personal items without informing the patient. Even the slightest repositioning of furniture or items can be totally confusing. This is one of the major complaints made by persons with low vision!

- Keep the largest pieces of furniture against walls and out of the paths of circulation, if possible.

Make sure that no furniture low to the ground (e.g., coffee tables) causes an obstruction in the path of circulation. These objects present a serious hazard, especially to individuals who have lost peripheral vision in the lower segment of the visual field. The lower the object, the greater the possibility of tripping over it.

- Make sure there are no hanging or protruding objects (e.g., hanging plants) at head or eye level. These objects present a serious hazard for individuals who have lost peripheral vision in the upper segment of the visual field or who have lost central vision.

- Check the furniture for sharp edges and corners and caution the patient.

- Keep all doors either completely open or completely closed. Doors can be a major hazard if left ajar.

- Eliminate throw rugs or check that all carpets and area rugs have skid-proof backings or are tacked to the floor. Loose carpeting on the stairs can be especially hazardous.

- Consider purchasing a portable phone, which can be taken from room to room to enable the individual with vision impairment to answer the telephone without rushing for it.

Navigation and Wayfinding Techniques

Although the O&M specialist and the rehabilitation teacher will focus on spatial relations and a variety of navigational techniques (e.g., trailing one's hand around the walls of a room to determine location), therapists and professionals who work with people with low vision should be, at the very least, familiar with how to use and teach the Sighted Guide Technique (see Figure 16.1).

The purpose of Sighted Guide Technique is to enable an individual with low vision to travel safely and efficiently with a sighted person within different environments and under varying conditions.

Grasp and position

1. The person with low vision should grasp the sighted guide's arm just above the elbow with the fingers on the inside and the thumb on the outside.
2. The patient keeps his or her upper arm vertical at his or her side with the forearm approximately parallel with the ground.
3. The patient is positioned a half-step behind and to the side of the guide.
4. If the guide has an unusually large arm, the patient can grasp the wrist, in which case the guide's arm remains at the side. When walking in a dangerous or obstructed area (e.g., a cafeteria or crowded hallway), the patient should walk on the side furthest from the obstacles.

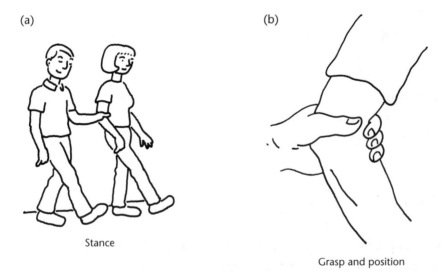

(a)

Stance

(b)

Grasp and position

Figure 16.1 Sighted Guide Technique, a) stance and b) grasp and position. Reprinted with permission.

Suggestions for the guide

1. Make physical contact with the visually impaired person by touching his or her arm before beginning to travel.
2. Briefly describe the environment before beginning to travel.
3. Always assist a person with low vision to make contact with some object or furnishing before leaving him or her in an unfamiliar place, and indicate when you are leaving.

Narrow passages and doorways

1. The guide moves arm back in toward center of his or her back as a signal of a narrow passage, doorway, or changing terrain.
2. The patient extends his or her arm to full length, placing him or herself one full step directly behind the guide. (It is important to maintain this distance behind the guide so as not to step on the guide's heels). Since this technique offers more protection than the regular sighted guide technique, it may also be used when the person with low vision is uncertain of the guide or his or her movements.

Closed doors

1. The guide pauses before a door, alerting the patient.
2. If the doorway is narrow, the patient follows a full step behind the guide.
3. The guide should indicate to which side the door will open (toward or away from you) and whether the door is self-returning.

Stairs

1. The guide should indicate that stairs are being approached and indicate whether they will go up or down. Guide should momentarily pause and instruct the patient to locate the stair edge with his or her foot.
2. The guide proceeds up or down one step ahead of the patient. The guide's upward or downward movement indicates that ascent or descent has begun.

3. The guide should pause momentarily on the last step to indicate the approach of the landing.

4. If available, a railing should always be used. The guide places the patient's hand on the railing to indicate location and direction (ascending or descending).

5. If there are two or more flights of stairs, the guide makes square corners (90° turns) when traveling from one flight to another.

Chair seating

The guide should put the patient in contact with some part of the chair and allow the patient to seat himself or herself as follows:

1. Place the patient's hand on back of chair first, and follow down the back to the seat of the chair.

2. Have the patient make a half circle on the seat with his or her hand to be sure the chair is empty and usable.

3. Before the patient sits down, have him or her turn around so that the back of his or her knees or legs touch the chair, and then sit down while maintaining contact with chair.

Psychosocial Aspects of Low Vision and Related Issues

The impact of blindness is to leave many people with the sense of abandonment. Feelings of discomfort result from asking family and friends for assistance. This discomfort frequently leads to avoidance. The person with a vision impairment wishing to avoid such embarrassment learns not to "make demands," not to expose oneself to further hurt or rejection. Isolation and loneliness then become a part of the impact of vision loss. (Freedman & Inkster, 1976, p.13)

According to Father Carroll, the seminal writer addressing the impact of vision loss in adults, the losses associated with sensory impairment include losses in psychological security, basic skills, communication, appreciation, occupation, and financial status, as well as a sense of wholeness (Carroll, 1961).

It should not be difficult for us as professionals to understand the feelings of frustration and anxiety experienced from the impact of vision loss, especially when the condition is first apparent to the patient. Feelings of depression are appropriate in the grieving for the loss of one's sight and one's former lifestyle. The impact of such feelings should not be minimized in terms of their influence on learning capacity, retention, and the ability to benefit from rehabilitation services.

Because it is difficult for the therapist to deal with these reactions, sometimes the tendency is to avoid confronting or discussing them directly. Instead, attention is placed on training and skills that will facilitate independent functioning. By addressing the individual's reactions and feelings directly and including these discussions as part of the rehabilitation process, the occupational therapist and other professionals will facilitate adjustment, particularly as new skills are learned that lead toward an increased feeling of competence and mastery.

Individuals may exhibit behaviors of such extreme magnitude or with such self-destructive potential that the therapist is alarmed or finds it difficult to continue therapy. As in all situations similar to this, referral for a psychological evaluation or counseling is appropriate. However, severe depression requiring medication or suicidal ideations are not the typical behavior of a person with a vision loss. It is more likely that the therapist will observe behaviors that range from sadness and anger to withdrawal, self-consciousness, and helplessness.

In addition to the impact of emotional and economic losses experienced by the person with low vision, relationships with family, friends, and the general community are altered. The need to ask for assistance can drastically change a person's self-perception, image, and sense of self-worth. For instance, asking for help in reading correspondence highlights the person's awareness of the loss both of ability and of privacy.

No one adjusts to change, to loss, or to impairment in a vacuum, or entirely independently. The success or failure of adjustment, and certainly the rate of adjustment, depends on individual coping strategies and the involvement and the reaction of significant others. . . . While the older visually impaired person's primary goal is to continue to be as independent as possible, of equal value is the ability to be interdependent with the family and within the social context. (Orr, 1991, p. 7)

The theoretical discussion is brought to life in direct conversation with people experienced with vision problems.

What have elders . . . told us of the experience of vision loss . . . ? First, loss of vision in old age is no small thing. It permeates all aspects of life. And it hurts a lot: anxiety, frustration, aggravation, caution, depression are frequent accompaniments. Time is not necessarily a healer. Due to changing life circumstances and the progressive nature of most vision impairments, attitude change may just as likely be for the worse as for the better. Elders look both from within and outside for support. Medical attention is important but it is recognized that it is not the only answer. Patience, doing what one can for oneself, keeping active, prayer, humor and tears may help. (Burack-Weiss, 1991, p. 23)

About VISIONS:
A Multidisciplinary Service Setting and Case Example

Prior to 1970, rehabilitation and social services were not readily available to the older adult blind and visually impaired population. Public and private funds were earmarked for the young and vocationally oriented. Owing to this lack of financial support, little was done to develop programs to meet the multifaceted needs of older adults with low vision. VISIONS/Services for the Blind and Visually Impaired, which includes a residential year-round Vacation Camp for the Blind, was a leader in the development of rehabilitation, recreation, volunteer services, senior center "mainstream" activities, and community education programs. VISIONS' office is located at 120 Wall Street, 16th Floor, New York, NY 10005-3904.

Since 1964, VISIONS programs have evolved as the demographics and needs of the clients have changed. The service delivery model is home- and community-based and makes use of a multidisciplinary team. Service plans are individualized and are based on the consumer's expressed and demonstrated needs. The goals of this model include skills training to promote independent ADL and lifestyle, and use of and equal access to community services and resources.

A Case Example

The following case study describes an adventitiously blind adult's experience with VISIONS' services.

Jane is a 76-year-old widow living alone at home. She has a history of glaucoma and cataracts and recently suffered a CVA with mild residual hemiplegia and spinal stenosis. She was introduced to VISIONS when the social worker from her clinic contacted the agency. She called on Jane's behalf because Jane had been diagnosed as legally blind by her ophthalmologist and was having difficulty completing daily household chores. Although instruction in these ADL tasks had been provided through traditional medical rehabilitation services following her stroke, Jane had made few gains. After an evaluation by VISIONS' intake worker, a certified rehabilitation teacher was assigned to work with Jane on a weekly basis. Through the use of adaptive techniques and nonoptical adaptive equipment introduced by the rehabilitation teacher, Jane's home became increasingly accessible to her. For example, raised dots on the stove and toaster oven enabled her to more easily identify temperature settings, so she no longer burned herself when preparing meals.

At the same time, she was referred by VISIONS for low vision services and training from a low vision optometrist and instructors. The low vision examination included a complete evaluation, testing of acuity, measurement of visual fields, refraction, and the introduction of various lenses to determine which ones allowed her to see most clearly. After testing a variety of optical aids and devices lent to her for home use, she returned to the low vision specialist for a follow-up visit and training in the use of the prescribed new equipment. Ultimately, she began to use a high-magnification screen enlarger to watch television, a hand-held monocular telescope to identify street signs when traveling outdoors, a high-powered stand magnifier for reading mail, a folding pocket magnifier for use when traveling or shopping, Noir UV shield glasses for outdoors (providing 100% UV and glare protection), and a halogen floor lamp with an adjustable arm, height adjustment, and weighted base.

An O&M specialist evaluated Jane for independent travel both indoors and outdoors. With Jane's approval, she began by covering Jane's traditional support cane in red and white reflective tape to identify her as a person with vision impairment. However, both the rehabilitation teacher and O&M specialist noted difficulties in completion of tasks as well as difficulty in orientation, balance, retention, and transfers. An occupational therapist was asked to complete an assessment.

Jane exhibited difficulty in the area of positioning, spatial awareness, and performance of ADL tasks. The occupational therapist began her participation in the rehabilitation process. After conducting an evaluation in the home, the occupational therapist observed Jane's inability to position her arms for protective techniques within her apartment; poor spatial and environmental concept development; ADL problems focusing on those tasks requiring motor planning and sequencing of steps, such as meal preparation; and visual field deficit and directionality required in simple sewing or total body involvement in such activities as bed making. Difficulties with dexterity and coordination were evident. In communication skills, she was unable to print her name, not only because she could not see the page but because she could not consistently find the left side of the paper, move the pen in the proper direction, or identify reference points on the page. Jane was found to have difficulty isolating body parts for purposeful movement or laterally flexing her neck or trunk owing to spinal stenosis and the results of the CVA. Proprioception and body concept were below average as was spatial awareness.

Transfers in bathing and toileting were observed and because of vestibular problems a high-color contrast grab bar and bath stool were installed in the shower and extensive training in safe transfers was provided. Tasks and positioning requiring simultaneous movements were incorporated along with many different motor-planning activities as an enhancement to the RT training. The latter began as very simple bilateral tasks and later included reciprocal patterns and more difficult bilateral skills.

One-to-one therapy included specific prehensile tasks to improve dexterity and coordination; introduction of signature and letter-writing guides and their placement to help her compensate for her left-side neglect; and work with the rehabilitation teacher on bilateral tasks, such as boiling water, pouring safely, reheating food safely on the top of the stove, and using a microwave.

Jane's writing became legible when she learned to use a specifically adapted writing, check-writing, and signature guide. In addition, she learned the Braille alphabet that she used primarily for marking labels, clothing, and medicine bottles. Instruction in the use of a large-print talking calculator helped Jane to manage her bookkeeping and checkbook.

At reevaluation, she showed improved fluidity of movement that significantly improved her ability to use the long cane and support cane simultaneously for outdoor travel. In addition, she learned complicated tasks with greater ease, suggesting improved motor planning.

An opportunity for recreation and social activities was offered to Jane, who was encouraged to join a nearby (two-block walk) senior center. The staff at the center received inservice training by VISIONS staff in adaptive techniques, and sensitivity training was offered to the seniors. The occupational therapist and the O&M specialist collaborated in an environmental assessment of the senior center. They evaluated the centers entrance, hallways, toilets, stairs, elevators, water fountain, and public telephone areas for safety, accessibility, and natural and artificial lighting conditions. They recommended environmental modifications to the center's director who facilitated their installation.

The O&M specialist conducted mobility lessons outdoors to enable Jane to walk with a cane to the center and once there to orient herself to the environment. The O&M specialist ensured that she was safe in navigating the new area. She now attends the center weekly. Jane was also given information and assistance in applying for Vacation Camp for the Blind, which she attended the following summer. There she made many new friends with whom she speaks throughout the year.

Summary

Objectives and accurate measures of the effects of treatment need to be more extensively applied on the functional performance of persons with low vision. Beginning efforts to measure outcomes do exist, including cost-benefit analyses and funding based on achievement of results (Persico, 1995).

The existing occupational therapy paradigm works for treatment of all aspects of the life of the person with disabilities. Rehabilitation with low vision patients offers occupational therapists an opportunity to exercise their wide range of talents from activity analysis to psychosocial adjustment while incorporating the specialized knowledge base from the field of low vision.

The ideal location for training is the patient's own home or residence. Rehabilitation goals become more relevant to the needs of the individual on a day-to-day basis if they are established and taught in a familiar setting. For the occupational therapist who is primarily a clinical practitioner, it must be recognized that the person with low vision may have difficulty transferring previous techniques and adaptations for independent living to the everyday environment because they were taught in the clinic, center, or hospital, and not in the home.

The nature of vision impairment, with its frequent result of isolation or withdrawal, translates into lack of access or involvement in the very services that could prevent isolation and increase independence. Outreach to all persons who can benefit from low vision and rehabilitation services and the provision of services to individuals in need, especially the elderly, remains an unmet goal.

Occupational therapists, by the nature of their training, use positive energy to help people help themselves and enable them to maintain the center of control. We are problem solvers and facilitators and, therefore, we are a critical resource for people with low vision.

However, to provide services needed by people with low vision, specialized knowledge is required, including ocular pathology, optics, functional use of magnification, specialized techniques, and adaptive devices specific to low vision. In addition, collaboration with the professionals in the traditional vision service network is essential. Occupational therapists will then be in a position to apply their unique expertise and expand the likelihood of positive outcomes for the growing numbers of people with low vision.

Note: The authors would like to thank Charles Fox, OD, PhD, for his invaluable and scholarly expertise and the generous time given to his review and recommendations on various sections of the chapter.

REFERENCES

American Foundation for the Blind. (1972). *An introduction to working with the aging person who is visually handicapped.* New York: Author.

Anderson, D. R. (1982). *Testing the field of vision.* St. Louis, MO: Mosby.

Branch, L., Horowitz, A., & Carr, C. (1989). The implications for everyday life of the incidence of self-reported visual decline among people over age 65 living in the community. *Gerontologist 29,* 359–365.

Burack-Weiss, A. (1991). In their own words: Elder's reactions to vision loss. In N. Weber (Ed.), *Vision and aging: Issues in social work practice* (pp. 15–23). Binghamton, NY: Haworth Press.

Carroll, T. (1961). *Blindness: What it is, what it does, and how to live with it.* Boston: Little, Brown.

Carter, K. (1983). Assessment of lighting. In R. Jose (Ed.), *Understanding low vision* (pp. 403–414). New York: American Foundation for the Blind.

Duane, T. D. (Ed.). (1990). *Clinical ophthalmology.* New York: Harper and Row.

Duffy, M., & Beliveau-Tobey, M. (Eds.). (1991). *New independence for older persons with vision loss in long-term care facilities.* New York: AWARE.

Faye, E. (1984). *Clinical low vision* (2nd ed.). Boston: Little, Brown.

Freedman, S., & Inkster, D. (1976). *The impact of blindness in the aging process.* New York: VISIONS CIL Publications.

Goodrich, G., & Mehr, E. (1986). Eccentric viewing training and low vision aids. *American Journal of Optometry and Physiological Optics, 63,* 119–126.

Kern, T. (1996). In B. Stancliff. (Ed.), Viewpoints on working with people with low vision. *OT Practice, 1,* 19.

Kern, T., & Shaw, C. (1985). *An interdisciplinary approach to training the adult blind client.* New York: VISIONS CIL Publications.

Lampert, J., & Lapolice, D. (1995). Functional considerations in evaluation and treatment of the client with low vision. *American Journal of Occupational Therapy, 49,* 885.

The Lighthouse. (1995). *National survey on vision loss.* New York: Author.

Ludwig, I., & Schneider, P. (1991). A model of comprehensive community-based services for older blind adults. In N. Weber, (Ed.), *Vision and aging: Issues in social work practice* (pp. 25–36). Binghamton, NY: Haworth Press.

Mulholland, M. (Ed.). (1993). Diabetes [Special issue]. *Journal of Visual Impairment and Blindness, 87,* 323–392.

National Eye Care Project. (1986). *Fact sheets.* San Francisco: The Foundation of the American Academy of Ophthalmology.

Orr, A. (1991). The psychosocial aspects of aging and vision loss. In N. Weber (Ed.), *Vision and aging: Issues in social work practice* (pp. 1–14). Binghamton, NY: Haworth Press.

Orr, A. (Ed.). (1992). *Vision and aging: Crossroads for service delivery.* New York: American Foundation for the Blind.

Persico, A. (1995). Targeting for results: An interview with Nancy D. Weber. *Innovating, 5,* 36–45.

Rogers, J. C. (1981). Gerontic occupational therapy. *American Journal of Occupational Therapy, 35,* 663–666.

Rosenbloom, A., & Morgan, M. (Eds). (1986). *Vision and aging: General and clinical perspectives.* New York: Professional Press Books/Fairchild Publications.

Sicurella, V. (1977). Color contrast as an aid for visually impaired persons. *Journal of Visual Impairment and Blindness, 71,* 252–257.

VISIONS/Services for the Blind and Visually Impaired. (1984). *Purpose and role of occupational therapy at VISIONS.* [Internal document].

Warren, M. (1995a). Including occupational therapy in low vision rehabilitation. *American Journal of Occupational Therapy, 49,* 857–860.

Warren, M. (Ed.). (1995b). Low vision [Special issue]. *American Journal of Occupational Therapy, 49.*

Watson, G., & Berg, R. (1983). Near training techniques. In R. Jose (Ed.), *Understanding low vision* (pp. 317–362). New York: American Foundation for the Blind.

Weber, N. (Ed.). (1991). *Vision and aging: Issues in social work practice.* Binghamton, NY: Haworth Press.

Woosley, T., Harden, R., & Murphy, P. (1985). *SPOTR: Screening for physical and occupational therapy referral.* Talladega, AL: Alabama Institute for Deaf Blind.

SELECTED READINGS

Bachelder, J., & Harkins, D. (1995). Do occupational therapists have a primary role in low vision rehabilitation? *American Journal of Occupational Therapy, 49,* 927–930.

Baker-Nobles, L., & Bink, M. (1979). Sensory integration in the rehabilitation of blind adults. *American Journal of Occupational Therapy, 33,* 559–564.

Boone, S., Watson, D., & Bagley, M. (1994). *The challenge to independence: Vision and hearing loss among older adults.* Little Rock: University of Arkansas Rehabilitation Research Training Center.

Colmery, A. (1979). *Aid for blind stroke victims.* Little Rock: University of Arkansas Department of Blind Rehabilitation.

Dickman, I. (1983). *Making life more livable: Simple adaptations for the homes of blind and visually impaired older people.* New York: American Foundation for the Blind.

Duane, T. D. (Ed.). (1981-1990). *Clinical ophthalmology.* New York: Harper and Row.

Fletcher, D. C., Shindell, S., Hindman, T., & Schaffrath, M. (1991). Low vision rehabilitation: Finding capable people behind damaged eyeballs. *Western Journal of Medicine, 154,* 554–556.

Fletcher, D. C. (1989). Vision loss: An ophthalmologist's perspective. In S. L. Greenblatt (Ed.), *Providing services for people with vision loss: A multidisciplinary perspective.* Lexington, MA: Resources for Rehabilitation.

Fox, C. (1993). Visual and vestibular function. In H. Cohen (Ed.), *Neuroscience for Rehabilitation.* Philadelphia: J. B. Lippincott.

Hazekamp, J., & Lundin, J. (Ed.). (1986). *Program guidelines for visually impaired individuals.* Sacramento, CA: State Department of Education.

Ingalls, J. (1972). *A trainer's guide to andragogy: Its concepts, experience and application.* Washington, DC: U.S. Department of Health Education and Welfare.

Jose, R. (Ed.). (1983). *Understanding low vision.* New York: American Foundation for the Blind.

Kirchner, C. (1988). *Data on blindness and visual impairment in the U.S.* (2nd ed.). New York: American Foundation for the Blind.

Lampert, J. (1994). Occupational therapists, O&M specialists, and rehabilitation teachers. *Journal of Visual Impairment and Blindness. 88,* 297–298.

Ruben, B. (1990). A new vision OT brings insight to the field of visual impairment. *OT Week, 4,* 4–5.

Wainapel, S. (1989). Severe visual impairment on a rehabilitation unit: Incidence and implications. *Archives of Physical Medicine and Rehabilitation, 70,* 439–441.

Warren, M., & Lampert, J. (1994). Considerations in addressing the daily living needs in older persons with low vision. In A. Colenbrander, & D. C. Fletcher (Eds.), *Low vision and vision rehabilitation: Ophthalmology clinics of North America, 7,* 194.

Williams, H., Webb, A., & Phillips, W. (1993). *Outcome funding: A new approach to targeted grantmaking* (2nd ed.). New York: Rensselaerville Institute.

Yeadon, A. (1978). *Toward independence: The use of instructional objectives in teaching daily living skills to the blind.* New York: American Foundation for the Blind.

RESOURCES

American Foundation for the Blind (AFB), 11 Penn Plaza, Suite 300, New York, NY 10001. 212-502-7600. Hotline: 800-232-5463. Maintains national directory of services, reference library, information services, and National Technology Center, including the latest computer and low vision adaptations, scholarships, and Kurzweil grants for persons in need.

American Foundation for the Blind. (1993). *AFB Directory of Services for Blind and Visually Impaired Persons in the United States and Canada* (24th ed.). New York: Author.

American Occupational Therapy Association, 4720 Montgomery Lane, PO Box 31220, Bethesda, MD 20824. 800-729-2682.

Association for Education and Rehabilitation of the Blind and Visually Impaired, 4600 Duke Street, Suite 430, PO Box 22397, Alexandria, VA 22304. 703-823-9690, e-mail: aernet@laser.net. Professional membership organization; conducts conferences and offers continuing education, publishes a newsletter and the journal *AER RE-View*; operates a reference information center; certifies rehabilitation teachers, O&M specialists, and classroom teachers.

Association of Radio Reading Services. c/o Elizabeth Young, WUSS Radio Reading Services, University of South Florida, WRB209, Tampa, FL 33620. 813-974-4193.

BlindFam Blindness and Family Life. Discussions of all aspects of family life as they are affected by blindness in one or more family member. To subscribe to BlindFam, send the following command to LISTSERV@SJUV M.BITNET in the body of e-mail: SUBSCRIBE BlindFam (your first name) (your last name).

Blind Rehabilitation Services, U.S. Department of Veterans Affairs, 810 Vermont Avenue, NW, Washington, DC 20420. 202-233-3232.

C Tech Catalog, *Products for the Blind and Low Vision Community,* c/o Chuck Cohen, PO Box 30, 2 North William Street, Pearl River, NY 10965-9998. 914-735-7907, 800-228-7798.

Dazor Manufacturing Corporation, 4483 Duncan Avenue, St. Louis, MO 63110. 800-345-9103. Largest manufacturer of adapted lighting and magnified lighting. Free catalog.

Descriptive Video Service (DVS) Home Video Catalog, WGBH-TV, 125 Western Avenue, Boston, MA 02134. Describes movies for people who have low vision. To listen using a Touch-Tone phone to a demonstration of DVS, hear a listing of home video titles, or request a catalog, call 800-333-1203. Orders: 800-736-3099.

Doubleday Large Print Home Library. Garden City, NY 11535-1104.

Duffy, M., & Beliveau-Tobey, M. (Eds.). (1991). *New Independence for Older Persons with Vision Loss in Long-Term Care Facilities.* Volume 1: Facilitator Guide; Volume 2: Learner Workbook; Volume 3: Resource Manual. Available from AWARE, PO Box 96, Mohegan Lake, NY 10547. 914-528-0567.

Glaucoma Research Foundation, 490 Post Street, Suite 830, San Francisco, CA 94102. 415-986-3162.

Joint Commission on Allied Health Personnel in Ophthalmology (JCAHPO), 2025 Woodlane Drive, St. Paul, MN 55125-2995. 612-731-2944. Certification of low vision technicians and low vision assisting. Publishes *Outlook* and newsletter.

Keitzer Writing Guides, K Enterprises, PO Box 1284, Lake Wales, FL 33853. 813-676-1805.

Library of Congress National Library Services for the Blind and Physically Handicapped. 1291 Taylor Street, NW, Washington, DC 20542. 202-707-5100 or 800-424-9100. Distributes free reading materials in Braille and on recorded disks and cassettes.

The Lighthouse, Inc., General Information and *Products for People with Impaired Vision Catalog,* 111 East 59th Street, New York, NY 10022. 800-829-0500.

Maxi Aids & Appliances for Independent Living Catalog, PO Box 3209, Farmingdale, NY 11735. 800-522-6294. Products for people who are blind, visually impaired, physically disabled, or hearing impaired and for senior citizens with special needs.

National Association for the Visually Handicapped, 22 West 21 Street, New York, NY 10010. 212-889-3141. Large-print reading material.

National Diabetes Information Clearinghouse, Box NDIC, Bethesda, MD 20892.

National Eye Health Education Program, 2020 Vision Place, Bethesda, MD 20892-3655. 301-496-5248.

Prevent Blindness America, 500 East Remington Road, Schaumberg, IL 60173. 312-843-2020.

Recording for the Blind and Dyslexic, 20 Roszel Road, Princeton, NJ 08540. 609-452-0606.

SPOTR Test, National Independent Living Skills Project, Alabama Institute for Deaf and Blind, PO Box 698, 205 East South Street, Talladega, AL 35160.

Telephone Services. Locate your local phone company in your local phone book and ask for the Center for People with Disabilities. Available free of charge: large-print number overlay (ring) for rotary phone; large print stick-on numbers for Touch-Tone phones; a dial "zero" overlay fits over push-button keypad and dials operator when any key is pressed; Braille or large-print phone bills; free dial-operator privileges and free directory assistance.

Vision Foundation, 818 Mt. Auburn Street, Watertown, MA 02172. 617-926-4232. Self-help, educational, and reference material.

VISIONS CIL publications series, titles include self-study audiobooks (tapes and large-print companion booklets): *Indoor Mobility, Housekeeping Skills, Personal Management, Sensory Development*; instructor manuals: *Basic Indoor Mobility, Personal Management, Sensory Development, Sewing*; special papers: *An Interdisciplinary Approach to Training the Adult Blind Client,* (1985) by Kern & Shaw; and *Vision and Aging: Issues in Social Work Practice,* (1991) by N. Weber, (Ed.), Haworth Press. Available from VISIONS, 120 Wall Street, 16th Floor, New York, NY 10005-3904. 212-425-2255, ext. 120, e-mail visions@sprintmail.com. Website ordering: www.cilpubs.com.

In New York State, the Commission for the Blind and Visually Handicapped, in conjunction with private, not-for-profit vision rehabilitation agencies, implemented an outcome-based model of service delivery with elderly people who are legally blind. Using a pretest and posttest questionnaire developed by The Lighthouse in New York City, the staff at VISIONS/Services for the Blind and Visually Impaired measure the actual changes in attitude and independent functioning experienced by older people with low vision who have completed a rehabilitation program. The program is based on patient-determined goals and outcomes ("consumer-driven rehabilitation plan"). The design includes a cost-benefit analysis and contract funding based on achievement of specified outcomes; it is funded by state monies combined with a federal demonstration grant. The project, *Integrated Rehabilitation Services for the Elderly (IRSE)*, consists of independent daily living skills taught by an occupational therapist and rehabilitation teacher, mobility and navigational skills taught by an O&M specialist, and use of low vision devices and adaptive equipment taught by all disciplines, combined with activities for social enrichment and benefits and entitlements. (For further information contact the authors.)

Index